Analysis of
Human Genetic Linkage

Analysis of Human Genetic Linkage

Third Edition

JURG OTT

Professor and Head, Laboratory of Statistical Genetics
The Rockefeller University
New York, New York

The Johns Hopkins University Press
Baltimore and London

The Johns Hopkins University Press
2715 North Charles Street
Baltimore, Maryland 21218-4363
www.press.jhu.edu

Library of Congress Cataloging-in-Publication Data

Ott, Jurg.
  Analysis of human genetic linkage / Jurg Ott.—3rd ed.
     p.   cm.
  Includes bibliographical references and index.
  ISBN 0-8018-6140-3 (alk. paper)
  1. Linkage (Genetics)   2. Human genetics.   I. Title. [DNLM: 1.
Linkage (Genetics)   QH 445.2 089a 1999]
QH445.2.088   1999
599.93′5—dc21
DNLM/DLC
for Library of Congress   98-37347

A catalog record for this book is available from the British Library.

To my wife, Salome

Contents

List of Illustrations   xiii

List of Tables   xv

Preface   xix

List of Symbols and Abbreviations   xxi

1. Introduction and Basic Genetic Principles   1

    1.1. Linkage Analysis and the Human Genome Project   1

    1.2. Mendelian Inheritance   2

    1.3. Crossing Over and Map Distance   9

    1.4. Recombination and Genetic Linkage   11

    1.5. Map Functions   17

    1.6. The Human Chromosomes   21

    1.7. Problems   23

2. Genetic Loci and Genetic Polymorphisms   24

    2.1. Nomenclature and Characterization of Genetic Loci   24

    2.2. Measures of Polymorphism   27

    2.3. DNA Polymorphisms   30

    2.4. Variants in Chromosome Morphology   32

    2.5. Genetic and Physical Maps   33

    2.6. Problems   36

3. Aspects of Statistical Inference   37

    3.1. Likelihood and Lod Score   38

    3.2. Maximum Likelihood Estimation   40

3.3. Statistical Properties of Maximum Likelihood Estimates   41

3.4. Significance Tests and *p*-Values   44

3.5. The Likelihood Method   47

3.6. Interval Estimation   48

3.7. Bayes Theorem   50

3.8. Problems   52

4. Basics of Linkage Analysis   53

4.1. A Brief Historical Review   53

4.2. Prior and Posterior Distribution of θ 59

4.3. The Lod Score Method   61

4.4. Testing for Linkage   65

4.5. Equivalent Numbers of Recombinants and
Nonrecombinants   70

4.6. Exact Tests in Simple Family Types   72

4.7. Multiple Comparisons   75

4.8. The Likelihood for Family Data   79

4.9. Some Special Methods   81

4.10. Problems   82

5. The Informativeness of Family Data   84

5.1. Measures of Informativeness   84

5.2. Expected Lod Score and Related Quantities   87

5.3. Expected Information and Variance   91

5.4. Mating Types   93

5.5. Double Intercross with Two Alleles   94

5.6. Double Intercross with More Than Two Alleles   98

5.7. Phase-Known Double Backcross   100

5.8. Phase-Unknown Double Backcross with Two
Offspring   100

5.9. Phase-Unknown Double Backcross with More Than Two
Offspring   104

5.10. Conditional ELODs: Maximum or Average Lod
Score?   106

5.11. Number of Observations Required to Detect Linkage   110
5.12. Problems   112

6. Multipoint Linkage Analysis   114

6.1. Notation and Terminology   115
6.2. Three-Point Analysis with Known Phase   118
6.3. Phase-Unknown Triple Backcross with Two Offspring   122
6.4. Interference in the Three-Point Cross   124
6.5. Crossover Distributions and Testing for Interference   128
6.6. Three-Point Locus Ordering   134
6.7. Mapping under Complete Interference   139
6.8. Map Construction and Gene Localization   144
6.9. Map Integration   148
6.10. Problems   150

7. Penetrance   151

7.1. Definitions of Penetrance   151
7.2. Cost of Incomplete Penetrance   153
7.3. Estimating Penetrance and Recombination Fraction   156
7.4. Factors Influencing Penetrance   160
7.5. Age-Dependent Penetrance and Segregation Analysis   161
7.6. Penetrance for Monozygotic Twins   168
7.7. Problems   169

8. Quantitative Phenotypes   171

8.1. Mixed Distributions   172
8.2. Parameter Estimation for Unrelated Individuals   173
8.3. Parameter Estimation in Family Data   175
8.4. Informativeness of Overlapping Distributions   175
8.5. Variance Components   177
8.6. Problem   178

9. Numerical and Computerized Methods   179

9.1. Calculating Lod Scores Analytically   179
9.2. The Elston–Stewart Algorithm   182

9.3. Computer Programs for Parametric Linkage Analysis   185
9.4. Special Applications of Linkage Programs   191
9.5. Linkage Utility Programs   196
9.6. Paternity Calculations   200
9.7. Computer Simulation Methods   201
9.8. Problems   210

10. Variability of the Recombination Fraction   211
10.1. Male and Female Recombination Fractions   211
10.2. Recombination Fraction and Age   214
10.3. Heterogeneity between Classes of Families   215
10.4. Heterogeneity due to a Mixture of Families   220
10.5. Hierarchical and Mixed Models of Heterogeneity   231
10.6. Covariates in the Test for Admixture   233
10.7. Problems   234

11. Inconsistencies   236
11.1. Ascertainment Bias   236
11.2. Misclassification   242
11.3. Misspecification of Penetrance   244
11.4. Misspecification of Heterogeneity   245
11.5. Pedigree and Genotyping Errors   247
11.6. Misspecification of Allele Frequencies   250
11.7. Other Model Misspecifications   251
11.8. Problems   252

12. Linkage Analysis with Mendelian Disease Loci   253
12.1. Mode of Inheritance   254
12.2. Number of Informative Meioses   258
12.3. Candidate Loci   260
12.4. Exclusion Mapping   262
12.5. Genetic Risks   263
12.6. Irregular Segregation   270
12.7. Problem   271

13. Nonparametric Methods 272

    13.1. Sets of Relatives 272

    13.2. Equivalence between ASP and Lod Score Analysis 279

    13.3. Exclusion Analysis 279

    13.4. Linkage Disequilibrium 280

    13.5. Haplotype Relative Risk and Related Methods 292

    13.6. Problems 295

14. Two-Locus Inheritance 297

    14.1. Two-Locus Models 298

    14.2. Parametric Analysis under Mendelian Inheritance 302

    14.3. Two-Locus Affected Sib-Pair Analysis 304

    14.4. Problems 305

15. Complex Traits 306

    15.1. Genetic Basis and Heritability 307

    15.2. Recurrence Risk in Relatives versus Population
            Prevalence 315

    15.3. Disease Phenotype 317

    15.4. Current Approaches 320

    15.5. Power Considerations 325

    15.6. Problems 328

Solutions to Study Problems 331

References 345

Index 377

List of Illustrations

1.1. Artificial family with assumed genotypes at two loci showing one recombinant and one nonrecombinant offspring   7

1.2. Schematic representation of two crossovers on a chromosome arm with three gene loci   10

1.3. Family showing inheritance of four closely linked markers on chromosome 1   12

1.4. Graphs of several mapping functions   20

4.1. Kinship L   54

4.2. Family 79   62

4.3. Lod score curve for 8 recombinants in 40 recombination events showing construction of support interval   68

5.1. Maximum lod score and observed information for an estimated recombination fraction from counts of recombination events   86

5.2. Graphs of the lod score curves associated with observed recombinants in three recombination events   87

5.3. Ratios of ELOD and expected information   99

5.4. Observed lod scores for double backcross matings with seven offspring each   105

5.5. Artificial small family with a dominant disease to show maximum possible lod score   107

6.1. Crossover events leading to the haplotype received by individual for different locus orders   117

6.2. Portion of family 21 showing segregation of haplotypes at three X-chromosomal marker loci   120

6.3. Regions of different locus orders with three gene loci   137

7.1. Restricted ranges of p_1 and p_3 in the estimation of f and θ 160

7.2. Age-of-onset curve from small sample of affecteds with Charcot–Marie–Tooth disease 168

7.3. Density and distribution function for age at onset assumed for familial osteoarthrosis 169

7.4. Diagram for risk calculations in Problem and Solution 7.2 338

9.1. A family showing linkage between the GM-CSF receptor gene and gender 192

9.2. Theoretical example for the linkage analysis between a pseudoautosomal locus and an X-linked locus 194

9.3. Artificial family for simulation of maximum and average lod scores 207

11.1. Apparent error rate as a function of the true error rate and number of alleles in marker system for families with two parents and one offspring 248

12.1. A family with a marriage among cousins demonstrating increased informativeness through homozygosity mapping 256

12.2. A family with dominant trait of late onset, one affected child and one young child 268

12.3. Risk distribution for counselee in Figure 12.2 based on results shown in Table 12.3 269

13.1. Nuclear families demonstrating identity by descent and identity by state for allele #5 277

13.2. Decay of disequilibrium over time for different values of the recombination fraction 284

13.3. *P*-value versus map distance between pairs of marker loci 290

13.4. Scheme for calculating risk in Problem 13.4 343

14.1. Examples of two-locus inheritance in nature 298

14.2. Mating with assumed genotypes at loci jointly underlying a two-locus threshold trait and all possible offspring genotypes 300

15.1. Biased correlation coefficients for quantitative observations in siblings 314

15.2. Effects of random stratification in analysis of 150 ASPs 325

List of Tables

1.1. Relation between genotypes and phenotypes (penetrances) at the *ABO* locus   5

1.2. Chromosome lengths in terms of male and female map distances and physical distances   11

2.1. Penetrances and expected phenotype and genotype frequencies at the *ABO* locus with four *ABO* alleles   26

2.2. Relation between LU genotypes and phenotypes (penetrances)   27

3.1. Calculation of expected value for three recombination events and known recombination fraction 0.1   43

3.2. Conditional probabilities of test results given state of nature   45

3.3. Example of calculation of inverse probabilities using the Bayes theorem   51

4.1. Lod score, likelihood ratio, and interval width at selected values of θ_i for the calculation of the posterior probability of linkage   60

4.2. Probability of a significant linkage result when double backcross families are investigated   73

4.3. Critical lod score for a genome-wide significance level of 0.05 and given marker spacing in affected sib pair analysis   78

5.1. Calculation of expected lod score for three meioses and expected Z_{max} under the true recombination fraction $r = 0.1$ 88

5.2. Offspring genotypes from mating *A1/B2* $\times$ *A1/B2*   95

5.3. Phenotypes of offspring from mating *A1/B2* × *A1/B2*   96

5.4. Offspring phenotypes with equal probabilities combined into one class each, mating *A1/B2* × *A1/B2*   97

5.5. Joint genotype probabilities of two offspring from a mating [*A1/B2* or *A2/B1*] × *A1/A1*   101

5.6. Joint offspring genotype probabilities from a phase-unknown double backcross mating   102

5.7. Phenotype classes of pairs of offspring from a phase-unknown double backcross mating   103

5.8. Possible offspring genotypes for pedigree in Figure 5.5, associated maximum lod scores and probabilities of occurrence for penetrance of 90%   108

5.9. Maximum lod scores and their probabilities of occurrence with penetrance of 90% for pedigree in Figure 5.5   109

5.10. Number of known recombination events required to find $Z_{\max} \geq Z_0$ with power ϕ 111

6.1. Numbering system for loci and map segments   116

6.2. Joint recombination probabilities and two-point recombination fractions for recombination and nonrecombination among loci *A, B,* and *C*   118

6.3. Conditional haplotype probabilities given phase, produced by a triply heterozygous parent   123

6.4. Offspring phenotype classes in phase-unknown triple backcross families with two offspring   123

6.5. Asymptotic standard error of coincidence coefficient estimates and number of meioses required for detecting positive interference   127

6.6. Offspring numbers from phase-known triple backcross matings interpreted under three locus orders   135

6.7. Lod scores under Kosambi interference for the observations in Table 6.6   138

6.8. Maximum lod scores and estimates of absolute map distances in the two intervals for different orders of three loci and for different map functions   139

6.9. Counts of gametes recombinant and nonrecombinant for loci *AB* and *BC*   142

7.1. Offspring phenotype probabilities in phase-known double backcross families with incomplete penetrance at the disease locus   154

7.2. Ratio of expected lod scores at true recombination fraction under incomplete penetrance versus full penetrance   155

8.1. Relative efficiency of the recombination fraction estimate with two overlapping distributions of the phenotype at the main trait   177

9.1. Four families from a linkage investigation of TCN2   180

9.2. Penetrances at an X-linked locus with an emulated autosomal inheritance pattern   193

9.3. Penetrances at a Y-linked locus with an emulated autosomal inheritance pattern   193

9.4. Example of determining the distribution of risks to a future child in a specific family   196

10.1. Sex-specific lod scores in a pedigree with dentinogenesis imperfecta and GC blood types   212

10.2. Two-point lod scores of polycystic kidney disease versus the marker 3'HVR and conditional probability of being of the linked type   218

10.3. Likelihood ratios and corresponding differences in log likelihood   219

10.4. $\log_e$ likelihoods for the 29 families in Table 10.2   222

10.5. $\log_e$ likelihoods for 35 families with respect to a mixture of three family types   228

10.6. Parameter estimates and evidence for heterogeneity in a mixture of osteogenesis imperfecta families   229

10.7. Asymptotic correlation between $\hat{\alpha}$ and $\hat{\theta}$ and standard error $\sigma(\hat{\theta})$ 231

11.1. Asymptotic bias of recombination fraction estimates and ELODs for some ascertainment schemes in phase-known double intercross families   239

11.2. General misclassification probability, incomplete disease penetrance, and probability of occurrence of phenocopies as special cases of penetrances   243

11.3. Relative ELOD of the recombination fraction estimate in the presence of misclassification   244

11.4. Probability of occurrence of recombinants and associated lod score in the presence of heterogeneity   246

11.5. Maximum Z of the expected lod score and value $\tilde{\theta}$ at which that maximum occurs   247

12.1. Increase in expected lod score at given true value of the recombination fraction due to adding one affected or one unaffected offspring   254

12.2. Lod scores obtained for a family as shown in Figure 12.1 with one or two affected offspring   256

12.3. All possible risks to counselee in pedigree shown in Figure 12.2   269

13.1. Counts of marker haplotypes A through D on CF and normal chromosomes   287

13.2. Comparison of two types of special populations suitable for disequilibrium mapping   290

13.3. Probabilities of transmitted and nontransmitted marker alleles for one parent with an offspring affected with a recessive trait   293

14.1. Examples of two-locus disease models: penetrances for given genotypes   299

14.2. A two-locus model predicting average numbers of 1.89 and 1.05 of alleles shared at loci *1* and *2*, respectively   301

14.3. IBD sharing probabilities for two-locus model in Table 14.2   301

15.1. Correlation coefficient among observations on unselected siblings and after ascertainment of proband's value   313

15.2. Haplotype frequencies between assumed marker and disease alleles   327

Preface

In the 8 years since the previous edition was written, so much progress has been made in human genetics that it is high time for a new edition. Dense human marker maps that essentially cover the entire genome are now available, and localizing a Mendelian trait gene on the human gene map has become almost a routine matter. What still poses major problems are complex traits such as diabetes, some cancers, and psychiatric conditions. Even though they may show high heritability, it has been difficult, if not impossible, to find locations of single genes contributing to these traits. This topic is now covered in a new chapter.

The first chapter presents basic genetic principles in a simple and intuitive manner. Crossing over (rather than recombination) is introduced and demonstrated in a simple example. Many sections in the first two chapters represent elementary introductions, and readers without any statistical knowledge should be able to understand them. For other sections and later chapters, some facility with equations and simple algebra will be beneficial. As in the first edition, no introduction to probability calculus is given. Readers without knowledge of probability laws will have to accept some statements at face value but should still be able to follow much of this book. On the other hand, an outline of some statistical methods, particularly significance testing, is provided in Chapter 3. Presentation of that material has been simplified considerably because there are good textbooks that cover statistical theory in detail.

No background is given on population genetics or genetic epidemiology because excellent treatments of these important topics exist (e.g., Cavalli-Sforza and Bodmer, 1971; Hartl, 1988; Maynard Smith, 1989; Khoury et al., 1993). Hartl (1988) also provided an introduction to molecular genetic aspects of population genetics, and Maynard Smith (1989) covered modern genetic concepts from an evolutionary standpoint. Mathematical and statistical treatments of a wide range of topics in classical and population genetics, including statistical methods for DNA sequence data, are presented in books by Weir (1996) and Lange (1997). For more general aspects of human genetics, the reader is referred to one of the human genetics texts, particularly the one by Vogel and Motulsky (1986). Theory and sampling in pedigree analysis may be found in Thompson (1986). Various facets of molecular genetics and sequencing are given in Strachan and Read (1996). For the reader who is rusty on probability calculus and statistics, an introduction to biostatistics has been written by Elston and Johnson (1994). A comprehensive book covering methods for human data and those on experimental organisms has been written by Lynch and Walsh (1998). A classic on many aspects of genetics is the book by Strickberger (1985).

This book is intended as an introduction to linkage analysis with emphasis on methodology rather than computer programs (although the latter are mentioned where appropriate). A companion book (Terwilliger and Ott, 1994) focuses on computer programs and provides step-by-step guidance on the use of LINKAGE and some other programs. Corrections to this and the companion book are updated on a continuing basis and may be found on the world-wide web at URL http://linkage.rockefeller.edu/ott/corr-ott.htm and http://linkage.rockefeller.edu/ott/corr-ter.htm.

I would like to take this opportunity to pay homage to an early pioneer in linkage analysis, James Renwick. He was the author of the first efficient linkage program for large human families. We never met, but shortly before his death, we had a long telephone conversation and he sent me the flow chart to his program. In remembrance of his work, I put this flow chart on my web page, http://linkage.rockefeller.edu/ott/renwick.html.

This book has also been written in memory of Ernst Hadorn, my former teacher in Zurich, who was a pioneer in experimental genetics (Nothiger, 1977). At one time in the mid-1960s, he introduced us students to a friend of his who was visiting him, Theodosius Dobzhansky. Although I was not a good zoology student and even flunked one of Dr. Hadorn's exams, he would enjoy seeing my work in human genetics.

Many readers have contributed to previous versions of this book by letting me know of errors and inaccuracies in the text. Also, I have greatly benefited from discussions with colleagues; for example, Robert Elston, Harald Göring, Lodewijk Sandkuijl, Joseph Terwilliger, Thomas Wienker, and many others. I very much welcome such comments. Readers are invited to submit them by e-mail (ott@rockefeller.edu), mail (see http://www.rockefeller.edu/), or fax (212-327-7996).

List of Symbols and Abbreviations

$[r]$ Nearest integer to the real number r. For example, $[2.4] = 2$, $[2.6] = 3$.

α Significance level (type I error) in a statistical test (lowercase Greek alpha); or
Proportion of a particular family type in a mixture of families

β Type II error in statistical test ($1 - \beta$ = power) (lowercase Greek beta)

γ Coefficient of coincidence

δ Indicator variable, $\delta = 0$ or $\delta = 1$ (lowercase Greek delta), identifying the intervals of a map, which constitute a given region A of the map; or
Difference operator

Δ Difference operator

ϵ Indicator variable, $\epsilon = 0$ or $\epsilon = 1$ (lowercase Greek epsilon), identifying the intervals of a map in which a crossover occurs

θ Assumed value of the recombination fraction as a variable in log likelihoods or lod scores (lowercase Greek theta); occasionally also the true value (r) of the recombination fraction when there is no danger of confusing it with the variable

θ_0, θ_1 Specific assumed values of θ. In the first edition of this book, θ_0 denoted the true value of the recombination fraction (now r)

$\hat{\theta}$ Maximum likelihood estimate of the recombination fraction

$\tilde{\theta}$ Asymptotic estimate of the recombination fraction; that is, the value of θ at which the expected log likelihood (expected lod score) attains its maximum

λ Exponent in power transformation of θ (lowercase Greek lambda); or

Risk ratio = recurrence risk in a relative divided by population prevalence

Λ Average of likelihood ratio (capital Greek lambda)

μ Mean (lowercase Greek mu)

ρ Correlation coefficient (lowercase Greek rho)

σ Standard deviation/standard error (lowercase Greek sigma)

Σ Summation operator (capital Greek sigma)

ϕ Power, probability of significant result (lowercase Greek phi)

ASP Affected sib pair

BMI Body mass index = body weight divided by the square of body height (kg/m^2)

df Degree(s) of freedom

E Expectation operator, $E(x)$, average of quantity x, where x may be a function

$E[Z(\theta)]$ Expected lod score, evaluated at θ

ELOD Expected lod score evaluated at its true value (i.e., $E[Z(r)]$)

EMLOD Expected maximum lod score (i.e., average of lod score maxima)

f Penetrance; or

Density of a random variable

F Distribution function of a random variable

G Joint or n-fold recombination fraction (as a function of e, section 6.1). Also,

Distribution function of age at disease onset

HRR Haplotype relative risk

HHRR Haplotype-based haplotype relative risk

i Expected Fisher information (average per observation)

I Total Fisher information for all observations

$\hat{\imath}$	Observed average Fisher information
$\hat{I}$	Observed total Fisher information
L	Likelihood
$L*$	Rescaled likelihood, or likelihood ratio
LD	Linkage disequilibrium
MCMC	Markov chain Monte Carlo (a particular method of computer simulation)
MELOD	Maximum of the expected lod score curve
ML	Maximum likelihood
MLE	Maximum likelihood estimate
p	Empirical significance level, p-value; or Allele frequency
QTL	Quantitative trait locus
r	True value of the recombination fraction (when used together with a formal θ parameter in the same context; otherwise, θ sometimes denotes the true recombination fraction)
R	Ratio, often likelihood ratio, or (relative) risk, or penetrance ratio, or linkage value (as a function of δ, section 6.1)
s	Reduction from full penetrance ($1 - s$ = penetrance), or misclassification probability, or conditional rate of false positives (sporadic cases) (s is typically a small value)
Z	Lod score, log likelihood ratio with respect to recombination fraction, $\log_{10}(R)$, $R = L(\theta)/L(\frac{1}{2})$

Analysis of
Human Genetic Linkage

1.

Introduction and Basic Genetic Principles

1.1. Linkage Analysis and the Human Genome Project

Genetic linkage analysis refers to the ordering of genetic loci on a chromosome and to estimating genetic distances among them, where these distances are determined on the basis of a statistical phenomenon (i.e., the crossover frequency occurring between two points on a gamete). Linkage was discovered by Morgan (1911) in *Drosophila,* and the first paper on gene mapping was written by Sturtevant (1913).

In human genetics, linkage analysis has seen much progress in statistical and computational methodology, which is reviewed in Section 4.1. Since 1980, molecular genetic and other techniques have become ever more important. Human gene mapping is now a field of science with many disciplines interacting to create genetic maps, physical maps, expression maps, and so on. The ultimate aim is to elucidate the sequence of human DNA, to understand mechanisms of genetic diseases, and, it is hoped, to prevent many of these diseases in the future. An important aspect of this research will be to recognize interactions between genes and the environment.

Although computers have long been important in linkage analysis as number crunchers, novel ways of electronic communication, the internet and world-wide web have had an increasing impact on human genetics (Lawrence and Giles, 1998). Pooling results through lod scores and perhaps pooling raw data have long been a common practice in human gene mapping. Now, several large databases exist to which researchers contribute and that are, in turn, proving fruitful for all of human genomics. For example, random complementary DNA clones (expressed sequence tags, or ESTs) are being sequenced, and the sequence made available in databases with the purpose of identifying new genes (Goodfellow, 1995). Sequences of cDNAs are being collected and databases recording different types of expression patterns for a variety of human cell types are being

1

established (Strachan et al., 1997). Although these techniques have liberated genetics from breeding experiments (Brenner, 1990), many "experiments" can now even be carried out on computers, and this work is likely to be gaining importance in the future (Schuler, 1997; Guigó, 1997; Claverie, 1997). Much information about these efforts may be obtained from the web pages of the National Center for Biotechnology Information (NCBI) at http://www4.ncbi.nlm.nih.gov/ or http://www.ncbi.nlm.nih.gov/. Several genomes are now completely sequenced; for a list of these, see http://linkage.rockefeller.edu/wli/seq/.

Among all these advances in molecular genetics and computer science, linkage analysis fulfills an important role. Disease gene mapping is still predominantly being done by linkage analysis although many disease genes have been localized by cytogenetic techniques. Currently, a hot debate is on the potential merits of linkage analysis for the localization of genes underlying complex traits, that is, diseases that are clearly heritable yet do not follow any of the known modes of inheritance and are thought to be due to the interaction of multiple genes (Chapter 15). This book presents the current status of human genetic linkage analysis with its most important theoretical underpinnings.

In the next section, mendelian inheritance, in which a gene is viewed as a point on the genome, will be briefly described. Several forms of inheritance have been discovered that are not adequately described by such a model. Some genes are quite long, with DMD being a prime example: with 79 exons spanning at least 2.3 Mb, it is the largest gene known (Tennyson et al., 1995). On the other hand, at least in bacteria, genes as short as 21 bp have been described (Gonsález-Pastor et al., 1994). In some genes, there is a tendency for trinucleotides to be repeated multiple times, with disease occurring when the number of repeats exceeds some threshold (Bulle et al., 1997; Koob et al., 1998). Examples of nonmendelian segregation are given in Section 12.6.

1.2. Mendelian Inheritance

In his textbook, Strickberger (1985) provides a nice introduction to genetics. For example, in Chapter 1 he points out that up until the 19th century, it was common to think that genetic material did not necessarily have to be transmitted between generations but could arise spontaneously. He also gives a detailed account of the mendelian principles and the history surrounding them. Below, only a brief outline is given.

In crossing experiments with peas, Gregor Mendel hypothesized what are now called Mendel's laws in 1865 (Mendel, 1866; Bateson, 1913).

After the rediscovery of these laws in 1900 by Correns, Tschermak, and de Vries, Sutton and Boveri in 1902 to 1904 formulated the chromosomal theory of inheritance. A proper understanding of chromosomes gave Mendel's laws the plausibility that they had been lacking. Below is a brief description of mendelian inheritance in current terminology. A more detailed introduction to genetics and cytogenetics may be found in the textbook by Strickberger (1985). Much of the material covered below refers to autosomal inheritance; that is, to inheritance related to autosomes (non-sex chromosomes). Sex-specific inheritance is mentioned in appropriate places.

Heritable characters are determined by *genes,* where different genes are responsible for the expression of different characteristics. In modern terminology, a gene is a specific coding sequence of DNA (Elandt-Johnson, 1971, p 3; Hartl, 1988), the unit of transmission, recombination, and function (Vogel and Motulsky, 1986). Estimates of the total number of genes range from 50,000 to 100,000 in the human, and 5000 in the fruitfly *Drosophila melanogaster* (McKusick and Ruddle, 1977; Schuler et al., 1996). A number of 1000 essential genes in *Drosophila* has also been quoted (Maynard Smith, 1989, p 59). As is well known, genes consist of coding regions (exons) with intervening sequences of noncoding DNA (introns). Mobile pieces of DNA (transposons) are also known that can "jump" from one genomic area to another. In fact, over 35% of the human genome is made up of transposon DNA (Kidwell and Lisch, 1998).

Each individual carries two copies of each gene, one of which was received from the mother and the other from the father. A gene may occur in different forms or states called *alleles,* each potentially having a different physical expression. For example, three major alleles of the ABO gene interact to determine the various ABO blood types. It is often difficult to distinguish whether different characteristics are caused by different genes or by different alleles of the same gene, and the solution to this question will be deferred to the next section. It should be mentioned here that some authors use a slightly different terminology—what here is called an allele is sometimes referred to as a gene.

Any heritable quantity that follows the mendelian laws is generally called a *locus* (plural, *loci*), where a gene is special type of locus, that is, a locus with a function (a gene product). For example, DNA polymorphisms are loci (generally without a function). Well-characterized loci with a clear mendelian mode of inheritance may serve as genetic *marker loci* (or *markers* for short). As in the case of genes, loci may also occur in different allelic forms. In the true sense of the word, "locus" refers to the position of a gene or any other mendelizing unit rather than to these quantities themselves. However, many authors treat "locus" as a synonym for any mendelizing quantity.

The relative frequencies in the population of the different alleles at a locus are called *gene frequencies* (this term is a reminder of the alternative meaning of "gene"), where each individual contributes two alleles (for an autosomal locus) to the population gene pool. For example, the three alleles, *A, B,* and *O,* of the ABO gene occur with approximate gene frequencies in Caucasians of $p_A = 0.28$, $p_B = 0.06$, and $p_o = 0.66$. A locus is called *polymorphic* when its most common allele has a population frequency of less than 95% (a less stringent criterion of 99% is sometimes used).

At a given locus, the pair of alleles in an individual constitutes that individual's *genotype*. With *n* alleles, $n(n + 1)/2$ possible genotypes may be formed. For example, at the ABO blood group locus ($n = 3$), the six genotypes are A/A, A/B, A/O, B/B, B/O, and O/O. The two alleles in an individual are either the same (A/A, B/B, and O/O), in which case a genotype is called *homozygous,* and the individual with such a genotype is said to be a homozygote, or they are different (A/B, A/O, and B/O), in which case the genotype is *heterozygous* and the individual with such a genotype is called a heterozygote. For loci on the X chromosome, the same terms are used in females, but in males the genotype is called *hemizygous* (e.g., A/*y*, where *y* stands for the Y chromosome). Finally, when the two alleles in a homozygous genotype are known to be copies of the same ancestral allele (identical by descent, or IBD), that genotype is termed *autozygous;* otherwise it is called *allozygous.*

The expression of a particular genotype is called a *phenotype*. At the ABO gene, the six genotypes determine four phenotypes (blood types)— type A, type B, type AB, and type O. The relation between genotypes and (qualitative) phenotypes for a particular gene is conveniently represented in the form of a table, in which the rows correspond to genotypes and the columns correspond to phenotypes. Each cell in the table then contains a *penetrance,* that is, the conditional probability of observing the corresponding phenotype given the specified genotype. In simple cases, penetrances are either 0 or 1; for many diseases, however, intermediate values of penetrances occur. A simple example with full penetrance is given in Table 1.1 for the ABO gene. The two genotypes A/A and A/O have the same phenotype (*A* blood type) or, as geneticists say, *A* is *dominant* over *O* (*A > O*), because the *A* allele is expressed irrespective of the presence of an *O* allele. Conversely, *O* is said to be *recessive* with respect to *A* because it has no effect on the phenotype in the presence of *A;* it is "seen" only in the genotype O/O, which leads to the *O* blood

Table 1.1. Relation between Genotypes and Phenotypes (Penetrances) at the *ABO* Locus

Genotype	Phenotype			
	Type A	Type B	Type AB	Type O
A/A	1	0	0	0
A/B	0	0	1	0
A/O	1	0	0	0
B/B	0	1	0	0
B/O	0	1	0	0
O/O	0	0	0	1

type. Also, *B* is dominant over *O*, whereas *A* and *B* are *codominant;* they are both expressed when present in the same genotype, A/B.

Dominantly inherited diseases tend to occur over several generations in large families. On the other hand, recessive traits generally occur only within a single sibship. Exceptions occur, for example, in isolated populations where many people are related. An example is a recessively inherited form of retinitis pigmentosa, which occurred in many sibships of a large kindred in the Dominican Republic (Knowles et al., 1994). The distinction between different modes of inheritance is sometimes blurred, depending on the phenotype considered. For example, aspartyl glucosaminuria (AGU, MIM number 20840) is one of the Finnish diseases (Vogel and Motulsky, 1986). While heterozygous carriers of the AGU gene do not express the disease, they can be identified through low activity of the enzyme aspartyl glucosaminidase (Grön, Aula, and Peltonen, 1990). Thus, AGU effectively becomes a codominant trait.

Many genetic terms have changed their meaning as they were being used by human or molecular geneticists. For example, *mutation* originally designated a process (a change from one allele into another) but now it is used as a synonym for *mutated allele.* In a similar vein, as outlined above, phenotype is simply anything we see. Recently there has been a trend to more narrowly define phenotype as ''what you see in a disease,'' as opposed to genotype, which is ''what you see in a marker locus.'' Clearly, this latter development is quite unfortunate and should not be supported.

Through the formation of gametes, each parent passes to each of his or her children one of the two alleles with probability ½. The allele received from the mother and that from the father constitute a child's genotype. For example, if two parents have the respective blood types AB and O (genotypes A/B and O/O), then half of their children are expected to have the genotype A/O, and the other half the genotype B/O. If the assumed mode of inheritance is correct, deviations from this 1 : 1 ratio will be due to chance fluctuations. When a new locus has been discovered and a particular mendelian mode of inheritance is hypothesized for it, it is common practice to predict for given parental matings the proportion of children with different phenotypes and to test whether observed and expected proportions agree. For example, Juneja et al. (1988) studied four alleles of the plasma $\alpha_1\beta$-glycoprotein gene. They grouped 57 families by their mating types (parental genotypes) and verified that the offspring genotypes were observed as predicted by mendelian inheritance. Two or more genotypes are termed genetically *inconsistent* or incompatible when they are not in agreement with the mendelian laws. For example, a mother's genotype A/B is inconsistent with an offspring's genotype O/O.

Under conditions of random mating and the absence of disturbing forces such as migration, mutation, and selection at the gene in question, a population is said to be in *Hardy–Weinberg equilibrium* (HWE), meaning that the genotype frequencies in the population depend only on the gene frequencies (Hartl, 1988). For example, $P(A/A) = p_A^2$, $P(A/B) = 2p_A p_B$. Notice that the genotype B/A is the same as A/B. A salient feature of the Hardy–Weinberg principle is that for autosomal genes, whatever the genotype distribution in the parental generation was, HWE will be obtained after one generation of random mating. In other words, the genotype frequencies in the children's generation depend only on the allele frequencies and not on the genotype frequencies in the parental generation. In a finite population, however, the genotype frequencies are not constant. By random fluctuation, allele frequencies in generation 2 may deviate somewhat from those in generation 1, and it is then the new allele frequencies in generation 2 that determine the expected genotype frequencies in generation 3. This random force of divergence is called *genetic drift* (Maynard Smith, 1989).

The existence of HWE is often taken to imply that mating is random. Although random mating implies HWE, the reverse is not necessarily true. Certain patterns of deviations from random mating (termed *pseudorandom mating*) have been shown to also lead to HWE in the offspring generation (Li, 1988).

Instead of a single locus, consider now two loci jointly, locus 1 with two alleles, A and a, and locus 2 also with two alleles, B and b. Figure 1.1 shows an artificial family in which the two grandparents are both doubly homozygous: the grandmother is homozygous for the alleles A (at locus 1) and B (at locus 2), and the grandfather is homozygous for the alleles a and b. In experimental organisms, such homozygosity can

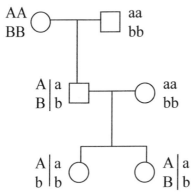

Figure 1.1. Artificial family with assumed genotypes at two loci showing one recombinant and one nonrecombinant offspring.

be achieved through successive inbreeding and selection of the desired genotypes. The father (son of the two grandparents) must have received alleles *A* and *B* from the grandmother and alleles *a* and *b* from the grandfather. The alleles (at different genes) received by an individual from one parent are called a *haplotype*. The father thus received the haplotype *AB* from his mother and the haplotype *ab* from his father.

In principle, a doubly heterozygous individual (*A/a, B/b*) received his or her *A* allele in coupling with either the *B* or the *b* allele from one parent. These two possibilities are distinguished as the two *phases* of a double heterozygote (more than two phases exist in individuals heterozygous at more than two loci). Depending on the alleles of interest, one of the two phases is called the *coupling,* or *cis* phase, and the other is called the *repulsion,* or *trans* phase. Often, the phase of a double heterozygote is unknown, that is, it is unclear which two alleles were received as a haplotype from one parent. For the father in Figure 1.1 (middle generation) the phase is known, which is indicated by the vertical bar in his genotype separating maternal (left side of bar) from paternal alleles. For genotypes in which at most one locus is heterozygous, the phase is always known because it is clear which alleles must have come as a haplotype from one of the parents, although one may be unable to indicate which haplotype came from which parent.

In analogy to the notion of gene frequency at a single locus, a population haplotype frequency may be defined. If n_i is the number of alleles at the *i*th locus, $i = 1 \ldots N$, the total number, *H,* of possible haplotypes at all *N* loci is given by the product, $H = n_1 \times n_2 \times \ldots$. The total number of different genotypes is then calculated as $H(H + 1)/2$, where multiple heterozygotes differing only in their phase are counted as different genotypes. For example, when three loci have 4, 2, and 3 alleles, respectively, there are 24 possible haplotypes and 300 possible genotypes. When alleles at different loci occur independently of each other in haplotypes, the population frequency of a haplotype is given by the product of the gene frequencies of its constituent alleles. Deviations from random occurrence of alleles in haplotypes are referred to as *allelic association* or *linkage disequilibrium* and will be covered in detail later (Section 13.3).

As is well known, in addition to the 22 pairs of chromosomes called *autosomes,* there exist two chromosomes, X and Y, called *sex chromosomes.* Of these, women carry two X and men carry one X and one Y. Everything said thus far about genes and chromosomes implicitly referred to autosomal genes. The X and Y chromosomes also carry genes that show characteristic *sex-linked* modes of inheritance, as boys (*X/Y*) receive their X from the mother and the Y from the father, and girls (*X/X*) receive one X each from mother and father. For an X-linked locus, each female contributes two alleles and each male contributes one allele to the total number of alleles in the population. Therefore, assuming equal numbers of females and males in a population, the population frequency of a particular allele at an X-linked locus is given by $(2p_f + p_m)/3$, where p_f is the gene frequency among females and p_m that among males. Under equilibrium conditions, $p_f = p_m$ (for $p_f \neq p_m$, HWE is not reached after one generation of random mating but only after a gradual stabilization). Well-known examples of X-linked genes are color blindness and hemophilia. For many autosomal genes, X-linked inheritance is mimicked in that the same genotype is expressed differently in males and females. This phenomenon, *sex-limited inheritance,* must not be confused with sex-linked inheritance. The vast majority of X-linked diseases are recessive, and the hallmark of recessive X-linked inheritance is a preponderance of males over females among affected individuals. Also, there is no father–son transmission for X-linked genes.

The above treatment of mendelian inheritance refers to genes residing on chromosomes, that is, in the cell nuclei. In addition to chromosomes, mitochondria also contain DNA (mtDNA). The phenotypes under the control of mitochondrial genes follow a *maternal mode of inheritance* (Wallace, 1989). The mitochondrial genome has been completely sequenced (Anderson et al., 1981). A well-known example of a maternally inherited disease, Leber disease, has been shown to be due to a single nucleotide change in the mitochondrial DNA (Wallace et al., 1988). It has been suggested that the mitochondrial DNA of all present-day human beings stems exclusively from one woman who lived about 200,000 years ago in Africa (Cann et al., 1987). Short pieces of mitochondrial DNA from Neanderthal fossil bones have been sequenced that indicate a period of roughly half a million years of independent evolution of Neanderthals and the line leading to modern humans (Ward and Stringer, 1997). In general, certain assumptions on the rate of DNA base pair substitutions have led to the concept of an evolutionary clock (Ayala, 1997).

As an aside, it may be mentioned that the chloroplasts of plants also contain genes. Mitochondria and chloroplasts are about the same size as bacteria and, like bacteria, have circular DNA genomes (Watson et al., 1987b), which suggests that they are derived from free-living bacteria (Palmer, 1997; Lang et al., 1997).

Gene expression not only depends on allelic status but also is determined by modifications of the DNA, higher order chromosome structure, and interaction among genes (*epistasis*). Many of these effects are due to methylation of DNA, and some are clearly heritable (*epigenetic inheritance*). A particular form of such effects is genomic imprinting (Section 12.6).

1.3. Crossing Over and Map Distance

In meiosis, that is, the cell division leading to the formation of gametes (egg or sperm cells), homologous chromosomes pair up. At that stage, each homolog consists of two strands (chromatids), so a chromosome pair consists of four strands. As meiosis progresses, the two homologous chromosomes separate from each other at most places but maintain one or more zones of contact known as *chiasmata* (Strickberger, 1985). They reflect the occurrence of crossing over (or *crossover*) between chromatids, where each crossover involves one chromatid from each of the two homologous chromosomes. Figure 1.2 schematically shows two crossovers, each involving two (possibly different) chromatids. The point on a gamete at which a crossover has occurred is called a *crossover point* (this terminology has been summarized in Ott, 1996). There always seems to occur at least one chiasma per pair of chromosomes; this may be necessary for an orderly separation of homologous chromosomes as meiosis progresses. While chiasmata can be observed under the microscope, crossovers may be observed in dense marker maps. An example is given in Figure 1.3, which is discussed in the next section.

When many genes along a chromosome are studied, one observes that crossovers occur more or less randomly along the chromosome in the sense that there is no observable constancy of time and location in their occurrence. This is not to say that their distribution along the

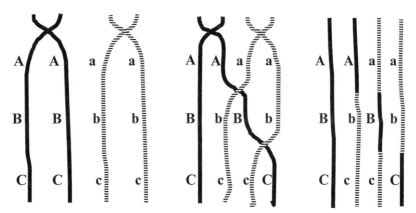

Figure 1.2. Schematic representation of two crossovers on a chromosome arm with three gene loci.

chromosome is uniform. On the contrary, crossover frequency varies with chromosomal regions and is, for example, almost totally suppressed in chromosomal inversions. An exception to the randomness of occurrence of crossovers is that the likelihood for a new crossover in the immediate vicinity of an existing crossover is much smaller than expected (*chiasma interference*). This is not of immediate concern here and will be discussed in more detail in Section 6.4.

Occurrence of crossovers is "semirandom" (Watson et al., 1987a), which is the basis for our ability to construct genetic maps (see below). Loci in close proximity of each other have only a small chance of experiencing a crossover between them. With increasing distance between two loci, an increasing number of crossovers is expected to occur between them. These considerations suggest that the number of crossovers between two loci could serve as a stochastic measure of distance between them. The genetic *map distance* (in units of Morgans) between two loci is defined as the expected (average) number of crossovers occurring on a single chromosome (in a gamete) between the loci. For example, the genetic length of chromosome 1 in females is 3.8 Morgans (Table 1.2). Thus, in gametes passed from parents to offspring, chromosome 1 exhibits an average of close to 4 crossover points.

Because chiasmata lead to crossovers and are cytogenetically observable, chiasma counts have early on provided estimates for the genetic length of the human genome. In male meioses, an average number of about 53 chiasmata has been observed over all of the autosomes. As each chiasma leads to a crossover point on half of the gametes, the average number of crossover points per gamete, and, thus, the total male autosomal

Table 1.2. Chromosome Lengths in Terms of Male and Female Map Distances and Physical Distances

Chromosome	Map Length (cM) Male	Map Length (cM) Female	Physical Length (kb)	Chromosome	Map Length (cM) Male	Map Length (cM) Female	Physical Length (kb)
1	221	376	263	13	107	157	144
2	193	297	255	14	106	151	109
3	186	289	214	15	84	149	106
4	157	274	203	16	110	152	98
5	149	267	194	17	108	152	92
6	142	222	183	18	111	149	85
7	144	244	171	19	113	121	67
8	135	226	155	20	104	120	72
9	130	176	145	21	66	77	50
10	144	192	144	22	78	89	56
11	125	189	144	X	—	193	160
12	136	232	143	Autos	2849	4301	3093

Source: Based on Collins et al., 1996a.
Note: Autos, sum over all autosomes.

map length, is estimated as 26.5 Morgans (Renwick, 1969) or 2650 centimorgans (cM). Based on higher chiasma frequencies in female than in male meioses, the female map length is approximately 1.5 times that of the male map (i.e., the female map length measures approximately 39 Morgans), and a sex-averaged autosomal map length of 33 Morgans may thus be quoted (Renwick, 1969). The "average" human chromosome is then 1.5 Morgans long; that is, it experiences an average of 1.5 crossovers. Newer investigations show that the human genome is somewhat larger with a sex-averaged total length of 36 Morgans (Table 1.2; see Section 1.6), but Renwick's predictions for genetic length some 30 years ago are remarkably accurate.

The concept of map distance has been covered here in a relatively simple manner, the emphasis being on application rather than theory. Mathematically inclined readers may be interested in a more thorough treatment of this subject, which may be found, for example, in Mather, 1938; Barratt et al., 1954; Bailey, 1961; Karlin, 1984; Liberman and Karlin, 1984; and McPeek and Speed, 1995. Crossovers and their chromosomal distributions will be covered more thoroughly in Sections 6.4 and 6.5.

1.4. Recombination and Genetic Linkage

In simple situations, it is possible to visualize crossovers between markers on a chromosome and to place a disease locus into a marker interval. For example, consider the small family in Figure 1.3, which shows three offspring affected with primary congenital glaucoma (Plášilová et al., 1998). Because this trait is recessively inherited, each parent is hetero-zygous at the disease locus and carries a disease allele on one of the two chromosomes. We can learn two things from this example. First, let's look at inheritance of the marker loci. The two haplotypes in the third offspring are the same as the corresponding ones in the parents. Also, one of the two haplotypes each (the one on the right side) in offspring 1 and 2 is the same as in the mother. However, the other haplotype in offspring 1 and offspring 2 each consists of two pieces, originating from different maternal haplotypes. In other words, in offspring 1, a crossover occurred between markers 2328 and 1356, while in offspring 2 a crossover occurred between markers 1788 and 1346.

The second lesson we learn from this example is to localize the disease locus to a map interval bounded by crossovers. In offspring 3, each of his two haplotypes carries a disease allele, and they identify the "disease" haplotypes in the parents. Thus far, the disease locus could be anywhere on these haplotypes or even outside the map spanned by the

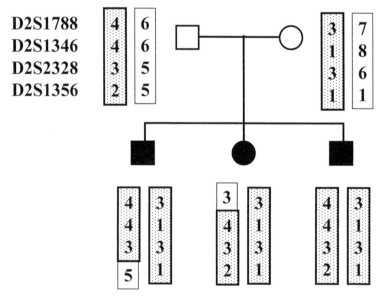

Figure 1.3. Family showing inheritance of four closely linked markers on chromosome 1. Individuals with solid symbols are affected with autosomal recessive primary congen-ital glaucoma. Shaded portions of haplotypes carry alleles. (Based on Plášilová et al., 1998.)

marker loci. However, the haplotype on the left side in offspring 1 demonstrates that the disease locus must be north of the crossover. As the crossover may have occurred anywhere in the interval between markers 2328 and 1356, all we can say is that the disease locus must be north of marker 1356. Analogously, the haplotype in offspring 2 carrying the crossover shows that the disease locus must be south of marker 1788. Thus, the two crossovers localize the disease gene to a position between markers D2S1788 and D2S1356.

This straightforward way of gene mapping is possible only under particularly favorable circumstances: no errors, known mendelian disease genotypes, and known dense marker map. Generally, however, crossovers cannot be observed directly in human families. Consider, for example, Figure 1.1, where it is assumed that the doubly heterozygous father is married to a doubly homozygous individual, *ab/ab,* who has the same genotype as one of the parents in the previous generation (one of the grandparents). Such a mating is called a *backcross,* a phase-known double backcross in this case. Based on what was said in the previous section, one might interpret an offspring genotype *Ab/ab* as showing occurrence of a crossover in the doubly heterozygous parent. However, consider Figure 1.2 and a parent with phase-known genotype, *AC/ac.* Two crossovers between two loci on a gamete lead to a haplotype, *ac,* that looks the same as if no crossover had occurred. In human families such as that depicted in Figure 1.1, we can only distinguish two types of offspring genotypes. The father potentially passes four haplotypes, *AB, ab, Ab,* and *aB,* to his offspring. Haplotypes *AB* and *ab* look the same as the ones he received from his parents (from the grandparents). Children receiving these are in classical genetics called *parental types* (e.g., the child on the right side of Figure 1.1). The other two haplotypes, *Ab* and *aB,* are unlike any haplotypes received by the father from the grandparents and contain one allele from each grandparent (a "re-combination" of grandparental alleles must have occurred in the father). In classical genetics, offspring carrying such haplotypes are designated as *nonparental types.* In human genetics, the nonparental types, *Ab* and *aB,* are called *recombinants,* and the other two haplotypes (*AB* and *ab*) are called *nonrecombinants.* A *recombination* between two genes denotes the event that two different grandparents contribute one allele at each of the two gene loci to a haplotype in an individual. On the other hand, a *nonrecombination* is said to have occurred when a haplotype in an individual contains two alleles (one at each gene locus) which originate from the same grandparent of that individual. An offspring is termed a recombinant or nonrecombinant if his phenotype indicates that a recombination or nonrecombination has occurred in one of the parents. Thus, in Figure 1.1, daughter 1 is a recombinant and daughter 2 is a nonrecombinant. The following relation between recombination and crossing over holds: An odd number of crossover points between two loci on a gamete leads to a recombination whereas an even number of crossover points leads to a nonrecombination. The proportion of recombinant haplotypes (or offspring) potentially produced by a doubly heterozygous parent is called the *recombination fraction,* which is also the probability of occurrence of a recombination. In human genetics, the recombination fraction is usually designated by a lowercase Greek theta, θ.

Which of the two homologous strands of a chromosome are involved in a crossover appears to be random and independent from one crossover to the next (absence of so-called chromatid interference). With only one crossover on a chromosome, the recombination fraction between two loci at opposite ends of a chromosome is 50% (because the crossover affects two of the four gametic products). Under absence of chromatid interference, the same result holds for any number of crossovers (Mather, 1938). With chromatid interference, θ may exceed 50%, but this theoretical possibility is not generally considered of importance in human genetics. For loci that are in close proximity of each other, at most one crossover occurs between them so that the recombination fraction is equal to the average number of crossovers on a gamete. Thus, for small intervals, the recombination fraction directly measures genetic distance.

Crossing over and recombination has been outlined above in a somewhat simplified manner. Consider again Figure 1.2, which shows three loci and two points of crossing over. An exchange of single strands between the parental chromosomes leads to the formation of a cross-bridged structure, the Holliday structure (see Strickberger, 1985, Figure 18–8). According to this recombinational model, the Holliday structure may be resolved by cutting of single strands, where the cuts can occur in two different directions, both leading to linear molecules (strands) but only one (shown in Figure 1.2) resulting in a recombination for outside gene markers. Meiosis results in the production of four sperm cells, or one egg cell and three polar bodies, each of which receives one chromatid of each chromosome. The exact relation between chiasmata and recombinant haplotypes is unclear; conventionally, it is assumed that one chiasma corresponds to two recombinant and two nonrecombinant haplotypes (see Section 1.5).

When two loci are inherited independently of each other, recombinants and nonrecombinants are expected in equal proportions among the offspring. For loci in close proximity of each other, one observes a consistent deviation from the 1:1 ratio of recombinant to nonrecombinant offspring: Alleles in a haplotype passed from a grandparent to a parent tend to be passed again as the same haplotype from the parent to the offspring. In other words, alleles at different gene loci appear to be genetically coupled, and this phenomenon is called *genetic linkage.* Two genes are completely linked when a doubly heterozygous parent can produce only nonrecombinant gametes, and linkage is absent (recombination is free), when a parent tends to produce both recombinant and nonrecombinant haplotypes in equal proportions (i.e., when $\theta = 0.50$). The following features characterize genetic linkage between two or more loci:

1. Because recombination events can be recognized only on the basis of haplotypes passed from parents to children, linkage analysis cannot be carried out with unrelated individuals but requires observations on relatives. Therefore, for linkage analysis, researchers collect phenotypic information on members of family pedigrees. A *pedigree* may be defined as a set of relatives with known relationships among individuals (for a graph-theoretic treatment of pedigrees, see Thompson, 1986). Pedigree members fall into two classes: *Founders* are individuals whose parents are not in the pedigree whereas *nonfounders* have their parents in the pedigree. For statistical reasons, each nonfounder is assumed to have both his or her parents in the pedigree. Founders are generally assumed to be unrelated and drawn randomly from the population, perhaps conditional on sampling schemes (e.g., that a pedigree should contain at least two individuals affected with the disease being studied).

2. Recombinant and nonrecombinant haplotypes produced by a parent cannot always be distinguished. Consider, for instance, the *Ab* haplotype produced by a parent with genotype *Ab/ab.* Because of homozygosity for the second gene, *Ab* could be a recombinant or a nonrecombinant haplotype. For these to be distinguishable, the parent must be doubly heterozygous. Only then is he or she potentially *informative for linkage,* as geneticists say. A mating is potentially informative for linkage between two specific genes when at least one of the parents is a double heterozygote.

3. For many pairs of loci, linkage analysis shows that the recombination fraction differs depending on the sex of the parent producing gametes. Therefore, one distinguishes a male recombination fraction, θ_m, and a female recombination fraction, θ_f. The distinction between the two refers to the gender of the parent in which recombination takes place and not to the gender of the children who may be counted as recombinant or nonrecombinant offspring. Sex dependency of the recombination fraction will be covered in greater detail in Section 10.1.

If locus 1 is genetically linked to locus 2, and locus 2 is linked to locus 3, then locus 1 may or may not be linked to locus 3. A *linkage group* is defined as a set of genes in which each gene is linked with at least one other gene in the same set. Thus, if locus 1 is unlinked with locus 3, the three loci considered here nonetheless form a linkage group. Experience shows that partitioning loci into linkage groups is unique in the sense that two loci belonging to different linkage groups are always unlinked. For early geneticists, the interpretation of the genetic phenomenon of a linkage group became clear with the observation that, in each (diploid) species investigated, the number of linkage groups coincided with the number of chromosome pairs. Linkage groups can now be interpreted as being the genetic equivalents of chromosomes on which loci are arranged in a linear order.

I will only briefly mention here that, in male meioses, the X and Y chromosomes also pair up. Recombination then takes place in small regions of homology between X and Y, the pseudoautosomal regions. Formal linkage analysis involving pseudoautosomal loci is covered in Section 9.4.

A phenomenon often related to recombination is that of *gene conversion:* When two alleles pair up at meiosis, one is "converted" to resemble the other (Maynard Smith, 1989). On the surface, this phenomenon is similar to mutation, but its characteristics are distinct from those of mutation. Details and genetic models of gene conversion may be found in Strickberger (1985). In some organisms, gene conversion is relatively frequent. For example, an apparent double recombination within a very short genomic segment may be caused by gene conversion. In humans, gene conversion has been demonstrated repeatedly, for example, by Giver and Grosovsky (1997).

As outlined above, the recombination fraction ranges from 0 for tightly linked loci to 50% for unlinked loci. In polyploid species, recombination fractions of 80% and more are regularly observed (Wright et al., 1983).

Loci located on the same chromosome are said to be *syntenic.* Synteny of a pair of loci has always been shown to imply that the two loci belong to the same linkage group, although they are not necessarily genetically linked. The converse, that nonsyntenic loci show linkagelike associations, has occasionally been observed and has been called *quasi-linkage* or affinity (Bailey, 1961). An example in the mouse and a discussion of various possible mechanisms may be found in Stockert et al. (1976).

The fact that two alleles at different loci occur in the same haplotype does not imply synteny of these loci. The vertical bar in the genotype of the father in Figure 1.1 simply indicates that phase is known, but this says nothing about the linkage or synteny relationship of the two loci involved. This situation is a source of confusion for many students of linkage analysis, and it is very important that these relationships are clearly understood before one proceeds.

The precise nature of the biochemical process of recombination is only partly understood. Recombination and its determinants are studied in experimental organisms, particularly yeast (Gangloff et al., 1994). The evolutionary significance of recombination is discussed in Chapter 12 of Maynard Smith (1989). Its major aspects seem to be twofold: Recombination increases variability and thus accelerates evolution by natural selection, and it is involved in repairing of DNA damage. A summary of the current research status has been given by Kanaar and Hoeijmakers (1998). In contrast to meiotic recombination covered thus far, there is also somatic (mitotic) recombination, but this is not pursued here (see Strickberger, 1985).

1.5. Map Functions

This section presents an overview with little mathematical complexity of various map functions (see also Section 6.5). As discussed above, when occurrence of multiple crossovers between two loci can be excluded (complete interference), the appropriate map function is simply

$$x = \theta, \tag{1.1}$$

because then, the probability, θ, of a recombination is equal to the expected number of crossovers between the two loci. This assumption is usually warranted for closely linked genes, say, when $\theta < 0.10$. For example, when the recombination fraction between two loci is $\theta = 0.06$, the map distance between them is approximately equal to 0.06 Morgan (i.e., a recombination fraction of 6% corresponds to ≈ 6 cM). When many closely linked loci are available on a chromosome and their order is known, then the simplest method of determining map distances among these genes is to estimate the recombination fraction in each interval of adjacent loci. The map distance between two more distant loci is then obtained as the sum of the map distances in the intervals between these loci (Sturtevant, 1913). Equation (1.1) is also known as *Morgan's map function* (Morgan, 1928).

When multiple crossovers occur between loci, recombination fractions in different intervals are no longer additive. For example, with three loci, 1, 2, and 3, and recombination fractions θ_1 and θ_2 in the corresponding two intervals, the recombination fraction between the flanking loci is generally smaller than the sum, $\theta_1 + \theta_2$. Under the assumption that crossovers in different intervals occur according to the Poisson probability law, Haldane (1919) expressed map distance as

$$x = \begin{cases} -\tfrac{1}{2}\ln(1 - 2\theta) & \text{if } 0 \le \theta < \tfrac{1}{2} \\ \infty & \text{otherwise,} \end{cases} \tag{1.2}$$

whose inverse is

$$\theta = \tfrac{1}{2}[1 - \exp(-2|x|)],$$

where exp denotes the exponential function (inverse of natural logarithm) and $|x|$ stands for the absolute value of x. For example, to convert a recombination fraction of 22% into a map distance according to the Haldane map function, $\theta = 0.22$ entered in equation (1.2) yields $x = 0.29$ Morgans or 29 centimorgans (cM). As a distance measure, x may in principle be taken to be positive or negative, which is why absolute signs are used above. In this book, however, map distance will generally be assumed to be positive. Below, for simplicity, it will be assumed that θ is smaller than 0.50 so the case $\theta = 0.50$ will not have to be considered separately.

Depending on the assumed mechanism by which interference operates, many other map functions have been derived. Here, only a few more shall be mentioned. By making particular assumptions on marginal interference to be covered in Section 6.4, Kosambi (1944) derived the map function

$$x = \tfrac{1}{2}\tanh^{-1}(2\theta) = \tfrac{1}{4}\ln\frac{1 + 2\theta}{1 - 2\theta} \tag{1.3}$$

with inverse

$$\theta = \tfrac{1}{2}\tanh(2x) = \tfrac{1}{2}\frac{\exp(4x) - 1}{\exp(4x) + 1}.$$

This map function has been widely used in genetics. Using the same example as above, $\theta = 0.22$ in equation (1.3) yields a map distance of 23.6 cM.

For the relatively strong interference in the mouse, Carter and Falconer (1951) made other assumptions on marginal interference and found the following map function to fit observed data rather well:

$$x = \tfrac{1}{4}[\tan^{-1}(2\theta) + \tanh^{-1}(2\theta)]. \tag{1.4}$$

Its inverse cannot be obtained in closed form, but the following equation allows an iterative computation of θ from x when the θ value is initially set equal to x:

$\theta = \frac{1}{2} \tanh[4x - \tan^{-1}(2\theta)]$.

The map functions considered thus far incorporate fixed assumptions on how interference operates. Interference is strongest in function (1.1), where no more than a single crossover is allowed, and is absent in (1.2). To provide for an adjustable level of interference, Haldane (1919) proposed the compound map function,

$$x = (1 - p)\theta - \frac{1}{2} p \ln(1 - 2\theta), \; 0 \le p \le 1. \tag{1.5}$$

It is a weighted average of the map functions (1.1) and (1.2) with weights $1 - p$ and p, where Haldane chose $p = 0.7$. For $p = 0$, (1.5) reduces to (1.1), and for $p = 1$, (1.5) is identical with the regular Haldane map function (1.2). Thus, the compound map function (1.5) allows any level of positive interference, but it is not generally used in human genetics.

Rao et al. (1979) extended this concept by defining a mapping parameter, p, such that x reduces to x_1, x_2, x_3, and x_4, given by (1.2), (1.3), (1.4), and (1.1), respectively, when p assumes the respective values 1, $\frac{1}{2}$, $\frac{1}{4}$, and 0. This map function is a weighted average, $x = \sum_{i=1}^{4} w_i x_i$, where $w_1 = p(1 - 2p)(1 - 4p)/3$, $w_2 = -4(1 - p)(1 - 4p)p$, $w_3 = 32(1 - p)(1 - 2p)p/3$, $w_4 = (1 - p)(1 - 2p)(1 - 4p)$, and $\Sigma w_i = 1$. The inverse of Rao's map function as well as that of (1.5) are unavailable in closed form but may be calculated by standard numerical methods.

Another map function with a variable level of interference has been given by Felsenstein (1979) as

$$x = \frac{1}{2(2 - k)} \ln\left[1 + \frac{2\theta(1 - k)}{1 - 2\theta} \right], \; 0 \le k < 2, \tag{1.6}$$

with inverse

$$\theta = \frac{1}{2} \frac{\exp[2x(2 - k)] - 1}{\exp[2x(2 - k)] + 1 - k}.$$

With $k = 1$, (1.6) is identical with the Haldane map function (1.2), and with $k = 0$ it is identical with the Kosambi map function (1.3). The strongest level of interference allowed by this map function is the one incorporated in Kosambi's function (1.3).

Postulating an obligatory chiasma and assuming additional chiasmata to be distributed at random, Sturt (1976) developed the map function

$$\theta = \frac{1}{2}[1 - (1 - x/L)\exp(-2x + x/L)], \; x < L, \tag{1.7}$$

where $L \ge \frac{1}{2}$ is the chromosome length in Morgans, with $\theta = \frac{1}{2}$ for $x = L$. For example, when two loci are 29 cM apart and are located on a chromosome of length 150 cM ($L = 1.5$), formula (1.7) predicts a recombination fraction of 23% between the two loci. The inverse of (1.7) may be obtained by standard numerical procedures and furnishes, for example, a map distance of $x = 0.25$ for $\theta = 0.20$ and $L = 1.5$. For $L = \frac{1}{2}$, the graph of (1.7) is a straight line, corresponding to (1.1). For large L, (1.7) becomes identical to the inverse of Haldane's map function (1.2).

All of the above map functions except (1.1) postulate a theoretically unlimited number of crossovers. If one assumes at most N crossovers, independently distributed in an interval of length x, with numbers occurring according to the binomial law (Karlin, 1984), one obtains the Binomial map function,

$$\theta = \tfrac{1}{2}[1 - (1 - 2x/N)^N], \quad x < N/2, \tag{1.8}$$

where $\theta = \frac{1}{2}$ for $x = N/2$. Its inverse is given by

$$x = \tfrac{1}{2}N[1 - (1 - 2\theta)^{1/N}]. \tag{1.9}$$

It follows from (1.9) that the map distance between unlinked loci is equal to $N/2$. Graphs of several map functions discussed above are shown in Figure 1.4.

Map functions incorporate different levels of interference, which may depend on map distance. Consequently, for three ordered loci, 1, 2, and 3, they yield different predictions of the recombination fraction, θ_{13}, between the flanking loci based on the recombination fractions θ_{12} and θ_{23} in the two intervals. For the Haldane map function, such an addition

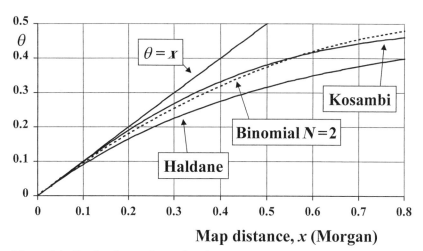

Figure 1.4. Graphs of several map functions.

formula is obtained as follows: To find θ_{13}, one must convert θ_{12} and θ_{23} into the respective map distances, x_{12} and x_{23}, which can then be summed to yield x_{13}. This, in turn, is then transformed back into a recombination fraction, θ_{13}. Equation (1.2) furnishes x_{12} and x_{23} so that one obtains $x_{13} = -\frac{1}{2} \ln[(1 - 2\theta_{12})(1 - 2\theta_{23})]$. Substituting x_{13} for x in the right side of the inverse of (1.3) gives the desired solution, $\theta_{13} = \theta_{12} + \theta_{23} - 2\theta_{12}\theta_{23}$. An interpretation of this formula is given in Section 6.4 on interference.

The MAPFUN computer program (Section 9.5) interactively calculates map distances from recombination fractions and vice versa for the map functions mentioned above. It allows, for example, numerical calculation of the predicted recombination fraction between the flanking loci based on the recombination fractions in the two adjacent intervals. In many multipoint computer programs, absence of interference is assumed for the calculation of haplotype probabilities. Researchers then often use the Haldane map function (absence of interference) to convert the estimated recombination fractions to map distances, but other map functions are employed as well. In fact, it seems preferable to use a map function with interference such as Kosambi's as it appears to produce more realistic map distance values than does Haldane's formula. For small distances, say, $\theta \leq 0.05$, any map function is appropriate.

If one wants to convert a map distance into a recombination fraction, one needs to know by what metric the map distance was obtained. Thus, it has been recommended (Keats et al., 1989) that map distances be identified through an appropriately modified symbol such as x_H, x_K, x_R, x_C, or x_F for the Haldane, Kosambi, Rao ($p = 0.35$), Carter–Falconer, or Felsenstein map function, respectively, or by labeling the measurement units as cM(H), cM(K), cM(R), cM(C), or cM(F). To compare genetic distance data based on different metrics, one must convert them into the same metric.

The map functions discussed above are those that a reader is most likely to encounter in practice. Some additional map functions, rarely used in human genetics, are mentioned in Section 6.5.

1.6. The Human Chromosomes

Map distance is a genetic distance, which need not correlate well with physical distance (measured in number of base pairs of DNA). The only unequivocal connection between them is that genetic and physical distances are monotonic, that is, an increase in map distance translates into a larger physical distance. However, the same map distance in different regions of the map may refer to different physical distances. Therefore, although recombination fractions are poor predictors of physical distances, it is recombination fractions and not physical distances that are relevant in genetic counseling.

Assuming a total genetic map length of 3000 cM (newer estimates of total map length are quoted at the end of this section) and a number of 3×10^9 bp in the haploid genome, a genetic distance of 1 cM approximately corresponds to 1000 kb or 1 million base pairs (1 megabase) (Donis-Keller et al., 1987). Such indirect estimates of the kb/cM ratio have been shown to vary considerably between species and between chromosomal regions within a species. For example, the region of the Duchenne muscular dystrophy (DMD) gene has been described as a hot spot for recombination (Grimm et al., 1989). Also, the X–Y pairing (pseudoautosomal) region appears to be a hot spot of recombination in males, presumably because of the requirement of one obligate crossover between the X and Y chromosomes occurring over a relatively short region.

As pointed out previously, the normal human karyotype comprises 22 pairs of autosomes and two sex chromosomes, X and Y. The morphology of the chromosomes is described by specific nomenclature rules (Mitelman, 1995). Each chromosome comprises two arms separated by a primary restriction, the centromere. The short arm is denoted by p (*petit* is French for small); the long arm by q. A secondary restriction (the centromere being the primary chromosomal restriction) is denoted by h. For example, 9qh designates the secondary restriction on the long arm of chromosome 9. The relative position of the centromere on a chromosome is indicated by the centromere index, $c = 100\ p/(p + q)$, where p and q refer to the arm lengths of the chromosome. Various staining methods show many different chromosome bands that allow unequivocal identification of each chromosome and of portions of chromosomes. The chromosome band nomenclature defines a *landmark* as a consistent and distinct morphologic feature, such as the ends of chromosome arms, the centromere, and certain bands. A *region* is defined as any area of a chromosome lying between two adjacent landmarks. Regions and bands are numbered consecutively from the centromere outward along each chromosome arm. For a detailed analysis, some bands are divided into subbands, whose numbers are separated from the band number by a decimal point. For example, the ABO blood group locus is at 9q34, that is, in band 34 on the long arm of chromosome 9.

Table 1.2 shows genetic and physical lengths of the human autosomes and the X chromosome. Genetic distances are given in units of centimorgans; physical distances are in units of megabases and have been determined (or estimated) by various methods (Collins et al., 1996a). The figures in Table 1.2 were obtained from the summary maps at URL http://cedar.genetics.soton.ac.uk/public_html/ (status 1 January 1998). Total male and female map lengths are 28 and 43 Morgans, respectively, with a sex-averaged genome length of 34 M. The female-to-male map distance ratio is equal to 1.51 over the whole genome. The same ratio applies more or less to each chromosome. However, there are known trends of this ratio along specific chromosomes (see Section 10.1).

1.7. Problems

Problem 1.1. Consider three gene loci numbered 1, 2, and 3, and assume that the recombination fractions in the two intervals are θ_{12} and θ_{23}. What is the recombination fraction, θ_{13}, between loci 1 and 3 in terms of θ_{12} and θ_{23} as predicted by the Kosambi formula?

Problem 1.2. Using the same assumptions as in Problem 1.1, derive the expression for θ_{13} in terms of θ_{12}, θ_{23}, and k, where k is the parameter in Felsenstein's map function (1.6). Then, solve the resulting equation for k, thus finding an estimator for the level of interference. Verify your results by setting $k = 1$, which should yield the results obtained for the Haldane map function.

Problem 1.3. Under complete interference, all chromosomes have equal genetic lengths. Why is this so, and what is this length?

2.

Genetic Loci and Genetic Polymorphisms

As we saw in Chapter 1, linkage analysis investigates genetic distance between loci, particularly the relationships between disease genes and *genetic markers,* that is, genetic entities known to follow a mendelian mode of inheritance (a narrower definition of genetic marker also requires that its map location be known). This chapter discusses specific aspects of human genetic loci. It involves few technical details and is intended only as a brief reference for linkage analysts.

2.1. Nomenclature and Characterization of Genetic Loci

Classically, the presence of genes has been recognized by the variability of their effects; that is, only polymorphic genes were readily detectable. Molecular genetics methods allow the recognition and location of genes based on the proteins they produce; the genes themselves may or may not be polymorphic. The estimated proportion of genes that are polymorphic varies from roughly 15% in fish to close to 50% in *Drosophila* (Hartl, 1988). In humans, the proportion of genes that are polymorphic has been estimated as 32% (Harris, Hopkinson, and Edwards, 1977).

Many of the known human genes have been mapped. A standing committee maintains rules for their nomenclature and assigns gene symbols (White et at., 1997; http://www.gene.ucl.ac.uk/nomenclature/). For DNA polymorphisms, special rules apply (see Section 2.3).

Probably the largest database of genes identified in humans is Professor McKusick's *Mendelian Inheritance in Man* (MIM). It was first published 1966 in book form and has been regularly updated. Its on-line version (OMIM$^{\text{(TM)}}$) is hosted by NCBI, the National Center for Biotechnology Information (http://www.ncbi.nlm.nih.gov/Omim/). OMIM describes disease genes as well as marker genes, each provided with a unique number (referred to as the MIM number). As of November 27, 1998, it comprises a total of 9993 genes (9344 autosomal, 560 X-linked, 29 Y-linked, and 60 mitochondrial genes).

Another source of information is the Genetic Data Base (GDB), which grew out of the Human Gene Mapping (HGM) workshops, but funding for it has ceased in 1998. As of November 22, 1998, the total number of genes mapped to chromosomal locations and stored in GDB is 6952 (http://www.gdb.org/gdbreports/CountGeneByChromosome.html).

Genetic loci that follow a dominant or codominant mode of inheritance are referred to as *factor–union systems* (Cotterman, 1969). Their phenotypes are reactions to some tests, and these reactions (called factors) are either positive (present) or negative (absent). Characterization of such phenotypes is particularly simple in factor–union notation (by a sequence of binary digits in which each element is either 1 or 0, where 1 stands for presence and 0 for absence of a particular factor).

Before the development of DNA variants (see Section 2.3), linkage analysts had at their disposition a battery of up to 60 classical marker loci. Many of these were polymorphic genes coding for blood cell antigens (Vogel and Motulsky, 1986). Here, only two of these genes are described, the ABO and LU systems.

The *ABO blood group* locus produces two major antigens, A and B, located on the surface of the red blood cells. These antigens can be probed with two antisera containing the respective antibodies, anti-A and anti-B. Cells with the A antigen will show a reaction (agglutination) to anti-A, and cells with the B antigen will react to the anti-B antiserum but not to the anti-A. It is convenient to code the presence or absence of an antibody–antigen reaction by the respective symbols 1 and 0 (factor–union notation). The reaction of the red blood cells of an individual to anti-A and anti-B is then coded as two digits. For example, 01 represents reaction to anti-B but not to anti-A; cells with this reaction carry the B antigen but not the A antigen on their surfaces. A total of four different reactions can be observed: 10, 01, 00, and 11, corresponding to the blood groups, A, B, O, and AB, respectively. It is a peculiarity of the ABO system that individuals always have in their blood serum the antibodies against those antigens not present on their red blood cells. For example, individuals showing reaction 10 (blood group A) have the A antigens on their red blood cells and the anti-B antibodies in their serum.

The genetic interpretation of the four phenotypes (blood groups) is that they are under the control of three alleles. Two alleles, *a* and *b,* produce the respective antigens A and B (codominant inheritance). A third allele, *o,* does not produce any antigens so that $o < a$ and $o < b;$ that is, *o* is recessive to *a* and *b*. These three alleles combine in pairs to form a total of six possible genotypes. The relations between genotypes and phenotypes are shown in Table 1.1. On the molecular level, the *a, b,* and *o* alleles differ in a few single-base substitutions (Yamamoto et al., 1990).

Blood type A may be subdivided into at least two subgroups called A_1 and A_2. Usually, the blood cells are first tested for a general A antigen. Those that respond negatively contain neither A_1 nor A_2. Those that respond positively are then tested for the A_1 antigen. A positive reaction indicates blood type A_1; a negative reaction, blood type A_2. Table 2.1 shows the relation between genotypes and phenotypes, assuming four different alleles at the ABO locus, a_1, a_2, *b,* and *o.* In Caucasian populations, their respective gene frequencies are approximately equal to 0.21, 0.07, 0.06, and 0.66, respectively. From these frequencies, under the assumptions of Hardy–Weinberg equilibrium, the expected frequencies of the genotypes and phenotypes can be calculated (Table 2.1). Associations between ABO blood groups and diseases are well known, and the world distribution of ABO gene frequencies suggests influences of natural selection (Vogel and Motulsky, 1986).

At the *Lutheran (LU) blood group* locus, two major alleles exist, *A* and *B,* with respective approximate allele frequencies of 0.04 and 0.96. The antigens may be detected by antibodies anti-A and anti-B, so that heterozygous *A/B* individuals are distinguishable from both types of homozygotes (codominant inheritance). Sometimes only anti-A is used in laboratories. In that case, *A* is dominant because *A/A* and *A/B* genotypes cannot be distinguished. Relations among LU genotypes and phenotypes are

Table 2.1. Penetrances and Expected Phenotype and Genotype Frequencies at the *ABO* Locus with Four *ABO* Alleles

Genotype	Phenotype						Genotype Freq.
	A_1	A_2	A_1B	A_2B	B	O	
a_1/a_1	1	0	0	0	0	0	0.0441
a_1/a_2	1	0	0	0	0	0	0.0294
a_1/b	0	0	1	0	0	0	0.0252
a_1/o	1	0	0	0	0	0	0.2772
a_2/a_2	0	1	0	0	0	0	0.0049
a_2/b	0	0	0	1	0	0	0.0084
a_2/o	0	1	0	0	0	0	0.0924
b/b	0	0	0	0	1	0	0.0036
b/o	0	0	0	0	1	0	0.0792
o/o	0	0	0	0	0	1	0.4356
Phenotype frequency	0.3507	0.0973	0.0252	0.0084	0.0828	0.4356	1

given in Table 2.2. The map location of the LU locus is on chromosome 19q, which was found only in the early 1980s. LU has long been known to be linked with the Secretor blood group. In fact, this was the first autosomal linkage detected in humans (Mohr, 1954).

Of particular importance in human genetics is the *HLA gene complex* (Lechler, 1994). Its antigens are located in the white blood cells and play a role in histocompatibility. This system consists of a set of several closely linked genes with a large number of different haplotypes. It is highly complex and extremely polymorphic. Some of its haplotypes show strong associations with diseases.

2.2. Measures of Polymorphism

The term *polymorphism* denotes the fact that a locus is polymorphic, but it is also used as a synonym for polymorphic locus. A general discussion of human polymorphisms may be found in Section 6.1.2 of Vogel and Motulsky (1986).

It was established in Chapter 1 that for a mating to be (potentially) informative for linkage between two gene loci, at least one of the two parents must be doubly heterozygous. Therefore, a marker's usefulness for linkage analysis depends on the number of its alleles and their gene frequencies (i.e., its degree of polymorphism) in the sense that an increased polymorphism leads to an increased probability of heterozygosity. Marker usefulness or informativeness is discussed here purely in terms of degree of polymorphism, but other characteristics of gene markers determine their usefulness in a more general sense. For example, a DNA polymorphism may have a large number of alleles that are recognized as bands on a Southern blot, but the bands may be so little separated from each other that unique identification of the different alleles is difficult, leading to phenotypic misclassification.

Table 2.2. Relation between LU Genotypes and Phenotypes (Penetrances)

	Phenotype				
	Using Anti-A, and Anti-B			Using Anti-A Only	
Genotype	A+ B−	A+ B+	A− B+	A+	A−
A/A	1	0	0	1	0
A/B	0	1	0	1	0
B/B	0	0	1	0	1

Two measures of the degree of polymorphism are generally used in human genetics. One is the *heterozygosity,*

$$H = 1 - \Sigma p_i^2, \tag{2.1}$$

where p_i is the population frequency of the ith allele, and H is simply the probability that a random individual is heterozygous for any two alleles at a gene locus with allele frequencies, p_i. For example, three alleles with frequencies of 0.28, 0.06, and 0.66 at the ABO locus yield a heterozygosity of 0.48 so that almost half of all individuals are expected to be heterozygous at the ABO locus. As defined above, equation (2.1) refers to the proportion of heterozygotes as predicted under HWE conditions (see Section 1.2) because genotype frequencies are determined by allele frequencies, p_i. Weir (1996) reserves the term heterozygosity for the proportion of heterozygotes in the population; that is, when inferences are made on genotypes rather than alleles. He refers to expression (2.1) above as gene diversity.

Assortative mating (matings occur preferentially between individuals with similar phenotypes) and inbreeding (mating between relatives) tend to reduce heterozygosity but do not change allele frequencies (Hartl, 1988). In human populations, these effects are not strong enough to reduce heterozygosity noticeably. Under inbreeding, the expected proportion of heterozygotes is $(1 - F)H$ (Hartl, 1988), where F is the inbreeding coefficient. Vogel and Motulsky (1986) give a lucid discussion of inbreeding and provide an extensive table of estimates of F for various human populations. The largest values found are around $F = 0.005$, but the values are in most cases much smaller than that. Therefore, predictions of the proportion of heterozygotes based on H [equation (2.1)] are not much biased by inbreeding. In isolated populations, higher inbreeding coefficients have been reported (e.g., an average value of $F = 0.04$ in the Hutterites) (Kostyu et al., 1989). Still, this reduces heterozygosity only by a factor of 0.96 (i.e., from 75% to 72%). This situation may be quite different for domesticated animal populations. For example, the inbreeding coefficient in pure-bred dogs may exceed 0.50 (Dorn and Schneider, 1976).

For a gene with a alleles, heterozygosity is largest with equally frequent alleles, $p_i = p_j = 1/a$. Then, heterozygosity takes the simple form,

$$H = 1 - 1/a. \tag{2.2}$$

For example, a locus with three alleles has a maximum heterozygosity of $H = 0.67$.

Solving (2.2) for a leads to $a = 1/(1 - H)$ which represents the number of equally frequent alleles (or the minimum number of alleles with any frequencies) required for a specified heterozygosity, *H*. For example, for a heterozygosity of 0.90, a gene must have at least 10 alleles, but its heterozygosity will be 0.90 only when each allele has a population frequency of 10%; otherwise, heterozygosity will be less than 0.90.

In human genetics, another measure of the degree of polymorphism often used is the polymorphism information content (PIC) value (Botstein et al., 1980). It was derived for the situation of a (rare) dominant disease in a nuclear family and a codominant marker. One of the parents is assumed to be affected (heterozygous for the disease allele). The PIC value is defined as the probability that the marker genotype of a given offspring will allow deduction of which of the two marker alleles of the affected parent it had received. PIC is calculated as

$$PIC = 1 - \sum_{i=1}^{a} p_i^2 - \sum_{i=1}^{a-1} \sum_{j=i+1}^{a} 2(p_i p_j)^2, \tag{2.3}$$

where p_i is the population frequency of the *i*th allele. For the ABO example used above, PIC is equal to 0.41.

As one can see from comparing (2.3) with (2.1), the PIC value is always smaller than the heterozygosity. For *a* equally frequent alleles, equation (2.3) reduces to

$$PIC = (a - 1)^2 (a + 1)/a^3 = 1 - 1/a - (a - 1)/a^3. \tag{2.4}$$

A comparison of equations (2.2) and (2.4) shows that, for large numbers *a* of alleles at a locus, heterozygosity and PIC become very close.

In Chapter 1, a gene was defined to be polymorphic when its most common allele has a population frequency of at most 95%. Equations (2.1) and (2.3) then imply that $H \geq 0.10$ and $PIC \geq 0.10$, respectively. Thus, a polymorphic gene has heterozygosity of at least 10%.

In practice, heterozygosity is a useful characterization of codominant loci only. For dominant loci, some heterozygotes and homozygotes cannot be distinguished so that heterozygosity specifies the unobservable proportion of heterozygotes.

Equation (2.1) is generally applied to *estimates* of allele frequencies rather than to allele frequencies known without error. Thus, the resulting value for heterozygosity is also an estimate. Although uncertainties in estimates are generally indicated with confidence intervals or standard errors, it is curious that this is rarely done for heterozygosity estimates.

Let *a* again be the number of alleles at a genetic marker system, and *n* the number of alleles sampled to estimate heterozygosity (the number of individuals sampled is then *n*/2). The observed proportions of alleles,

$\hat{p}_i$, are then maximum likelihood estimates (MLEs) of the population allele frequencies, p_i, and, in analogy to (2.1), the MLE of heterozygosity is given by

$$\hat{H} = 1 - \sum_{i=1}^{a}\hat{p}_i^2, \tag{2.5}$$

which is the formula generally used. However, (2.5) is biased (see Section 3.3) and yields an estimate of H that is somewhat too small (Weir, 1996). An unbiased estimate is given by

$$\hat{H}_U = \hat{H}n/(n - 1). \tag{2.6}$$

The bias, $b = -H/n$, is noticeable only for small sample sizes. For example, consider a locus with $a = 4$ equally frequent alleles so that heterozygosity is equal to 0.75. When 10 individuals ($n = 20$ alleles) are sampled, the expectation of the conventional estimate $\hat{H}$ is equal to 0.71 whereas that of $\hat{H}_U$ is equal to 0.75.

The sampling variance of the biased estimate (2.5) was derived by Nei and Roychoudhury (1974) as

$$V(\hat{H}) = \frac{2(n - 1)}{n^3}\left[(3 - 2n)\left(\sum_{i=1}^{a}p_i^2\right)^2 + 2(n - 2)\sum_{i=1}^{a}p_i^3 + \sum_{i=1}^{a}p_i^2\right]. \tag{2.7}$$

Based on (2.6), the variance of the unbiased estimate is given by $V(\hat{H}_U) = V(\hat{H})n^2/(n - 1)^2$, which is slightly higher than that of the biased estimate. For equal allele frequencies, $p_i = 1/a$, expression (2.7) reduces to $V(\hat{H}) = 2(n - 1)(a - 1)/(n^3a^2)$. Comparisons of the precision of biased and unbiased estimates are often made in terms of the mean square error (MSE), which is the variance plus the square of the bias. At least for equally frequent alleles, it is easy to show that for all sample sizes $n > 2$, the MSE of the unbiased estimate (i.e., its variance) is always smaller than the MSE of the biased estimate. Thus, for the estimation of heterozygosity, expression (2.6) is preferable over (2.5). A 95% confidence interval for H is easily obtained as $\hat{H}_U \pm 1.96\sqrt{V(\hat{H}_U)}$. All these calculations may be carried out with the aid of the HET program (Section 9.5).

2.3. DNA Polymorphisms

The rapid progress in molecular genetics has been a boon to human linkage analysis. In a seminal paper, Botstein et al. (1980) proposed to treat differences in the DNA sequence as genetic markers for gene mapping. Based on a technique described by Southern (1975), such differences can be made visible by the use of restriction enzymes, which cut DNA at specific sequences (the recognition sites) resulting in DNA fragments of various lengths. If the DNA sequence at a cutting site is different in a homologous chromosome, DNA will not be cut there so that fragments of different sizes occur. The size differences will then lead to differential migration in electrophoresis and can be made visible as different banding patterns. Details of this technique are found in many textbooks. Polymorphisms obtained in this manner are appropriately called restriction fragment length polymorphisms (RFLPs).

RFLPs are generally based on single nucleotide changes and, therefore, often have heterozygosities below 50%. In addition to these markers, various other DNA polymorphisms have been developed. For example, a type of polymorphism results from a variable number of tandem repeats (VNTRs) of a relatively short oligonucleotide sequence (Nakamura et al., 1987). VNTRs are much more polymorphic than RFLPs.

Multiple occurrences of very short sequences, so-called minisatellites, often differ in the number of these repeats and thereby may serve as extremely useful polymorphic marker loci (for example, CA repeats; Weber and May, 1989). These short stretches of DNA can be amplified directly with the polymerase chain reaction (PCR) technique so that a large number of copies of these DNA segments are synthesized; they can then be put on a gel and subjected to electrophoresis. In addition to these dinucleotide repeats, trinucleotide and tetranucleotide repeats have been developed and are generally easier to score than dinucleotide repeats. Many thousands of genetic markers are now available.

More recently, single nucleotide polymorphisms (SNPs) have been gaining momentum. These PCR-based markers can be developed in large quantities and processed on DNA chips (Collins et al., 1997). Although each of these markers has only two alleles, their sheer number and the possibility for automation make them very attractive (Wang et al., 1998).

DNA polymorphisms generally have no physiologic function. Thus, they can be expected not to interfere with the phenotypic expressions at other loci and to be free of the influences of selection. Researchers developing new polymorphisms or investigating polymorphisms in a new population often compare observed numbers of genotypes with those expected under Hardy–Weinberg equilibrium (see Section 1.2). For example, Väisänen et al. (1988) investigated four RFLPs in the type II collagen gene in the Finnish population and found satisfactory agreement between observed and predicted genotype distributions.

In many cases, the two alleles at a DNA polymorphism in an individual are recognized without error. Consequently, molecular geneticists tend to call them genotypes. However, it is not always easy to identify alleles uniquely. Also, various errors tend to occur at rates up to 1% (see Section 11.5). Thus, whatever is observed on an individual should be called his phenotype, which may or may not correspond to the underlying (unobservable) genotype.

Names for DNA polymorphisms are assigned according to strict rules. They all begin with the letter D (and are thus called D numbers) followed by the number of the chromosome on which they are located. After that, a letter indicating the complexity of the DNA sequence and a unique sequential number are assigned. As mentioned in Section 2.1, a standing committee is responsible for unique D numbers.

Probes recognizing repetitive sequences at not one but several loci are extremely polymorphic (Jeffreys, Wilson, and Thein, 1985; Strachan and Read, 1996). However, the resulting banding patterns are difficult to interpret and alleles cannot generally be recognized. Such probes furnish a genetic "fingerprint" that is practically unique for each individual and is, among other things, often used before linkage analyses as a preliminary test of paternity. However, an occasional crossover or DNA slippage during replication might lead to unexpected differences between parents and offspring, and this may occur at a rate of one in several hundred (Vogel and Motulsky, 1986, Section 6.1.2).

Like many genetic loci, DNA polymorphisms undergo mutations at certain rates. In population genetics, some arguments show that higher heterozygosity of a polymorphism is associated with a higher mutation rate. Under the so-called infinite-alleles model and the assumption of an equilibrium between mutation rate and random genetic drift, heterozygosity is given by $H = 1 - 1/(4N\mu + 1)$, where μ is the mutation rate per generation and N is population size (Hartl, 1988). In other words, the mutation rate is proportional to $H/(1 - H)$. Mutation rates also seem to vary with the type of DNA polymorphism. It has been shown that among non–disease-causing microsatellite loci, dinucleotides appear to have mutation rates 1.5 to 2 times higher than the tetranucleotides, and trinucleotides have mutation rates intermediate between the di- and tetranucleotides; disease-causing trinucleotides have mutation rates 3.9 to 6.9 times larger than the tetranucleotides (Chakraborty et al., 1997).

2.4. Variants in Chromosome Morphology

Chromosomes exhibit a fair degree of morphologic variability. Not infrequently, such variants were observed in parents and offspring, so that inheritance had to be assumed. For example, Cooper and Hernits (1963) described an elongated chromosome 1 in a mother and daughter.

They were unable to decide whether the elongation was due to the presence of an extra segment in the long arm, near the centromere, or whether it was the consequence of an alteration in the coiling structure at that place. They nonetheless regarded the unusual spot on chromosome 1 as a chromosome marker and carried out linkage studies between it and nine genetic markers. The Duffy blood group was consistent with linkage, although the small size of the family did not permit any definite conclusions. In contrast to other researchers, these authors tended to believe that the occurrence of the chromosome variant and the phenotypic abnormality in the proband was fortuitous because chromosome studies were carried out preferentially on phenotypically abnormal individuals.

Donahue et al. (1968) and Ying and Ives (1968) independently reported families segregating apparently the same chromosome variant, and both found good evidence for linkage to the Duffy blood group. This established the first assignment of a human gene to an autosome. The particular chromosome variant (a secondary restriction) occurs in about 0.5% of the population and is dominantly inherited (Vogel and Motulsky, 1986).

On many chromosomes, *fragile sites* have been observed. These are chromosome sites showing an increased risk of breakage, particularly under special cell culture conditions. Most of them do not seem to be associated with any phenotypic abnormalities. A well-known exception is the fragile site at Xq27.3 (gene symbol FRAXA), which is associated with a characteristic form of mental retardation, the mar(X), Martin–Bell, or fragile X syndrome (Vogel and Motulsky, 1986). It is inherited as an X-linked dominant condition with incomplete penetrance (Sherman et al., 1985). In addition to these (rare) fragile sites, *common (induced) fragile sites* have been described; they may play a role in disease etiology (Simonic and Gericke, 1996; Wang et al., 1997).

2.5. Genetic and Physical Maps

A genetic map consists of a set of ordered loci with known (i.e., estimated) genetic distances between adjacent loci. The majority of loci in human genetic maps comprises genetic markers. As outlined above, these are loci, usually without any function, whose mode of inheritance is clearly mendelian. Physical maps are ordered loci that have been constructed by physical means (i.e., by means other than genetic mapping). Examples of physical mapping techniques are radiation hybrid mapping and ordering loci through pulse-field gel electrophoresis. Below, such maps and some of their characteristics are discussed.

Soon after the first development of RFLPs in humans, Professor Dausset in Paris proposed and implemented the idea that a human *genetic map* should be constructed on the basis of reference families. DNA from family members would be made available to researchers world-wide so that the whole genetics community could participate in this effort. A foundation in France supported this idea, and a set of originally 40 (later expanded to 64) such families from France and Utah formed what became known as the CEPH families (for Centre d'Etudes du Polymorphisme Humain). Each family consists of one pair of parents, an average of 8.3 offspring, and up to four grandparents (Dausset et al., 1990). With the advent of highly polymorphic markers, most gene mappers no longer use all 40 families but only a specific subset of 8 or 9 of them. Also, a few individuals from these families are regularly used as controls for the sizing of repeat polymorphism alleles. Techniques of map construction will be discussed in Section 6.8. Results of mapping efforts have regularly been published in proceedings of the HGM workshops. Earlier, workshop participants handled all organizational aspects of human gene mapping, but with the enormous growth of the map various tasks have been delegated to special committees (http://www.gdb.org/gdb/hugoEditors.html). For example, the chromosome 1 committee maintains a web page (http://linkage.rockefeller.edu/chr1/) with relevant information on this chromosome. Genetic maps have been published, for example, by Dib et al. (1996). These authors also provided maps of recombination events that occurred in seven of the CEPH families.

Reference families have been set up for various organisms. For example, gene mapping is carried out in dogs (Werner et al., 1997) and dog families serve as reference pedigrees. However, unlike the situation in humans, no cell lines are available on these reference animals as dog cells cannot be transformed.

In their fundamental paper mentioned above, Botstein et al. (1980) proposed that a rather small number of genetic markers could span the whole human genome. They assumed equally spaced markers with a constant interval length of $2d = 20$ cM so that any gene to be mapped will be within $d = 10$ cM of the nearest marker. Then, with a genome length of 33 Morgans, the required number of markers is given by 3300/20 = 165. For a long time, of course, markers were not equidistant but found randomly on the genome.

In the early days of human linkage mapping, the number of genetic markers (mostly blood groups and enzyme polymorphisms) was severely limited and, even with excellent family data, linkage analyses had little prospect of success. Mohr (1964) was interested in the a priori probability of success assuming a varying number, *m,* of markers, even though at the time only 16 useful autosomal marker systems were available. He posed the question: Given a map length of *L* Morgans, what is the probability of an arbitrary locus being no more than $d = 20$ cM from the nearest known marker system? (This probability is 1 when all markers are spaced 40 cM apart.) Using computer simulation, assuming a map length of $L = 28.57$ Morgans and randomly placed marker and disease loci, he found, for example, a probability of 32% for 30 markers and 54% for 60 markers.

This question was treated analytically by Elston and Lange (1975) and Lange and Boehnke (1982). Here, a simple approximation is given as follows: Assume a relatively dense map of randomly placed markers. Total map length is *L,* for example, $L = 3300$ centimorgans. Disregarding the possibility that markers are located toward the ends of chromosomes, the probability that a gene is within a distance, *d,* of a random marker is given by $2d/L$. For *m* markers, assuming independence, the probability that a gene is *not* within a distance *d* of any of them is equal to $(1 - 2d/L)^m$. Therefore, the gene is within a distance *d* of at least one of the *m* markers with probability

$$P = 1 - (1 - 2d/L)^m. \tag{2.8}$$

For example, assume that a disease gene is detectable only when a (random) marker is no more than a recombination fraction of 30% away from it. With the Kosambi map function, this recombination rate corresponds to a map distance of 35 cM. With a map length of 3400 Morgans (see Section 1.6), the probability of detectable linkage is then equal to $P = 2\%$ for one marker (Elston and Lange [1975] quote the same figure). For 100 markers, the probability that at least one of them is within detectable distance from the disease gene is 88%. Equation (2.8) may be solved for the number of markers,

$$m - \log(1 - P)/\log(1 - 2d/L). \tag{2.9}$$

For example, for a probability of $P = 90\%$ that a gene be located within $d = 1$ cM of a marker, approximately $m = 3800$ randomly placed markers are required. If a higher certainty of 99% is postulated, about 7600 markers are required. Approximately, the number of markers required increases linearly with total map length *L* and with the inverse of the postulated distance *d* between gene and marker.

Radiation hybrid maps rest on the randomness of chromosome breaks inflicted by X irradiation, where these breaks are analogous to crossovers in genetic maps. A particular human chromosome is irradiated by x-rays such that it breaks into several fragments. These are recovered in rodent cells, and the rodent–human hybrid cells are cloned. For example, consider two markers on a chromosome. The breakage probability, θ, is the probability of at least one chromosome break occurring between the two markers. The distance between the markers is then obtained as $d = -ln(1 - \theta)$ and is measured in Rays (Lunetta et al., 1996). For small θ, $d \approx \theta$. In radiation maps, loci need not be polymorphic, which represents a major difference between radiation hybrid and genetic mapping.

2.6. Problems

Problem 2.1. For a marker locus with a equally frequent alleles, what is the difference between heterozygosity, H, and polymorphism information content, PIC, expressed in terms of a? What is the minimum number of alleles such that this difference is no greater than 0.01?

Problem 2.2. A chromosome of length 100 cM should be covered with m marker loci such that, with probability $P = 95\%$, a gene with unknown location on this chromosome will be at most 5 cM from the nearest marker. What is the minimum number m of markers required?

3.

Aspects of
Statistical Inference

This chapter provides a selection of technical statistical tools for readers with little background in statistics. Knowledge of this material is not absolutely necessary for a fruitful study of the remainder of this book, although a deeper understanding of linkage analysis, especially of the methods to be presented in Chapter 4, requires familiarity with basic principles of statistical inference. Of course, researchers who want to carry out independent and original work in gene mapping methods need to know much more than is presented here. Also, knowledge of computer programming is essential for anyone doing methodological work.

The discussion in this chapter is not intended as a rigorous outline of statistical methods or as a historical overview. The modest goal is to define some statistical terms and to explain the rationale for and technique of a selection of statistical methods. As will be seen in the next chapter, in linkage analysis, elements from more than one "school" of thought are in current use. I see nothing wrong with that. Some statistical approaches are better than others at solving a particular problem, and the situation may be reversed for another problem. In this chapter, what is largely missing is a discussion of Bayesian inference methods—a reflection of my personal bias. Of course, where useful prior information is available, it should not be disregarded, and using Bayes' theorem does not make one a Bayesian. However, translating ignorance on a parameter into a uniform distribution for it and the arbitrariness inherent in rules of assigning prior distributions (Rao, 1973, Section 5b.3) do not appeal to me.

A brief discussion of the concepts of prior and posterior probability of linkage is given in Chapter 4. Readers interested in a broader outline of statistical methods than presented here are referred to the literature (e.g., Smith, 1959; Edwards, 1989, 1992; Elston and Johnston, 1994). Interesting aspects of statistical methodology are also discussed in Cohen (1990). Lod scores are briefly introduced in this chapter; a more detailed discussion follows in Chapter 4.

As pointed out in the preface, no introduction to probability calculus is provided in this book. Outlines of probability calculus are given, for example, in the appendix of Thompson (1986) and in Elston and Johnson (1994).

3.1. Likelihood and Lod Score

This section is statistically somewhat detailed. For the reader who is not interested in statistical detail, this first paragraph provides a heuristic explanation of lod scores as follows: Likelihood and lod score are measures of plausibility of the observed data (they differ from each other in their scale—the lod score is on a log scale). Their values depend on assumed values of θ. If a number of θ values are tried and the likelihood (or lod score) computed for each of them, the plausibility of the data will be largest for one specific θ value, which is then taken to be the best estimate (the maximum likelihood estimate) of θ. If there is linkage, the maximum lod score tends to increase with an increasing number of families. Once it reaches or exceeds 3, linkage is generally considered significant. Below and in Section 4.3, more detailed introductions to likelihood and lod scores are given.

To ''explain'' a particular phenomenon in nature, scientists build a *model* (also called a *hypothesis*) of the phenomenon, that is, a description that accounts for as many of the phenomenon's known properties as possible. Models may be of a biochemical, physical, statistical, or other nature. Good models are those that explain and accurately predict a large number of properties. For example, the mendelian laws are a model for the inheritance of genetic markers and many diseases. Consider a gene locus with two alleles, *A* and *a*, where *A* is dominant over *a*. The three genotypes, *A/A, A/a,* and *a/a,* give rise to two phenotypes, A+ under *A/A* and *A/a,* and A− under *a/a.* Assume that two parents each have phenotypes A+ and that their genotypes are known to be *A/a* each (see Problem 3.1). A child of such an *A/a* × *A/a* mating is predicted to have phenotype A+ with probability ¾ and phenotype A− with probability ¼. Once the first child is born, the same probabilities hold for each subsequent child because, according to Mendel's laws of inheritance, one child's phenotype does not influence that of another. In other words, with given parental genotypes, offspring phenotypes are mutually independent. Among a large number of children, one expects to find a proportion of roughly 75% to be of phenotype A+. On the basis of these assumptions, using probability calculus, one may make further predictions. For example, the probability that among two children at least one has the A+ phenotype (which is the same as saying that not both children are A−) is given by $1 - (\frac{1}{4})^2 = 0.9375$, or the probability that both children are either A+ or A− is $(\frac{3}{4})^2 + (\frac{1}{4})^2 = 0.625$.

Hypotheses are verified on the basis of observations. The better the data are in agreement with a hypothesis, the more readily we accept it as being "true." But how are we to measure how well observations agree with a hypothesis, or whether observations agree better with hypothesis H_1 or H_2? The statistical quantity that seems most suitable to serve as a measure for our belief in a particular hypothesis is the likelihood (Fisher, 1970; Edwards, 1992). The *likelihood* for a hypothesis H given a set of observations F is defined as the probability, $L(H) = P(F; H)$, with which the observations have occurred, this probability being calculated under the targeted hypothesis. For example, using the hypothesis of the previous paragraph, if the parents have three children, the first two with A+ phenotypes and the third with an A− phenotype, the likelihood is calculated as $(\frac{3}{4}) \times (\frac{3}{4}) \times (\frac{1}{4}) = 9/64$ (see Problem 3.3).

As will be seen in the next paragraph, it is often different values of an unknown parameter (rather than different hypotheses) whose likelihoods are of interest. Thus, the distinction between likelihood and probability is that the former is as a function of a parameter (an unknown constant) whereas the latter is a function of an event (Weir, 1996). The two quantities, likelihood and probability, thus have different properties and follow different laws (Fisher, 1970), but both are calculated by the laws of probability calculus.

When comparing hypotheses (or values of an unknown parameter), the absolute values of their likelihoods are not generally meaningful so that they are often scaled by suitable constants. The *odds* in favor of hypothesis H_1 versus H_2 are expressed by the likelihood ratio, $R = L(H_1)/L(H_2)$, often written as $R:1$. For example, in gene mapping of several linked markers, the hypotheses of interest may be different locus orders (e.g., O'Connell et al., 1987). The natural logarithm of the likelihood, $S(H) = \ln[L(H)]$, is referred to as the *support* for hypothesis H (or for a particular value, H, of an unknown parameter).

In linkage analysis for two loci, the two basic hypotheses are free recombination (H_0) and linkage (H_1). They are defined through the value of the recombination fraction, free recombination corresponding to $\theta = \frac{1}{2}$ and linkage to $\theta < \frac{1}{2}$. Conventionally (see Section 4.1), the common (decimal) logarithm of the likelihood ratio, the so-called lod score

$$Z(\theta) = \log_{10}[L(\theta)/L(\frac{1}{2})], \tag{3.1}$$

is used as the measure of support for linkage versus absence of linkage.

For example, if observations consist of k recombinants and $n - k$ nonrecombinants, the corresponding lod score is given by

$$Z(\theta) = \begin{cases} n\log(2) + k \log(\theta) + (n - k)\log(1 - \theta) & \text{if } \theta > 0 \\ n\log(2) & \text{if } \theta = 0 \text{ and } k = 0 \\ -\infty & \text{if } \theta = 0 \text{ and } k > 0, \end{cases} \quad (3.2)$$

where the domain is usually $0 \leq \theta \leq \frac{1}{2}$. A step-by-step introduction to lod scores is given in Section 4.3.

3.2. Maximum Likelihood Estimation

Many models or hypotheses contain variables, called *parameters,* whose values are unknown and have to be estimated on the basis of observations. In the example used above, the population gene frequency p of allele A is such a parameter. In statistical terminology, observations are random variables. Any function of random variables, which does not depend on unknown parameters, is termed a *statistic.* In particular, *estimates* or *estimators* are functions of observations and are constructed to estimate unknown parameter values. For instance, consider a sample of individuals of size n, k of whom are of phenotype A+ (genotypes A/A or A/a), the remaining $n - k$ being of phenotype A− (genotypes a/a). Under Hardy–Weinberg equilibrium, the proportion of A− individuals in the population is expected to be equal to $q = (1 - p)^2$. The commonly used estimate of that proportion is simply the observed proportion of A− individuals in the sample, $(n - k)/n = 1 - (k/n)$.

Various statistical methods of parameter estimation exist. A very general one is the method of maximum likelihood (Fisher, 1922a). It is based on the likelihood function of a parameter, which is, as defined above, the probability of the observations used as a function of the unknown parameter(s). For example, take the sample of n observations considered in the previous paragraph, k of whom are A+ (occurring with probability $1 - q$) and $n - k$ of whom are A− (occurring with probability q). The log likelihood is then proportional to $S(q) = \ln[L(q)] = (n - k) \ln(q) + k \ln(1 - q)$. The *maximum likelihood estimate* (MLE) $\hat{q}$ of q is defined as that value of q which maximizes $S(q)$. An MLE of a parameter is usually symbolized by the parameter symbol with a hat on top. Maximization of S may be carried out analytically by taking the first derivative, dS/dq, of S and setting it equal to zero. When $dS/dq = 0$ (the so-called likelihood equation) is solved for q, it results in the MLE, provided that the solution represents a maximum rather than a minimum. For the present example, this procedure leads to the estimate, $\hat{q} = 1 - (k/n)$, which shows that the intuitive estimate mentioned above is an MLE.

In linkage analysis, as will be seen later, the likelihood cannot generally be maximized analytically. Instead, MLEs must be found numerically by varying the values of the parameters of interest and recomputing the likelihood for many trial values of the parameter until an approximate maximum is found. An outline of numerical methods is given in Chapter 9.

A particular situation applies in the estimation of a parameter, s, when the likelihood can only be calculated if values of another parameter, t, are also specified. Assume that a test of the hypothesis, $s = 0$, is to be carried out. One approach might be to assume that t is known and to compute the test statistic, $L(\hat{s}, t)/L(s = 0, t)$. This likelihood ratio has 1 df as the difference in numbers of parameters estimated in numerator and denominator is equal to one. However, t may be unknown and no good estimate of t may be available. An alternative approach is then to treat t as a *nuisance parameter,* that is, to separately estimate t in numerator and denominator. Thus, the likelihood ratio, $L(\hat{s},\hat{t})/L(s = 0, \tilde{t})$, is formed, which again has 1 df. A common intermediate approach is to replace t in the former likelihood ratio by an estimate. When the two parameter estimates are correlated, this tends to lead to an increase or a decrease of the likelihood ratio relative to the likelihood ratio with nuisance parameters, depending on whether the common estimate of t was obtained jointly with $\hat{s}$ or under the assumption of $s = 0$, respectively. In the former case, for example, the numerator of $L(\hat{s}, \hat{t})/L(s = 0, \hat{t})$ is as large as it can be while this is not so for the denominator (the $\hat{t}$ in the denominator is the same as that in the numerator).

3.3. Statistical Properties of Maximum Likelihood Estimates

Maximum likelihood estimates have certain well-known properties, some of which are briefly discussed here. For a more detailed treatment of this subject, see Elandt-Johnson (1971) or Weir (1996).

Function of a Parameter. It is often easier to find the *MLE of a function of a parameter* rather than of the parameter itself. In the example of the previous section, the MLE of the proportion q of A$-$ individuals was simply given by $1 - (k/n)$, the observed proportion of A$-$ individuals in the sample. It is a function of the parameter of interest, the gene frequency p: $q = (1 - p)^2$. For any monotonic function (one-to-one transformation), $p = f(q)$, if $\hat{q}$ is the MLE of q, then $\hat{p} = f(\hat{q})$ is the MLE of p. Thus, because $p = 1 - \sqrt{q}$, the MLE of p is given by $\hat{p} = 1 - [1 - (k/n)]^{1/2}$. As another example, assume that in a genetic counseling situation one needs to know the probability, θ^2, that a recombination has occurred in each of two parents. An MLE, $\hat{\theta} = k/n$ (the proportion of recombinants out of n phase-known meioses), is available for θ. The MLE estimate of θ^2 is then given by $(k/n)^2$ because θ^2 is monotonic for $\theta \geq 0$.

Bias. Maximum likelihood estimates are often *biased*. In repeated samples of the same data type, the MLE can assume a number of values. For example, consider the estimate of the recombination fraction, $\hat{\theta} = k/n$, where k is the number of recombinants and $n - k$ is the number of nonrecombinants. This estimate can assume $n + 1$ values ($0/n$, $1/n$, etc.), and the probability of each outcome is given by the binomial formula $\binom{n}{k}\theta^k(1 - \theta)^{n-k}$. In general, if θ_i denotes the ith outcome of a particular MLE of θ, and p_i is the probability with which it occurs, then the weighted average,

$$E(\hat{\theta}) = \Sigma p_i \hat{\theta}_i, \tag{3.3}$$

is the expected value or *expectation* of the estimator $\hat{\theta}$ (an example is calculated below). If (3.3) is equal to the (true) parameter value θ, then $\hat{\theta}$ is said to be unbiased. The quantity,

$$b(\hat{\theta}) = E(\hat{\theta}) - \theta, \tag{3.4}$$

is called the bias of $\hat{\theta}$. For binomial and multinomial proportions, the observed class frequencies are unbiased estimators of the class proportions (probabilities), but estimates of nonlinear functions of the class probabilities are generally biased. In the example given above, the frequency $(n - k)/n$ is an unbiased estimate of the proportion q of A$-$ individuals, but the estimate of the gene frequency $p = 1 - \sqrt{q}$ must be biased. Bias reduction techniques for this case were proposed by Huether and Murphy (1980). A general method for bias reduction is the jackknife procedure (see discussion in Weir, 1996). Bias reduction techniques have rarely, if at all, been applied in human linkage analysis.

Bolling and Murphy (1979) demonstrated strong biases in the estimate of the recombination fraction from certain family types. These biases are at least partly due to truncation: If θ is estimated from k recombinants and $n - k$ nonrecombinants, then $\hat{\theta} = \frac{1}{2}$ if $k > n/2$. For example, with $n = 3$ and an assumed known recombination fraction of 0.1, Table 3.1 demonstrates the calculation of $E(\hat{\theta})$ and shows that it is different from θ. As will be seen later, in linkage analysis, the statistical bias due to truncation is not a matter of concern; the really serious biases are those arising from selected sampling when only a portion of the data is analyzed.

Generally, if T is the value of θ in the interval (0, 1) at which

Table 3.1. Calculation of Expected Value $E(\hat{\theta}) = 0.095$ for $n = 3$ Recombination Events and Known Recombination Fraction 0.1

k	P(k)	$\hat{\theta}$	$\hat{\theta} \times P(k)$
0	0.729	0	0
1	0.243	⅓	0.0810
2	0.027	½	0.0135
3	0.001	½	0.0005
Sum	1		0.0950

Note: k = number of recombinants. $P(k)$ = binomial probabilities.

the log likelihood is maximized, the recombination fraction estimate is defined as

$$\hat{\theta} = \begin{cases} T \text{ if } T < \frac{1}{2} \\ \frac{1}{2} \text{ otherwise.} \end{cases}$$

For phase-known data, T is unbiased so that $\hat{\theta}$ is clearly biased because $T > \frac{1}{2}$ is truncated to ½. However, because $\theta \leq \frac{1}{2}$, the *mean square error* of $\hat{\theta}$ is smaller than that of T: $E[(\hat{\theta} - \theta)^2] < E[(T - \theta)^2]$ (Rao, 1973).

In linkage analysis, the recombination fraction θ is generally a complicated function of multinomial proportions and is thus usually biased (for examples, see end of Sections 6.3 and 7.3). This statistical bias has not received much attention, probably because it tends to vanish with increasing sample size (see following paragraph).

In general, MLEs are *asymptotically unbiased,* that is, their bias tends to vanish when the number of observations becomes large, where *observations* refers to either the number of families or the number of individuals within a family (Bailey, 1961).

Consistency. MLEs generally are *consistent,* that is, they are asymptotically unbiased, and their variances approach zero in the limit for a large number of observations. In other words, the accuracy of MLEs increases with increasing sample size; they "close in" on the true parameter value, so to speak. In the presence of ascertainment biases, as will be seen in Chapter 10, MLEs are often inconsistent. This is a most unfortunate situation because with the accumulation of more and more data, one will find an increasingly precise estimate of a quantity that is different from the one to be estimated.

If an MLE is consistent, the maximum of the expected support function occurs at the true parameter value, under which the expectation is calculated (see inequalities 5f.2.1 on p. 364 in Rao, 1973). This property provides a simple method to prove or disprove consistency (see Chapter 10). A simple numerical example may be found in Section 5.2. MLEs are also asymptotically normally distributed, which allows the calculation of asymptotic variances (see Section 5.3).

Classes of Data. In many situations, observations (phenotypes) occur in a number m of classes, with class probabilities being functions of some parameters, where the number of parameters to be estimated by ML is much smaller than m. Analytical expressions for the MLEs of these parameters are often unavailable. For the special case that the number of parameters is equal to the number of degrees of freedom (e.g., $m - 1$), MLEs may simply be obtained by equating observations to their expected values (Bailey's rule, page 63 in Weir, 1996). This method is used at various places in this book.

3.4. Significance Tests and *p*-Values

The object of estimating an unknown parameter is often to prove a hypothesis that a researcher suspects is correct. For example, in linkage analysis, a researcher is convinced that two loci are genetically linked. The investigation of five recombination events in one family showed that one was a recombination whereas four were nonrecombinations. The estimated recombination fraction is thus 20%. Is this convincing evidence for linkage? Statistical tests discussed below are designed to answer such questions. Two hypotheses may be distinguished, the null hypothesis, H_0, and the alternative hypothesis, H_1, where H_1 is the one a researcher would like to prove. The principle of significance testing is to assume that H_0 is true until one has good evidence to the contrary. A researcher thus must make an effort to *dis*prove H_0.

On the basis of an experiment, a significance test (a decision rule, to be discussed below) will either reject H_0 (the investigator accepts H_1) or will fail to reject H_0. In the first case, the experiment is said to have furnished a significant result, and in the second case, the result is said to be nonsignificant. Depending on the state of nature (i.e., whether H_0 or H_1 is true), the test result is associated with one of two types of errors whose conditional probabilities of occurrence are displayed in Table 3.2. A *type I error* (false-positive result) occurs when the test rejects H_0 although H_0 is true, with $\alpha = P$ (test is significant$|H_0$) being the probability of occurrence of a type I error. A *type II error* (false-negative result) occurs when the test fails to reject H_0 although it is false, with $\beta = P$ (test is not significant$|H_1$) being the probability of occurrence of a type

Table 3.2. Conditional Probabilities of Test Results Given State of Nature

State of Nature	Test Rejects H_0		Sum
	No	Yes	
H_0	$1 - \alpha$	α	1
H_1	β	$1 - \beta$	1

II error. The power $1 - \beta$ of the test is the probability that it rejects H_0 when it is false. The probability of a type I error is also known as the *significance level* of the test. Significance tests are carried out assuming H_0 is true. Hence, if a test is nonsignificant, one cannot say that it accepts H_0. The result may be nonsignificant because H_0 is in fact true or because of low power.

In descriptive statistics, two terms are often used to measure the effectiveness of a test procedure, for example, in diagnosing a disease (Elston and Johnston, 1994). They are somewhat related to the conditional probabilities of test results discussed above: *Sensitivity* is the conditional probability that the test is positive given the disease is present, and *specificity* is the conditional probability that the test is negative given that the disease is absent.

Hypotheses are often defined by the values of an unknown parameter. A hypothesis specified by a single parameter value (e.g., $\theta = \frac{1}{2}$) is called a simple hypothesis, whereas a hypothesis admitting a whole range of parameter values (e.g., $\theta < \frac{1}{2}$) is a composite hypothesis. In the following few paragraphs, simple hypotheses for the recombination fraction are discussed as these were important in the early days of statistical linkage analysis.

Simple Hypotheses. Consider two simple hypotheses, the null hypothesis $H_0 : \theta = \frac{1}{2}$ of free recombination and the alternative hypothesis $H_1 : \theta = \theta_1$, where $\theta_1 < \frac{1}{2}$ is some fixed value of the recombination fraction such as 0.1. To test H_0 on the basis of observations, one may use the likelihood ratio, $T(\theta_1) = L(\theta_1)/L(\frac{1}{2})$, as a test statistic. If H_0 is true, one expects small values of T, but if H_1 is true, a tendency toward larger T values is expected. The statistical test consists of the decision rule to reject H_0 if T exceeds a critical point, T_c, and not to reject H_0 if T falls below T_c. Any test such as this, based on the likelihood ratio, is called a *likelihood ratio (LR) test.*

To determine the error probabilities associated with this test, one must work out the distribution of the test statistic, T, where $\alpha = P(T \geq$

$T_c|H_0)$ and $\beta = P(T < T_c|H_1)$. If the assumed distribution for T deviates from its true distribution, the assumed or nominal significance level, α_N, may be different from the actual significance level, α. A test is called *conservative* if $\alpha < \alpha_N$ (i.e., if the actual type I error is smaller than anticipated) and nonconservative or anticonservative if $\alpha > \alpha_N$. In the latter case, under H_0, the test will be significant more often than one anticipates on the basis of the assumed wrong distribution of T.

Not knowing the distribution of the test statistic, one can give an upper bound to α (Haldane and Smith, 1947; Smith, 1953). Let $T(\theta_1) \geq 0$ be the likelihood ratio defined above; under H_0, its average value is equal to 1 (Haldane and Smith, 1947). With this, probability calculus leads to the Chebyshev-type inequality (Johnson and Kotz, 1970):

$$\alpha \leq 1/T_c, \quad T_c > 1, \tag{3.6}$$

where T_c is the critical limit of the likelihood ratio above which the test for $\theta = \theta_1$ is declared significant. For example, assume a critical limit of $T_c = 1000$ (corresponding to a lod score limit of 3). The type I error associated with this limit is at most $1/1000 = 0.001$.

In the tests considered thus far, the number of observations is viewed as a fixed constant (this is also the case in general likelihood ratio tests discussed in the next paragraph). In the *sequential probability ratio test* (SPRT), which was developed by Wald (1947) in connection with acceptance sampling, data are accumulated until a stopping criterion is met. The number of observations is thus a random variable. With this test, one tries to discriminate between two simple hypotheses, $H_0 : \theta = \theta_0$ (e.g., $\theta_0 = \frac{1}{2}$) and $H_1 : \theta = \theta_1$ (e.g., $\theta_1 = 0.2$). Observations are gathered one at a time. After each new observation, the likelihood ratio $T = L(\theta_1)/L(\theta_0)$ is formed for all observations, and one of the following three actions is taken:

1. Continue sampling if $B < T < A$
2. Accept H_1 (reject H_0) if $T \geq A$
3. Accept H_0 (reject H_1) if $T \leq B$,

where A and B are suitably chosen constants, for example, $A = 1000$ and $B = 0.01$ (see Section 4.1). Approximately, for A large ($A \gg 1$) and B small ($B \ll 1$), the following relationships hold between the constants A, B and the error probabilities α, β defined above:

$$A \approx (1 - \beta)/\alpha, \, B \approx \beta/(1 - \alpha).$$

Setting $A - B \approx A$, $1 - B \approx 1$, and $A - 1 \approx A$ leads to

$$\alpha \approx 1/A, \quad \beta \approx B. \tag{3.7}$$

Composite Hypotheses. The upper bound (equation 3.6) on the significance level is useful when H_0 is tested against a simple alternative hypothesis. In practice, of course, one wants to consider not just a single alternative but the whole range of values, $0 \le \theta < \frac{1}{2}$. A possible solution proposed by Haldane and Smith (1947) is to use as a test statistic the average value, $\overline{T}$, of the likelihood ratio between 0 and $\frac{1}{2}$. For this test statistic, too, inequality (3.6) holds when $T(\theta_1)$ in (3.5) is replaced by $\overline{T}(\theta_1)$, but, presumably, a test based on $\overline{T}$ is not very powerful and will often miss a true linkage. It is not used in current linkage analysis and is mentioned here only for historical reasons.

In the general LR test, a number n of parameters may be estimated under the alternative hypothesis, H_1. These parameters may be viewed as spanning an n-dimensional space. The null hypothesis, H_0, generally represents a subspace of H_1, formed by a number d of linear restrictions on the parameters. To test H_0 versus H_1, the LR criterion $T = L(H_1)/L(H_0)$ is constructed, where the likelihoods are evaluated at the MLEs of the parameter values considered. Asymptotically, the random variable $2ln(T)$ follows a chi-square distribution with d degrees of freedom (df) (Rao, 1973). Most tests in general use (e.g., t test, F test) are LR tests. The lod score method as used today (see Section 4.3) falls into this category of tests.

Tests of a hypothesis $H_0: \theta = r_0$ may be carried out in a one-sided or two-sided fashion. The test is two-sided when deviations from H_0 in either direction (low or high values of θ) can be significant. In linkage analysis, the test of $H_0: \theta = \frac{1}{2}$ is carried out in a one-sided manner; one usually does not even look at estimates of θ larger than $\frac{1}{2}$ (but see Sections 4.5 and 5.9).

In significance tests, one often does not set a rigorous critical boundary for the test statistic. Instead, with an observed value, T_{obs}, of the test statistic, one calculates the smallest value of α for which T_{obs} is still significant and calls it the p value or *empirical significance level,* $p = P(T \ge T_{obs} | H_0)$. Notice that p is not the probability that H_1 is true; rather, it represents the probability, given that H_0 is true, that T turns out as large or larger than T_{obs}.

3.5. The Likelihood Method

The support (log likelihood) function may be used for finding an MLE (see Section 3.2), in which case only its properties at the MLE of the parameter are of interest. LR testing also makes use of the support function. In the so-called likelihood method, however, one uses likelihoods for inference directly (Edwards, 1992). The whole support function is meaningful, not just its maximum.

No significance test is carried out in the likelihood approach; rather, hypotheses (or parameter values) are compared with respect to their associated relative likelihoods. In general likelihood ratio testing, only the null hypothesis is relevant for the distribution of the test statistic (which is the likelihood ratio or some function of it); in the likelihood method, the likelihoods under either of the hypotheses are compared directly. A further difference between the various approaches is that, in maximum likelihood estimation, estimates for the same quantity obtained from different sources are combined by forming a weighted mean, the weights usually being the inverse of the variances. In the likelihood method, on the other hand, support functions are pooled (Edwards, 1992).

Each of these approaches has advantages and disadvantages. The results of significance testing can be formulated in terms of probabilities, which is not possible in the likelihood method. On the other hand, hypotheses can be compared by the significance testing method only when they have a hierarchical structure (the null hypothesis must correspond to a subspace of that of the alternative hypothesis), whereas no such restrictions exist in the likelihood method.

As we will see in Chapter 4, human linkage analysis uses elements from more than just a single method.

3.6. Interval Estimation

A *confidence interval* is a statistical construct that is intimately tied to the concept of significance tests (Rao, 1973). Its definition is more complex than is generally appreciated by nonstatisticians, the reason being that confidence intervals refer to a set of parameter values, but one cannot make simple direct probability statements about parameters (they are not random variables). Imagine a statistical test of the hypothesis, $H_0 : p = p_0$, that some parameter p has the value p_0. Further assume that an estimate, $\hat{p}$, of p has been obtained which may or may not have resulted in a significant result of the test of H_0. Now, consider a set of hypotheses, $H_i : p = p_i$. Each of these may be tested using the same estimate $\hat{p}$ of p. The confidence interval of p is defined as consisting of all those points, p_i, for which the corresponding hypothesis H_i is nonsignificant (Fisher, 1960; Chotai, 1984). When these hypothesis tests are carried out under a significance level α, the associated confidence interval is said to have confidence coefficient of $100(1 - \alpha)\%$.

As an example, given an estimate, $\hat{p} = k/n$, constructing an exact confidence interval for the parameter, p, of the binomial distribution may proceed as shown below (Pfanzagl, 1966; see also Armitage and Berry,

1987, Section 4.7). The test shall be two-sided, resulting in a lower (p_L) and an upper (p_U) bound of the confidence interval, where the two bounds are associated with the respective (one-sided) significance levels, α_L and α_U. These define an associated overall confidence coefficient of $100(1 - \alpha_L - \alpha_U)\%$. Consider now a value p_L, $p_L < \hat{p} = k/n$. The test of the hypothesis, $p = p_L$, against $p > p_L$ will be significant for large values of k. That is, the critical region of the test consists of all those values of i, $k \leq i \leq n$, whose probability of occurrence is (less than or) equal to α_L. Therefore, p_L is obtained as the solution of the equation,

$$\alpha_L = \sum_{i=k}^{n} \binom{n}{i} p_L^i (1 - p_L)^{n-i}. \tag{3.8}$$

Analogously, solving

$$\alpha_U = \sum_{i=0}^{k} \binom{n}{i} p_U^i (1 - p_U)^{n-i} \tag{3.9}$$

for p_U will yield the upper endpoint of the desired confidence interval. The BINOM program, which solves (3.8) and (3.9) numerically, may be used to determine confidence intervals for binomial proportions. For example, assume that, in a count of recombination events, 2 recombinants and 18 nonrecombinants were observed, furnishing an estimate of the recombination fraction of $\hat{\theta} = 2/20 = 0.10$. Disregarding any considerations of prior probability of linkage (see Section 4.2), the 99% confidence interval on the (true but unknown) recombination fraction is $(0.005, 0.387)$, and the 95% confidence interval is $(0.012, 0.317)$.

For $k = 0$ and $k = n$, equations (3.9) and (3.8) may be solved analytically as follows: When $k = 0$ is observed, the $100(1 - \alpha)\%$ confidence interval for the proportion p consists of all those values for which the probability of the observations, $(1 - p)^n$, is larger than α. The endpoint of the confidence interval is thus obtained by solving $(1 - p)^n = \alpha$ for p (equation [3.9]) so that the confidence interval is given by $(0, 1 - \alpha^{1/n})$. For example, with $\alpha = 0.05$ and $n = 100$, the 95% confidence interval associated with $k = 0$ is equal to $(0, 0.03)$. Analogously, for $k = n$, solving $p^n = \alpha$ for p yields the confidence interval $(\alpha^{1/n}, 1)$. This material is covered here in such detail as it is not often found in statistics textbooks.

As we will see later, in linkage analysis, determining a proper confidence interval on θ is usually impossible because the distribution of the MLE is unknown. Often, "approximate" p values are calculated on the basis of the asymptotic distribution of the LR criterion, but in many applications (such as multipoint linkage analysis) the accuracy of this approximation is unknown and may be quite unsatisfactory. However, binomial confidence intervals are easy to obtain and are important in computer simulation. For example, the power of a test is approximated by the proportion of replicates with significant results. The methods described above may then be applied to construct confidence limits on the true power (see Section 9.7).

Another route often taken is to construct *support intervals.* For a unimodal likelihood curve with an interior maximum, the *m*-unit support limits for a parameter are the two parameter values astride the estimate at which the support is *m* units less than the maximum (Edwards, 1992). Generally, for *n* parameters, the *m*-unit support region is that region in the parameter space bounded by the $n - 1$ dimensional region on which the support is *m* units less than the maximum. The value $m = 2$ has been recommended (Edwards, 1992). In linkage analysis, it is customary to construct a similar support interval (see Section 4.4).

3.7. Bayes Theorem

Consider two nonindependent events, E and F, for example, the genotype E and phenotype F of an individual. It is often easy to specify the conditional probability, $P(F|E)$, and difficult to find $P(E|F)$, but the latter is what may be of interest. For example, models of inheritance spell out the penetrance $P(\text{phenotype}|\text{genotype})$, but often one would like to draw inferences on an underlying genotype, given an observed phenotype. Bayes theorem allows the calculation of such "inverse" probabilities as follows:

$$P(E|F) = \frac{P(F|E)P(E)}{P(F)} = \frac{P(F|E)P(E)}{P(F|E)P(E) + P(F|E^c)P(E^c)}, \tag{3.10}$$

where E^c stands for the complement of E, "not E." Equation (3.10) may be generalized to a set of mutually exclusive events, E_i, whose conditional probabilities of occurrence are to be calculated, given that an observation F has been made. In analogy to (3.10), the conditional probability of the kth event E_k is then given by

$$P(E_k|F) = P(F|E_k)\,P(E_k)\,/\,\textstyle\sum_j P(F|E_j)\,P(E_j). \tag{3.11}$$

A streamlined form of the Bayes theorem is often presented in a table with columns that correspond to the different events E_i of interest, the rows being formed by the various unconditional and conditional probabilities (Murphy and Chase, 1975). Some of the rows are often labeled "prior" and "posterior," but this is not done here, as no connection to bayesian inference shall be implied. As an example, consider a rare dominant disease with population frequency p of the disease allele. Two parents, one of whom is affected, have a number of children, and the two events of interest are E_1 and E_2 denoting homozygous and heterozygous disease status of the affected parent, respectively. Barring phenotypic differences between heterozygous and homozygous affected individuals, the unconditional (sometimes called "prior") probability that the affected parent is homozygous is given as follows: the population frequency of homozygous affecteds is p^2 and that of heterozygous affecteds is $2p(1 - p)$. The relative frequency of the former is thus $P(E_1) = p^2/[p^2 + 2p(1 - p)] = p/(2 - p)$, and that of the latter is $P(E_2) = 2(1 - p)/(2 - p)$. These two probabilities are unconditional with respect to our observation F, but they are, of course, conditional on that parent's being affected. Assume now that all n children are affected, which represents the observation F. What is then the conditional (sometimes called "posterior") probability $P(E_1|F)$ that the affected parent is homozygous?

Table 3.3 shows the relevant calculations. At the top, one lists the set of mutually exclusive events E_i, for which "inverse" conditional probabilities are to be computed. The first line simply gives the relative unconditional probabilities of these events. On the second line, one computes the probabilities of the observation F ("n affected children") given each of the events E_i. In this case, for $E_1 = $ "affected parent is homozygous," all children are affected with probability 1. For $E_2 = $ "affected parent is heterozygous," each of the children is affected with probability $\frac{1}{2}$. The answer to our question is obtained as the first expression in the last line. For example, given three affected children, the affected parent

Table 3.3. Example of Calculation of Inverse Probabilities Using the Bayes Theorem (Probabilities P Explained in Text)

	E_1	E_2	Sum
Unconditional P	$p/(2 - p)$	$2(1 - p)/(2 - p)$	1
Conditional P	1	$(\frac{1}{2})^n$	—
Joint P^a	$p/(2 - p)$	$\dfrac{(1 - p)(\frac{1}{2})^{n-1}}{2 - p}$	$\dfrac{p + (1 - p)(\frac{1}{2})^{n-1}}{2 - p}$
Inverse cond. P^b	$\dfrac{2^{n-1}p}{2^{n-1}p + 1 - p}$	$\dfrac{1 - p}{2^{n-1}p + 1 - p}$	1

[a] Multiply the two rows above.
[b] Divide column above by sum on its right side.

has an "inverse" conditional probability of $4p/(3p + 1)$ of being homozygous as compared with the unconditional probability of $p/(2 - p)$. For small p (disease rare), the two probabilities are approximately equal to $4p$ and $\frac{1}{2}p$, respectively, so having three affected children increases the chances of the affected parent being homozygous by a factor of 8. Of course, these calculations may be carried out directly, using Bayes theorem without resorting to the scheme shown in Table 3.3, but such a table may be helpful for researchers without a solid background in probability calculus.

3.8. Problems

For Problems 3.1 through 3.3, assume a gene with two alleles, A and a, and gene frequency $p = P(A)$, where genotypes A/A and A/a determine the phenotype A+, and a/a determines the phenotype A−. (This example was used at the beginning of Section 3.1.) Genotypes are assumed to be in Hardy–Weinberg equilibrium.

Problem 3.1. For an individual with phenotype A+ who has no children, how could we be certain that he or she has genotype A/a? Hint: Consider the parents' phenotypes.

Problem 3.2. Assume two parents with phenotypes A+ each, where the parents of these two individuals are unknown. What is the probability of their having a child with phenotype A+? Does this probability stay the same for each subsequent child, irrespective of the known phenotypes of children already born?

Problem 3.3. In the example of the three children with phenotypes A+, A+, and A−, whose parents both have genotypes A/a, the likelihood (probability of children's phenotypes) was calculated as $L_1 = (\frac{3}{4}) \times (\frac{3}{4}) \times (\frac{1}{4}) = 9/64$. Another way of looking at this situation is to compute the probability that, of three children, two have phenotype A+ and one has phenotype A− (only these two phenotypes are possible). According to the binomial formula, this probability is given by $L_2 = 3 \times (\frac{3}{4})^2 \times (\frac{1}{4}) = 27/64$. Why are L_1 and L_2 different? What is the significance of this difference? Which is the correct likelihood?

Problem 3.4. Assume that, in 10 opportunities for recombination, no recombination has been found so that $\hat{\theta} = 0$. What is the)90% confidence interval for the true recombination fraction based on this result?

4.

Basics of Linkage Analysis

This chapter is intended to introduce the reader to the basic principles of human linkage analysis between two loci (methods involving more than two loci are introduced in Chapter 14). A brief historical review is provided below but is by no means complete and only touches on some of the earlier approaches to linkage analysis. For the novice in linkage analysis, it will be important to carefully follow the analysis presented for the pedigree shown in Figure 4.1. Readers not interested in statistical detail may just want to read Section 4.3, which describes the lod score method, and Section 4.7 that deals with the problem of multiple comparisons, particularly the question of locus-specific versus genome-wide p-values. Because of their practical importance, nonparametric (e.g., affected sib pair) methods are covered separately (Chapter 13).

4.1. A Brief Historical Review

In this section, the main stages of development of human linkage analysis are briefly sketched. Not restricted to human genetics, Edwards (1996) has given an account of the history of the estimation of linkage from a more statistical standpoint.

Direct Method. An early approach to human linkage analysis was what became known as the *direct method*. It consists of directly observing and counting recombinants and nonrecombinants. The total of these recombination events is often referred to as the number, n, of opportunities for recombination, or meioses. If the number of observed recombinations is denoted by k, then a "natural" estimate of the recombination fraction is given by $\hat{\theta} = k/n$.

The direct method is appealing because one can see all recombination events. Many researchers, particularly in the past, have trusted no other method. However, with unknown phase, incomplete penetrance, and other factors clouding a direct view of genotypes through phenotypes, the direct method often extracts only a limited amount of information from real data, sometimes even in a biased manner. A pedigree in which the direct method extracts all linkage information is shown in Figure 4.1 and discussed in the next paragraph. In this case, the estimate, $\hat{\theta} = k/n$ is the maximum likelihood estimate of the recombination fraction.

In Figure 4.1, dark symbols represent individuals affected with the autosomal dominant trait Charcot–Marie–Tooth neuropathy (CMT1), also called hereditary motor and sensory neuropathy type 1. On the left side of Figure 4.1, the ABO blood types are shown. The first step in this analysis is to find out as much as possible about the genotypes, which may proceed as follows (results are shown on the right side of Figure 4.1): Individuals 2.1 and 3.2 are both homozygous normal; that is, they have the genotype d/d at the trait locus, whereas 3.1 must be heterozygous, D/d, because he inherited a normal allele from his mother and a disease allele from his father. As the disease is rare, the grandfather may be assumed to be heterozygous at the disease locus, but this assumption is not crucial for the present analysis. At the ABO locus, by his phenotype, 3.1 could be A/A or A/O, but the presence of O children as well as the O genotype of the grandmother excludes the A/A genotype; thus, 3.1 must

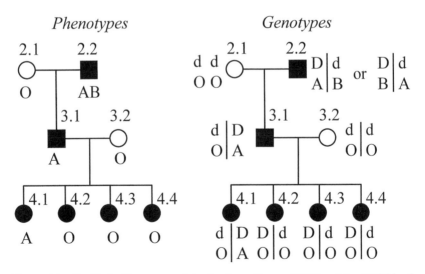

Figure 4.1. Kinship L. Phenotypes of the dominant disease CMT1 and the ABO blood types are shown on the left side, genotypes on the right side. (Based on Dyck et al., 1983, Fig. 2.)

be doubly heterozygous. Furthermore, knowing that the alleles *d* and *O* came from his mother determines his phase, which is thus *dO/DA*, as shown on the right side of Figure 4.1. Because 3.2 is doubly homozygous, each of the four children carries a *dO* haplotype. The remaining haplotypes must be *DA* in 4.1 and *DO* in each of 4.2 through 4.4. The father has therefore produced one nonrecombinant (*DA*) and three recombinant gametes, leading to the estimate ¾ = 0.75 for the recombination fraction. As the true value of the recombination fraction is assumed to range from 0 through ½, the result, k/n = ¾, is generally interpreted as $\hat{\theta}$ = ½.

Scoring recombination events in Figure 4.1 is carried out by inspection of the children's phenotypes. A child is thus usually called a "recombinant" or a "nonrecombinant" depending on whether or not recombination occurred in a parent.

Knowing the parental genotypes (including phase) is a necessary condition for direct linkage analysis. It is, however, not sufficient in all cases. For example, as will be seen later, two phase-known doubly heterozygous parents can have children, which do not unequivocally reveal recombination events in the parents. The direct method is particularly useful for loci on the X chromosome, for which males are hemizygous so that alleles are always in coupling (except for loci in the pseudoautosomal region).

Y Statistics. Consider the situation that the grandparents in Figure 4.1 are unknown. This leaves the phase in the father (3.1) unknown so that the children cannot unequivocally be scored as recombinants or nonrecombinants. Each child is either a recombinant, given one of the phases, or a nonrecombinant, given the other phase. Early geneticists were under the impression that such pedigrees did not yield any information on linkage. The German physician Bernstein (1931) was the first to point out a possible type of indirect analysis, using the following approach: When k is the number of recombinants, given one of the phases in the doubly heterozygous parent, then k may be small or large depending on the assumed phase. However, the product $y = k(n - k)$ is the same in either phase. Furthermore, the average value of this y *statistic* depends on the recombination fraction and is largest for θ = ½ and zero for θ = 0. For several types of matings, Bernstein (1931) published mean values of y for different sibship sizes and values of the recombination fraction, which enabled researchers to estimate recombination fractions and gauge whether linkage might be present. One of these tables is reproduced in Stern (1973). However, y statistics are less efficient than maximum likelihood estimates; that is, they waste some of the information contained in the data.

Sib-Pair Method. Introduced by Penrose (1935), this method is based on the relative frequencies of pairs of siblings being alike or unlike for two traits whose linkage relationship is to be investigated. Its original form is relatively inefficient. The sib-pair method is further discussed in Section 13.1.

Maximum Likelihood Method. Fisher's (1922a, 1922b) development of maximum likelihood as a general statistical estimation procedure method allowed fully efficient estimation of recombination fractions and superseded previous ad hoc methods. However, it was tedious to apply to human families. Bell and Haldane (1937) analyzed known multigenerational pedigrees segregating hemophilia and color blindness by computing the likelihood with respect to gene frequency, recombination fraction between the two loci, and mutation rate at the hemophilia locus. They even discussed such modern concepts as germline mosaicism although not under this name. Ten years later, Haldane and Smith (1947) calculated the likelihood for 17 pedigrees with hemophilia and color blindness, a task judged ''very laborious'' by the authors, although calculation of the likelihood is simpler in X linkage than in autosomal linkage. Based on the likelihood, these authors applied several analysis techniques. The maximum likelihood estimate of the recombination fraction between hemophilia and color blindness was equal to 9.5%.

u **Scores.** For the linkage analysis of two-generation families, Fisher (1935a) implemented a systematic scheme of the maximum likelihood method in the form of *u scores*. These are functions of the observed frequencies of offspring phenotype classes such that with a transformation of the recombination fraction, the likelihood (probability of occurrence of the observations) can be represented in a particularly simple form, although this involves some approximations. The whole procedure is quite elaborate, taking into account various mating types and modes of ascertainment. It was later extended by Finney but this is not pursued here. The interested reader is referred to Smith (1953) or Bailey (1961). This method is applicable to two-generation data and is fully efficient only for loose linkage.

Lod Scores for Small Families. Morton (1955) put forward the use of *sequential test procedures* in the linkage analysis between two loci, recognizing that the typical method of sampling small families was in fact sequential. Applying Wald's (1947) sequential probability ratio test (see Section 3.4) of the null hypothesis $\theta_0 = \frac{1}{2}$ versus a fixed alternative value, $\theta_1 < \frac{1}{2}$, and postulating a power of 0.99 and a significance level of 0.001, he proposed to keep sampling families as long as

$$Z_1 < Z(\theta) < Z_0 \mid Z_0 = 3, Z_1 = -2, \tag{4.1}$$

where $Z(\theta)$ is Barnard's (1949) *lod or lod score*, $Z(\theta) = \log_{10}[L(\theta_1)/L(\theta_0)]$, summed over all families in the sample at the given value, θ_1, of the recombination fraction (for a simple step-by-step introduction to lod scores, see Section 4.3). Sampling is terminated when either of the two bounds in (4.1) is reached or exceeded. When $Z(\theta)$ is equal to or larger than the upper bound, $Z_0 = 3$, the hypothesis of free recombination is rejected, and when $Z(\theta)$ reaches or drops below the lower bound, $Z_1 = -2$, the hypothesis of free recombination (absence of linkage) is accepted. The values of the two bounds in (4.1) are a consequence of Morton's (1955) requirement of a power of 0.99 at $\theta = \theta_1$ and a significance level of 0.001 in the sequential test (see Section 3.4). The significance level was chosen to be this small because of the low prior probability of linkage for autosomal loci. For X-linked loci, as outlined in Section 4.4, a less stringent critical lod score limit $Z_0 = 2$ is deemed sufficient.

Morton (1955) also defined a "posterior type I error,"

$$P(H_0|s) = P(s|H_0)P(H_0)/[P(s|H_0)P(H_0) + P(s|H_1)P(H_1)], \tag{4.2}$$

where s stands for the event that the test is significant ($s =$ "Z_{max} exceeds 3"), $P(s|H_0) = 0.001$ is the significance level, $P(s|H_1)$ is the average power for different values of θ, and $P(H_1) = 0.05$ is the approximate prior probability of linkage. Morton's (1955) choice of power and significance level was dictated by the aim that the posterior rate of false positive results (4.2) stay below 5%. For example, assuming an average power of 0.50, equation (4.2) yields $P(H_0|s) = 0.04$.

Nowadays, the sequential test is no longer carried out in its original form (current procedures are described in Sections 4.3 and 15.4). In particular, one no longer tests for linkage under a fixed value of the recombination fraction. Several of Morton's (1955) original recommendations, however, are still in current use.

In addition to proposing a sequential test for linkage, Morton (1955) streamlined its application by recommending that researchers accumulate and publish results of linkage analyses in the form of lod scores at a fixed set of θ values covering the range from 0 through $\frac{1}{2}$. This simple concept proved to be very effective. For two-point analyses, it is still in general use today. For many types of two-generation families, Morton (1955) and others published lod score tables that are reminiscent of the tables of *y statistics* published by Bernstein (1931). The ease with which Morton's lod score concept could be applied represented a breakthrough in linkage analysis.

Peeling Methods. A very general approach to the analysis of pedigree data, proposed by Elston and Stewart (1971), set the stage for many of the currently used maximum likelihood estimation and likelihood ratio test procedures. Although not restricted to linkage analysis (Elston et al., 1992), this area is the one in which it probably proved most fruitful (Stewart, 1992). This approach allows the representation of the likelihood, or lod score, for pedigrees with any number of generations and for qualitative as well as quantitative data. Missing information is dealt with in a very elegant manner. Furthermore, Elston and Stewart (1971) presented a recursive method, the *Elston–Stewart algorithm* (see Section 9.2), for fast and exact calculation of likelihoods in large pedigrees.

Based on this algorithm, I developed the LIPED computer program (for *li*kelihood in *ped*igrees) for linkage analysis between pairs of loci (Ott, 1974a). Although it is restricted to two-point analysis (it works with two loci at a time), it is still in use by some researchers because it has been error free for over 25 years. Details of the program are discussed in Section 8.3.

In the 1970s, methods of somatic cell genetics and cytogenetics became widely available, allowing the localization of genetic markers to single chromosomes and specific chromosomal segments. Toward the end of the decade, the seemingly old-fashioned "family method" seemed doomed to disappear. At the beginning of the 1980s, the introduction of molecular genetics methods to human genetics made genetic linkage analysis suddenly very interesting again and led to an ever-increasing importance of these techniques.

The increasing availability of DNA polymorphisms as genetic markers called for the introduction of multipoint analysis methods, which can analyze more than just two loci jointly (see Chapter 6). Probably the most widely used general multipoint analysis programs are the LINKAGE program package (Lathrop et al., 1984), which is based on extensions of the Elston–Stewart algorithm, and GENEHUNTER (Kruglyak et al., 1996; Kong and Cox, 1997). For details on this and other linkage programs, see Chapter 9.

Most of the newer methods for linkage analysis are based on particular novel representations of the pedigree likelihood (see Section 4.8). For example, the Lander–Green (1987) algorithm permits the simultaneous consideration of many loci. One of the most recent accomplishments is an algorithm (VITESSE) that permits much faster evaluation of likelihoods than previously known methods (O'Connell and Weeks, 1995). Whereas VITESSE is, in principle, an extension of the Elston–Stewart algorithm, the most recent and widely used extension of the Lander–Green algorithm is implemented in the GENEHUNTER program, which combines both parametric and nonparametric linkage analysis at many loci.

4.2. Prior and Posterior Distribution of θ

This section briefly discusses Bayesian approaches to linkage analysis. It is somewhat technical and may be omitted by readers less interested in statistical details.

As will be seen in Section 4.3, in this book the recombination fraction is treated as an unknown parameter that is to be estimated by maximum likelihood techniques. Other approaches exist, however, and one of them is briefly discussed here (for a "rough and ready" determination of the posterior probability of linkage, see Section 4.4). It assumes that the recombination fraction θ (or the event that two loci are a distance θ apart) is a random variable with a prior density function, $f(\theta)$. The prior density is then modified by the observations, F, leading to a posterior density, $f(\theta|F)$. This approach is generally referred to as the Bayesian method of linkage analysis. Related questions of prior probability of linkage and the number of markers required to span the human genome were discussed in Section 2.7. The mathematically less inclined reader may want to skip the derivation presented in the subsequent paragraph and turn directly to the example in the next paragraph.

Smith (1959) assumed a mixed prior density for θ, which is uniform $f(\theta) = 1/11$ on $\theta < \frac{1}{2}$, and a point mass of 21/22 at $\theta = \frac{1}{2}$. The prior probability of linkage, therefore, is taken to be $1/22 \approx 0.05$. With F standing for the observed family data, for $0 \le \theta < \frac{1}{2}$, the posterior density of θ is obtained by the Bayes theorem as

$$f(\theta|F) = \frac{f(F|\theta)}{\int_{0 \le t < 0.5} f(F|t)f(t)dt + f(F|\theta = 0.5)P(\theta = 0.5)}. \tag{4.3}$$

In this expression, $f(F|\theta)$ is the pedigree likelihood, $L(\theta)$, for a given value of θ. Dividing it by $L(0.5)$ leads to the likelihood ratio, $L(\theta)/L(0.5)$, which is the antilog of the lod score, $Z(\theta)$. If numerator and denominator in (4.3) are divided through by $L(0.5)$ and by the prior probability of linkage, $P(0 \le \theta < \frac{1}{2}) = 1/22$, then the integral in the denominator becomes the expectation of the likelihood ratio, that is, the average height, Λ, of the (observed) likelihood ratio curve. Thus, one has $f(\theta|F) =$

22 $[L(\theta)/L(0.5)] f(\theta)/(\Lambda + 21)$. Integrating this over the range $0 \le \theta < \frac{1}{2}$ furnishes the posterior probability of linkage,

$$P(\theta < \frac{1}{2}) = \Lambda/(\Lambda + 21). \tag{4.4}$$

In practice, one divides the interval $0 \le \theta < \frac{1}{2}$ into a number of segments, depending on the number of θ values at which lod scores were calculated. The ith segment, $i = 1. \ . \ . \ s$, of length b_i, then contains the likelihood ratio, $L(\theta_i)/L(0.5)$, where $b_1 = \frac{1}{2}(\theta_2 + \theta_1)$, $b_i = \frac{1}{2}(\theta_{i+1} + \theta_i) - \frac{1}{2}(\theta_i + \theta_{i-1}) = \frac{1}{2}(\theta_{i+1} - \theta_{i-1})$, $b_s = 0.5 - \frac{1}{2}(\theta_s + \theta_{s-1})$; $\Sigma b_i = 0.5$. The average height of the likelihood ratio is then approximated by

$$\Lambda \approx 2 \Sigma [L(\theta_i)/L(\frac{1}{2})] b_i, \tag{4.5}$$

that is, the area underneath the likelihood curve divided by the length, $\frac{1}{2}$, of the θ axis.

As a numerical example, assume that, in a linkage analysis between two loci, 1 recombinant was observed out of 12 opportunities for recombination, so that the antilog of the lod score is given by $L(\theta)/L(\frac{1}{2}) = 2^{12}\theta(1 - \theta)^{11}$. Using the values shown in Table 4.1, the average height of the likelihood ratio, approximated by (4.5), is then obtained as 53.47, resulting in a value of 0.72 for Smith's (1959) posterior probability of linkage (4.4). Although a priori the chance that the two genes are located on the same chromosome is only about 5%, after only 1 recombinant in 12 opportunities is observed, this "chance" or belief is increased to 72%. For definite evidence of linkage, this method usually requires a posterior probability of linkage of 95% or higher.

The mathematically inclined reader may be interested in the exact solution to the calculations approximated above. Because the likelihood ratio is known analytically, one need not divide the θ axis into segments but rather solves the beta integral, $\int_{0 \le \theta < \frac{1}{2}} \theta(1 - \theta)^{n-1} d\theta = [1 - (n + 2)(\frac{1}{2})^{n+1}]/[n(n + 1)]$. With appropriate adjustments, this leads to a figure of

Table 4.1. Lod Score $Z(\theta_i)$, Likelihood Ratio $L^*(\theta_i)$, and Interval Width b_i at Selected Values of θ_i for the Calculation of the Posterior Probability of Linkage

i	θ_i	b_i	$Z(\theta_i)$	$L^*(\theta_i)$
1	0.01	0.025	1.56	36.7
2	0.05	0.050	2.07	116.5
3	0.10	0.075	2.11	128.5
4	0.20	0.100	1.85	70.4
5	0.30	0.100	1.38	24.3
6	0.40	0.150	0.77	5.9

0.73 for the posterior probability of linkage. The approximate method of computation is thus quite reliable.

4.3. The Lod Score Method

In this section, the lod score method of linkage analysis for pairs of loci is introduced with as little mathematical detail as possible. For the statistically minded reader, I would just like to point out that the statistical techniques used in current linkage analysis are mostly based on maximum likelihood estimation and likelihood ratio testing. Occasionally, methods from other fields are also used, which may be irritating to the reader looking for a methodologically pure approach, but I am trying to present linkage analysis the way it is actually carried out. Statistical properties of the various procedures, where known, will be dealt with in later chapters. A scholarly review from a statistical viewpoint of the lod score method and some of its predecessors was given by Chotai (1984).

Under favorable circumstances, the phenotypes in a pedigree imply the underlying genotypes in such a way that recombination events can be scored unambiguously. An example is shown in Figure 4.1, in which the phase of the doubly heterozygous father is known. In that example, one counts 3 recombinants and 1 nonrecombinant, leading to an estimate of the recombination of ¾, which is usually interpreted as $\hat{\theta} = \frac{1}{2}$.

A complication arises when parental phase is unknown. As an example, consider family 79 in Bodmer et al. (1987) segregating the autosomal dominant disease familial adenomatous polyposis (APC, adenomatosis polyposis coli, chromosomal location 5q21-q22). The family is displayed on the left side of Figure 4.2. The phenotypes are affection statuses (filled symbols for *affected*, open symbols for *unaffected*) and typing results (allele numbers) for a chromosome 5 marker identified by the probe C11p11. In the parental generation, the two rightmost individuals are identical (monozygotic) twins. Genetically, they represent two independent expressions of a single zygote so that, for this marker, only one typing result is shown (in the analysis, they count as one individual). The affected females' spouse is unknown and is thus not shown—a customary abbreviation. Presumably, that spouse was unaffected.

The genetic interpretation of family 79 in Bodmer et al. (1987) is shown on the right side of Figure 4.2. The grandmother is dead but is known to have been affected. Because she has unaffected offspring, she must be heterozygous *F/f* at the disease locus, where *F* stands for the disease allele and *f* for the normal allele. The grandfather is homozygous for both the disease and the marker genes and thus always passes an *f 2*

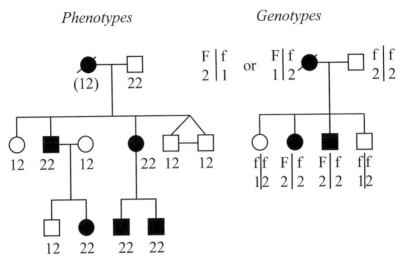

Figure 4.2. Family 79. Phenotypes of familial adenomatous polyposis (dominant) and a chromosome 5 gene identified by the probe C11p11 are shown on the left side, the relevant genotypes on the right side. (Based on Bodmer et al., 1987, Fig. 1.)

haplotype (gamete) to his children. The grandmother is untyped, but her marker type can be inferred to be *1 2,* because some children received a *1* allele and others a *2* allele from her. Genotypes that can be unambiguously inferred are generally given in parentheses. However, her phase is unknown, the two possible phases being indicated by *I* and *II.* The two affected parents in the parental generation (middle generation on the left side of Figure 4.2) are both homozygous at the marker locus. Thus, they are uninformative for linkage; that is, their children cannot reveal recombination events between marker and disease in the parents (for a formal demonstration of this fact, see Section 5.1) and are thus not shown on the right side of Figure 4.2.

   If the grandmother's phase is *I,* her offspring reveal 4 nonrecombinations, and, if it is *II,* there are 4 recombinations, the two cases having equal a priori probabilities. Therefore, one cannot count recombinants and nonrecombinants in this family. Estimating the recombination fraction is then carried out by the method of maximum likelihood (see Section 3.2). In this method, one calculates the likelihood (i.e., the probability of occurrence of the data) for a variety of assumed values of θ and selects that θ value associated with the highest likelihood as the best estimate. It is designated by the symbol $\hat{\theta}$.

   In abbreviated form, the likelihood for this family is calculated as follows: Given phase *I*, there are 4 nonrecombinants, each of which occurs independently with probability $1 - \theta$, so that the likelihood for the 4 nonrecombinants is equal to $(1 - \theta)^4$. Analogously, given phase *II*, the likelihood is θ^4. Combining these results and allowing for the fact that each phase has a probability of occurrence of ½ lead to the likelihood for family 79 in Bodmer et al. (1987) of

$$L(\theta) = \tfrac{1}{2}[(1 - \theta)^4 + \theta^4]. \tag{4.7}$$

This expression disregards terms due to allele frequencies and includes only those terms relevant for the recombination fraction. Strictly speaking, (4.7) is proportional to the likelihood rather than equal to it, but terms not relevant to the recombination fraction will cancel in the likelihood ratio to be formed below, which is why they may be omitted. For any value assumed for θ, the corresponding likelihood can now be calculated. For the proper likelihood, the result is always between 0 and 1, but its numerical value is not generally of interest because it very much depends on the size of the family—the larger the family, the smaller the likelihood.

A more relevant quantity is the likelihood ratio that is obtained by dividing $L(\theta)$ by its value under free recombination,

$$L^*(\theta) = L(\theta)/L(\tfrac{1}{2}). \tag{4.8}$$

This likelihood ratio has loosely been called odds for linkage as it indicates, for a given value of $\theta < \tfrac{1}{2}$, how much higher the likelihood of the data is under linkage than under absence of linkage. Generally, however, the term *odds* refers to a ratio of probabilities and not of likelihoods (Armitage and Berry, 1987). Notice that, by construction, $L^*(\tfrac{1}{2}) = 1$. For family 79, one obtains $L^*(\theta) = 8[(1 - \theta)^4 + \theta^4]$.

It is usually convenient to work not with the likelihood ratio but with its logarithm (to base 10), the so-called *lod* or *lod score* (Barnard, 1949)

$$Z(\theta) = \log_{10}L^*(\theta) = \log_{10}[L(\theta)/L(\tfrac{1}{2})]. \tag{4.9}$$

By construction, $Z(\tfrac{1}{2}) = 0$. Now, our estimate of the recombination fraction is that value of θ at which $Z(\theta)$ is highest. For family 79, the lod score is given by the expression $\log(8) + \log[(1 - \theta)^4 + \theta^4]$. For example, at $\theta = 0, 0.01, 0.05$, and 0.10, one obtains the respective lod scores 0.903, 0.886, 0.814, and 0.720. The θ estimate is thus $\hat{\theta} = 0$, the same as if phase *I* had been assumed to be known, but this is not generally the case (see Problem 4.2). Phase *I* is more plausible than phase *II* in the following sense: Under phase *I*, the offspring (4 nonrecombinants) have probability of occurrence $(1 - \theta)^4$ which, at $\hat{\theta} = 0$, is equal to 1. Under phase *II*, the offspring (4 recombinants) occur with probability θ^4 which, in the range $0 \leq \theta \leq \tfrac{1}{2}$, attains its maximum value of $(\tfrac{1}{2})^4 = 0.0625$ at

$\theta = \frac{1}{2}$. The conditional likelihood, given phase *I*, is thus considerably higher than that given phase *II*.

Because of a variety of complicating factors such as incomplete penetrance, missing information, unequal male and female recombination fractions, and so on, lod scores are rarely calculated analytically as in the model case discussed above. Instead, one has computer programs carry out this arduous job (see Chapter 8).

In Section 1.2, parents were said to be potentially informative for linkage when they are doubly heterozygous. A family or set of families is called *informative for linkage* when the lod score $Z(\theta)$ is different from zero for at least one value of $\theta < \frac{1}{2}$. Similarly, offspring are termed informative for linkage when their phenotype reveals linkage information.

As observations in different families are statistically independent, lod scores at a fixed θ value can simply be added over families, assuming homogeneity (see heterogeneity in Chapter 9). In publications, linkage analysis results are usually presented in a table with rows referring to different families and columns referring to different θ values. The body of such a table then contains the lod scores for the *i*th family at the *j*th θ value. The bottom row usually contains the sum of the lod scores for the different families at the corresponding θ values.

As is pointed out in Chapter 8, linkage programs permit relatively easy calculations of lod scores. However, in addition to computing lods, one should also inspect the data for any unusual features that may not be reflected in the lod score. A case in point is skewed segregation. For example, the sex distribution among children is expected roughly to follow a binomial distribution with mean $\frac{1}{2}$, or a parent is expected to pass each of his or her two alleles to an offspring with probability $\frac{1}{2}$. Marked deviations from these expectations can be indicative of errors in the data. These deviations strongly reduce the likelihood of the data, but the reduction occurs both in the numerator and in the denominator of the likelihood ratio and thus cancels, so that skewed distribution does not show in the lod score. I vividly remember a case in which a parent seemingly had passed the same allele to all of her eight offspring; after many days of deliberations, a mix-up of samples in the laboratory was detected and retesting that nuclear family no longer resulted in any unusual segregation. On the other hand, cases of irregular segregation are known to occur and to have a biological basis (see Section 11.9).

It has been recommended (Conneally et al., 1985) that two-point lod scores (i.e., between pairs of loci) be reported at the following fixed set of θ values: 0, 0.001, 0.05, 0.1, 0.2, 0.3, and 0.4. Generally, lod scores are calculated at fixed values of θ between 0 and $\frac{1}{2}$, often in steps of

0.05. Some computer programs (e.g., ILINK in the LINKAGE program package) find the maximum of the log likelihood for the whole range, $0 \leq \theta \leq 1$. The reason for this is that a value of $\theta > \frac{1}{2}$, if associated with a high lod score, may be indicative of problems in the data, which is valuable to know.

Another of the recommendations issued at the Helsinki workshop (Conneally et al., 1985) was to report lod scores with an accuracy of two decimal places. This accuracy is certainly sufficient to represent the maximum lod score as evidence for linkage. However, some analyses such as tests for heterogeneity and computation of standard errors of the recombination estimate employ lod scores for further calculations, in which case two decimal places for the lod scores are insufficient for good accuracy of the final result. Lods should therefore be published with (at least) three decimal places.

4.4. Testing for Linkage

In the previous section, the maximum likelihood method of estimating the recombination fraction was described, where the particular form of that method used in human genetics is known as the lod score method. Here, questions of significance of the result of a linkage analysis are addressed.

Positive lod scores indicate evidence in favor of linkage, and negative lods indicate evidence against linkage. When linkage in fact exists, as one accumulates more families, lod scores tend to become larger and larger. The maximum of the lod score, denoted by $Z(\hat{\theta})$ or $Z_{\max}$ or $\hat{Z}$, serves as a measure for the weight of the data in favor of the hypothesis of linkage. When that maximum reaches or exceeds a certain critical value, Z_0, the data are said to convey *significant evidence for linkage*. The critical value generally adhered to is the one originally proposed by Morton (1955), $Z_0 = 3$, for autosomal loci, and $Z_0 = 2$ for X-linked loci. Note that these critical limits are appropriate for a given pair of loci, for example, a disease and a marker locus. Slightly different limits apply in genome screens when a disease locus is tested against a battery of marker loci (see Section 4.7).

Declaring a linkage result significant when $Z_{\max} > 3$ amounts to carrying out a likelihood ratio (LR) test with fixed sample size, which is conceptually quite different from Morton's (1955) sequential test procedure. The theory of LR tests predicts that asymptotically, under the null hypothesis of absence of linkage, $4.6 \times Z_{\max}$ follows a chi-square distribution with 1 degree of freedom (df). Consequently, owing to the critical level of $4.6 \times 3 = 13.8$ for chi-square, the asymptotic (two-sided) significance level, α, of this likelihood ratio test is equal to 0.0002. In practice, the test is only then declared significant when $\hat{\theta} < \frac{1}{2}$ but not when it exceeds $\frac{1}{2}$, that is, the test is carried out in a one-sided manner. Under the null hypothesis of no linkage ($\theta = \frac{1}{2}$), $\hat{\theta}$ is symmetric about $\frac{1}{2}$ so that the actual significance level of the test for linkage is equal to $\alpha/2 = 0.0001$. However, depending on the family type and the number of families investigated, the null distribution of Z_{max} can be quite different from chi-square (see Section 4.6 for some examples).

Some computer programs furnish *p*-values rather than maximum lod scores. Also, when multiple testing is taken into account, results are often presented in the form of an overall *p*-value. Many geneticists have a better "feel" for maximum lod scores than for *p*-values as statistics in the linkage test. Thus, one may convert a significance level, *p*, into an associated maximum lod score, *Z*, by finding the normal deviate, *x*, which corresponds to the upper tail probability *p* of the normal distribution. The desired maximum lod score is then given by $Z = 0.5x^2/\ln(10)$. The NORINV program (one of the Linkage Utilities) provides *Z* for given *p*. It is ironic that *p*-values should be converted to lod scores for better interpretation of results but in human linkage analysis, lod scores simply are more appreciated than *p*-values.

Thus far, the tacit assumption has been that recombination in male parents occurs with the same frequency, θ_m, as that in female parents, θ_f. A possible difference between the two rates will be discussed more fully in Section 9.1, but its statistical aspect is best covered in the present context. If male and female recombinations fractions are estimated, the lod score is a function of two parameters, $Z(\theta_m, \theta_f)$. Consider the two hypotheses, $H_0: \theta_m = \theta_f = \frac{1}{2}$; and $H_1: \theta_m < \frac{1}{2}, \theta_f < \frac{1}{2}, \theta_m \neq \theta_f$. Assume that the test of H_0 against H_1 is declared significant if the maximum lod score exceeds 3. Asymptotically, if H_0 is true, $4.6 \times Z_{max}$ follows a chi-square distribution on 2 df, where Z_{max} is the maximum lod score, $Z(\hat{\theta}_m, \hat{\theta}_f)$. The asymptotic significance level of this test is thus equal to $\alpha = 0.0010$. In practice, only those values of $\hat{\theta}_m$, and $\hat{\theta}_f$ are considered that lie in the quadrant ($\theta_m < \frac{1}{2}, \theta_f < \frac{1}{2}$). Assuming that $\hat{\theta}_m$ and $\hat{\theta}_f$ are uncorrelated, the actual significance level is equal to $\alpha/4 = 0.00025$, which is higher than the corresponding significance level of 0.0001 when male and female recombination fractions are taken to be equal. Therefore, when the same critical limit for Z_{max} is applied, allowing for different recombination rates in males and females is somewhat less conservative than assuming $\theta_m = \theta_f$. To achieve the same asymptotic significance level, $\alpha/4 = 0.0001$, when allowing for different male and female recombination fractions, the critical lod score must be set at 3.40 (this is equivalent to a chi-square limit of 15.65 on 2 df, which is associated with a significance level of $\alpha = 0.0004$).

An interesting test for linkage has been proposed, which allows for differences in sex specific recombination fractions yet is associated with only 1 df (Cleves and Elston, 1997). The null hypothesis, $H_0 : \theta_m + \theta_f = 1$, is tested against the alternative, $H_1 : \theta_m + \theta_f < 1$. Under some conditions, particularly a large excess of θ_f over θ_m, this test is more powerful than the classical approach.

For tests against a single alternative value of θ, inequalities (3.5) and (3.6) provide an upper bound for the significance level. Morton (1978) stated that these inequalities also hold in the generalized likelihood ratio test (where θ is estimated rather than fixed in advance), that is,

$$\alpha = P[Z_{max} \geq Z \,|\, H_0] \leq 10^{-Z}, \tag{4.10}$$

and Chotai (1984) furnished a statistical proof for that assertion, where Z is any critical level for the maximum lod score. An heuristic explanation for this statement might be that power and significance level are highest in fully informative matings and with a true recombination fraction of zero. In this case, as shown in Section 4.6, equation (4.10) with equality between the left and right sides provides the exact significance level. Consequently, the critical lod scores, $Z_0 = 3$ and $Z_0 = 2$ (in the X-linked case), have associated significance levels of no more than $10^{-3} = 0.001$ and $10^{-2} = 0.01$, respectively. Analogously, an observed maximum lod score, Z_{max}, has an associated empirical significance level, which is at most equal to $10^{-Z_{max}}$.

Equation (4.10) has a practical application in small families for which asymptotic results are unlikely to hold. It then provides an upper bound to the significance level associated with a maximum lod score although that significance level is likely to be conservative (too high). As a particular application, assume that a researcher wants to replicate a linkage finding in a set of small families. He does not want to find a new locus and, thus, is satisfied with a resulting significance level of 0.05. Solving (4.10) for Z leads to $Z \leq -\log(\alpha)$. With $\alpha = 0.05$, one finds $Z = 1.3$ as the corresponding critical lod score.

The significance level of the test for linkage is much smaller than the significance levels of 0.05 or 0.01 customarily used in statistical tests. The reason for the low value of α was given by Smith (1953) along the lines of arguments given below (more formal considerations follow from equation 4.2, above). Assume that one tests for linkage at a significance level of 5%. This means that, when no linkage exists, one will nonetheless declare the test for linkage significant at the (false-positive) rate of 5%. Consider now a test with 100% power, one that will detect every linkage whenever it is present. The a priori chance that a pair of loci will be on the same chromosome is about 5%, so our perfect test will "detect" as many nonexistent linkages as real ones (true positives). With less than perfect power, of course, the situation is even worse. The remedy lies in lowering the significance level to the much smaller values currently used.

Another way of interpreting the low formal significance level is in terms of a somewhat loosely defined "posterior probability of linkage." Although the prior probability of two random loci being on the same chromosome is about 0.05, the chance they are within measurable distance of each other is only $P(H_1) = 0.02$ (see Section 2.5). The posterior probability of linkage may then be expressed as

$$P(H_1|F) = P(F|H_1)P(H_1)/[P(F|H_1)P(H_1) \\ + P(F|H_0)P(H_0)] = R/(R + 49),$$

where $R = P(F|H_1)/P(F|H_0)$ is the likelihood (odds) ratio. The conventional critical odds ratio, $R = 1000$, is then seen to correspond to a posterior probability of linkage of 95%.

In human linkage analysis, accuracy of the estimate $\hat{\theta}$ is assessed via a specific support interval. An example is graphically depicted in Figure 4.3, which shows the lod score curve for 8 recombinants out of 40 recombination events. The curve reaches its maximum, $Z_{max} = 3.348$, at $\hat{\theta} = 8/40 = 0.20$. As recommended by Conneally et al. (1985), the $Z_{max} - 1$ *support interval* is obtained by drawing a horizontal straight line

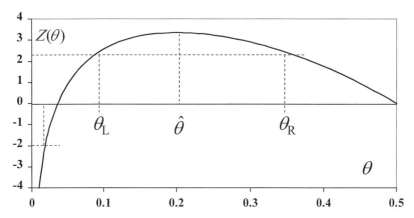

Figure 4.3. Lod score curve for 8 recombinants in 40 recombination events showing construction of support interval.

at 1 unit of lod score below Z_{max} (here at $Z = 2.348$), provided that $Z_{max} \geq 3$ (otherwise, no support interval is constructed). The points of intersection of this line with the lod score curve, when projected onto the θ axis, mark the endpoints θ_L and θ_R of the support interval. Of course, when the lod score curve keeps increasing toward $\theta = 0$, only the upper bound of the support interval is defined in this way, the lower bound being at $\theta = 0$.

Testing a null hypothesis, $\theta = \theta_0$, such that the test is significant when chi-square exceeds 4.6 (1 lod score unit converted into chi-square units by multiplying it by 4.6), corresponds to an asymptotic significance level of 0.032. Therefore, the support interval defined in the last paragraph is sometimes interpreted as an asymptotic confidence interval, for it consists of all those points θ_0 which render the test nonsignificant (see Section 3.6). The asymptotic confidence coefficient of said confidence interval is better than 95%. According to inequality (4.10), the actual confidence coefficient is at least 90%.

A point of logical inconsistency should be noted in applying the $Z_{max} - 1$ support intervals. Generally, in statistical tests, there is a one-to-one correspondence between confidence intervals and test results in that the test is nonsignificant when the confidence interval contains the parameter value specified by the null hypothesis. In linkage analysis, the null parameter value is $\theta = \frac{1}{2}$, which would be included in the confidence interval only when $Z_{max} < 1$. On the other hand, the test is declared significant when $Z_{max} \geq 3$. As pointed out above, this discrepancy has been resolved by the recommendation (Conneally et al., 1985) that a confidence (support) interval should not be constructed while Z_{max} stays below the critical limit of 3. The logically consistent solution, however, is to construct a confidence interval as consisting of all those points with log likelihood larger than $Z_{max} - 3$; when this confidence interval contains $\theta = \frac{1}{2}$ the customary test for linkage is not significant.

In Morton's (1955) sequential test for linkage, the null hypothesis of free recombination ($\theta = \frac{1}{2}$) is not rejected when the lod score at the predetermined value $\theta = \theta_1$ dips below -2. In today's likelihood ratio test approach, that concept is sometimes invoked for constructing a set of "excluded" θ values, although it is incompatible with the support interval defined above. Specifically, all values of θ at which $Z(\theta) < -2$ are said to be definitely excluded. For the case of 8 recombinants in 40 recombination events shown in Figure 4.3, values smaller than 0.015 are excluded by this criterion. This method of defining regions of exclusions or implausibility for θ is preferentially used in the process of mapping a disease gene by testing it against many marker genes and thereby excluding one chromosomal segment after another (see Section 11.7 on exclusion mapping).

4.5. Equivalent Numbers of Recombinants and Nonrecombinants

While the maximum lod score serves as an indicator for the evidence for linkage provided by a set of families, one would often like to know how many meioses and how many recombinants the data set contains. Approximate methods have been developed to obtain such numbers based on fitting the lod score function for known recombinants and nonrecombinants to the observed lod score curve. Two such methods are described below.

Edwards' Method. In their analysis of color blindness and hemophilia, Bell and Haldane (1937) approximated the likelihood of different families by a function, $\theta^k(1 - \theta)^{n-k}$, where n and k are not necessarily integers, and interpreted n as the number of gametes investigated and k as the number of crossovers found. Edwards (1971, 1976) extended this concept in the manner outlined below.

Generally, the lod score curve for large pedigrees has no simple interpretation. For a rough comparison of an observed lod score curve with that for known recombination events, and for an intuitive interpretation of the information content of family data, Edwards (1976) suggested equating the observed Z_{max} with that corresponding to known recombination events and deducing an equivalent number of recombinants and nonrecombinants. If k denotes the number of recombinants out of n opportunities, then $\hat{\theta} = k/n$ is the maximum likelihood estimate of the recombination fraction, and the maximum of the lod score is known to be equal to

$$Z_{max} = \begin{cases} n[\log(2) + \hat{\theta}\log(\hat{\theta}) + (1 - \hat{\theta})\log(1 - \hat{\theta})] & \text{if } \hat{\theta} > 0 \\ n\log(2) & \text{if } \hat{\theta} = 0. \end{cases} \quad (4.11)$$

Working backwards from these expressions, one obtains the equivalent numbers

$$n = \begin{cases} Z_{max}/[\log(2) + \hat{\theta}\log(\hat{\theta}) + (1 - \hat{\theta})\log(1 - \hat{\theta})] & \text{if } 0 < \hat{\theta} < \frac{1}{2} \\ Z_{max}/\log(2) & \text{if } \hat{\theta} = 0, \end{cases} \quad (4.12)$$

and

$$k = n\hat{\theta},$$

where $Z_{max} > 0$ is the maximum lod score obtained for the family data investigated and $\hat{\theta}$ is the θ value at which the maximum of the lod score occurs. This method is not applicable to recombination fraction estimates of ½ as this leads to $n = 0$. The equivalent number n of opportunities for recombination may serve as a measure of information content in the data. The equivalent numbers, n and k, may be obtained in this way from the EQUIV program.

As an example, consider the analysis of familial adenomatous polyposis (APC) discussed in the previous section. In 6 families, testing APC versus the gene identified by probe C11p11, Bodmer et al. (1987) obtained $Z_{max} = 3.26$ at $\hat{\theta} = 0$. This result corresponds to equivalent numbers of $k = 0$ and $n = 10.83$. Inspection of the data showed that in some matings phase was known and in others phase was unknown. Assigning the most probable genotypes in all cases, the data were consistent with an interpretation of no recombinants among 24 meioses (Bodmer et al., 1987). As 24 is much higher than the equivalent number of meioses of about 11, assigning plausible phases and genotypes when these are only partially known is seen to overestimate the amount of information in the data. Looking at this situation from a different angle, the difference between the number of meioses (24) and the equivalent number of meioses (10.83) reflects the loss of information through not having data on phase (Edwards, 1971). The maximum lod score, 3.26, of course, properly reflects all of the information in the data to the extent that gene frequencies and linkage disequilibrium are known and specified.

Edwards' equivalent number n of meioses is useful for comparing observed lod score maxima with those expected for known recombination events at the same θ values. However, k and $n - k$ do not provide the actual number of known recombinants and nonrecombinants in a pedigree unless the data are mostly phase-known. Also, the numbers k and n must be used only for illustration purposes and *not*, for example, in chi-square or other statistical tests as if they corresponded to actual numbers of observations.

Two-Point Method. While Edwards' method works only for positive maximum lod scores, the method described here is applicable to any lod score curve. It is based on the lod score function for k known recombinants and $n - k$ nonrecombinants, $Z(\theta) = n \times \log(2) + k \times \log(\theta) + (n - k) \times \log(1 - \theta)$. For very small θ, the last term in this expression becomes so small that it may be omitted. Then, a comparison between the lod scores at two small θ values is used to reconstruct k and n as follows:

1) $\theta = 0.0010 \Rightarrow Z(0.0010) = n \times \log(2) - 3k$

2) $\theta = 0.0001 \Rightarrow Z(0.0001) = n \times \log(2) - 4k.$

Subtracting line 2 from line 1 directly yields $k = Z(0.0010) - Z(0.0001)$, and inserting this result in line 1 leads to $n = 3.322 \times [Z(0.0010) + 3k]$, where the lod scores at $\theta = 0.0010$ and 0.0001 are obtained by a computer program.

4.6. Exact Tests in Simple Family Types

The lod score method as outlined above serves two purposes: (1) estimation of the recombination fraction, θ, and (2) carrying out of a statistical test of the null hypothesis of free recombination ($\theta = \frac{1}{2}$) versus the alternative hypothesis of linkage ($\theta < \frac{1}{2}$). Important characteristics of a statistical test are its significance level and its power. In this section, these characteristics are briefly investigated for small numbers of families of a simple structure (asymptotic, i.e., large sample size properties have been discussed above). Results will be relevant for sample size considerations; in a more general setting, questions of sample size are covered in Section 5.10. The statistically less interested reader may want to skip the remainder of this section.

As outlined in Section 3.4, the significance level (or type I error or rate of false-positive results) is the probability, $\alpha = P(s; \theta = \frac{1}{2})$, that the test is significant (indicated by s) when there is no linkage. The rate of false-negative results or type II error, $\beta = P(\text{not } s; \theta < \frac{1}{2})$, is the probability that the test is not significant although there is linkage. Its complement is the power, $1 - \beta = P(s; \theta < \frac{1}{2})$, that is, the probability of detecting linkage when it exists. By convention, as outlined above for autosomal loci, the test for linkage is declared significant when the maximum, Z_{max}, of the lod score exceeds the bound $Z_0 = 3$.

Two family types are investigated here: (1) the phase-known double backcross, and (2) the phase-unknown double backcross (see Section 5.7). In either family type, one has a pair of parents, one being doubly homozygous and the other being heterozygous at both loci considered, and a number m of offspring per family. The number of families is denoted by n.

Phase Known. The phase-known double backcross allows unambiguous counting of recombination events. It is thus unimportant how the offspring are distributed over the different families; the only relevant quantity is the total number, nm, of recombination events. For simplicity, it will be assumed in the derivation of the formulas that n families with 1 offspring each are available.

With n phase-known families, there are $n + 1$ possible outcomes, $k = 0...n$, where k is the number of families with a recombinant off-spring. Each outcome has a probability of occurrence, $P(k; \theta)$, which may be obtained from the binomial formula, with θ being the true recombination frequency. Furthermore, for each outcome, the associated maximum lod score Z_{max} may be obtained from equation (4.11). The probability, $P(s; \theta)$, of a significant result is thus given by the sum of the probabilities of all of those outcomes, k, for which $Z_{max} \geq Z_0$, and depends on the true recombination fraction. Notice that $P(s; \theta)$ is the significance level for $\theta = \frac{1}{2}$ and the power for $\theta < \frac{1}{2}$.

For $Z_0 = 3$ and phase-known families, one finds that for $n < 10$, Z_{max} never reaches or exceeds 3. For $n = 10 . . . 15$, $k = 0$ is the only outcome leading to $Z_{max} \geq 3$. Therefore, $P(s; \theta) = P(k = 0; \theta) = (1 - \theta)^n$, $n = 10 . . . 15$. Similarly, when $n = 16 . . . 19$, Z_{max} exceeds 3 when either 0 or 1 family contains a recombinant child, so $P(s; \theta) = (1 - \theta)^n + n\theta (1 - \theta)^{n-1} = (1 - \theta)^{n-1}[1 + (n - 1)\theta]$. For selected values of θ, numerical values are shown in the second and third columns of Table 4.2. For $n = 10$ and $n = 16$, the respective significance levels associated with the critical limit $Z_0 = 3$ are 0.001 and 0.00026.

The *empirical* significance level p associated with an observed maximum lod score, Z_{max}, is the probability of obtaining a result as

Table 4.2. Probability, $P(Z_{max} > Z_0; \theta)$, of a Significant Linkage Result when n Double Backcross Families with m Offspring Each Are Investigated

| | $Z_0 = 3$ | | | | $Z_0 = 2$ | | |
| | Phase Known | | Phase Unknown ($n = 10$) | | Phase Known | Phase Unknown | |
θ	$nm = 10$	$nm = 16$	$m = 2$	$m = 3$	$nm = 7$	$n = 7$, $m = 2$	$n = 4$, $m = 3$
Power							
0	1	1	1	1	1	1	1
0.01	0.904	0.989	0.819	0.966	0.932	0.869	0.886
0.05	0.599	0.811	0.369	0.572	0.698	0.497	0.541
0.10	0.349	0.515	0.137	0.202	0.478	0.249	0.284
0.20	0.107	0.141	0.021	0.015	0.210	0.067	0.073
0.30	0.028	0.026	0.004	0.001	0.082	0.022	0.019
0.40	0.006	0.003	0.001	0.00008	0.028	0.010	0.006
Significance Level							
0.50	0.001	0.00026	0.001	0.00003	0.008	0.008	0.004

extreme or more extreme than the one observed. For counts of recombination events, with k observed recombinants in n informative meioses, the empirical significance level is given by the binomial probability $p = P(x \leq k; r = \frac{1}{2})$, where x denotes the possible number of recombinants (binomial random variable) and r denotes the assumed true recombination fraction. For any k and n, p may easily be calculated using the BINOM program. For example, $k = 2$ recombinants in $n = 20$ meioses represent an empirical significance level of 0.0002. With no recombinants observed, $k = 0$, one obtains $p = (\frac{1}{2})^n$. In this case, the maximum lod score occurs at $\theta = 0$ and attains a value of $Z_{max} = n \times \log(2)$. Applying equation (4.10) with this value of Z_{max} leads to $p = (\frac{1}{2})^n$, that is, in this case the significance level attains the upper bound predicted by (4.10). For $k > 0$, the upper bound of the significance level is not reached (see Problem 4.4).

The above examples show that a constant critical limit of the maximum lod score leads to tests of different sizes, that is, tests associated with different significance levels (line $\theta = 0.50$ in Table 4.2). In significance testing, this is an undesirable situation (Elston, 1994), but a lod score threshold rather than a critical p-value has become customary in human genetics. In principle, the empirical significance level associated with an observed maximum lod score could be calculated, or at least approximated, by computer simulation. This has not often been done in practice but may become more widespread in genome screening.

Phase Unknown. For phase-unknown families, one must keep track of the number m of offspring per family. For example, as outlined in Section 5.9, families with $m = 3$ offspring fall into two distinct classes, a class 1 family occurring with probability $3\theta(1 - \theta)$. Evaluation of all possible outcomes and associated values of Z_{max} in $n = 10$ families shows that $Z_{max} > 3$ when the number of class 1 families is either 0 or 1. This leads to $P(s; \theta) = [1 - 3\theta(1 - \theta)]^9[1 + 27\theta(1 - \theta)]$.

One can read off Table 4.2 that 10 recombination events are sufficient for detecting linkage with a power of 90%, but only when the linkage is very tight ($\theta \leq 0.01$). With 16 recombination events available, one is able to detect a slightly looser linkage although, at $\theta = 0.05$, power has already dropped to 80%. Generally, it is much harder (requires more observations) to detect loose than tight linkage.

Table 4.2 shows that the significance level depends very much on the type of family and ranges from 0.001 down to 0.00003. Computing it for increasing numbers n of phase-known families with one offspring each, one finds that α oscillates around the limiting value of $0.0001 = 10^{-4}$, the deviations quickly becoming small; for $n > 10$, $0.3 \times 10^{-4} < \alpha < 2.6 \times 10^{-4}$.

4.7. Multiple Comparisons

For a given body of data, an investigator often carries out a multitude of tests in an attempt to find linkage between a marker and a disease locus underlying the trait studied. For example, various classification schemes are tried for defining who is affected and who is unaffected; several different analysis methods are applied; in the lod score method, several sets of penetrances are tried; many marker loci are tested for linkage with a disease locus; and so on. In the end a rather large number of tests are carried out on the same body of data. Without linkage, there is a small chance (probability of a type I error) that each test will lead to a significant result. With multiple such opportunities, if success is scored when any one of these tests is significant, the overall type I error must be higher than that for each single test—this phenomenon is known as the multiple comparisons or multiple testing problem. As outlined below, corrections have been developed so that the overall type I error stays at some predefined level. This problem is well known in biostatistics but seems somewhat difficult to grasp for nonstatisticians.

I have heard people say: ''My tests are all independent of one another. I don't need a correction for multiple testing.'' Quite the opposite is true! The problem is most severe when the various tests are independent of each other. On the other hand, if test results are correlated, for example, if a positive outcome of one test makes it likely that other tests will also be positive, then the multiple testing problem is less acute because each new test does not really provide an independent opportunity for a type I error. The ''effective'' number of independent tests is then smaller than the actual number of tests carried out, so to speak.

A particular multiple testing problem exists in genomic screening (''genome screens'') for a disease locus. In many linkage investigations, the relation between a putative disease locus and a number, g, of marker loci is analyzed. For this discussion, assume that pairwise (two-point) linkage analyses are performed, test locus versus each of the marker loci.* The test result is then considered significant when at least one of the

---

*For linked markers, multipoint rather than two-point linkage tests may be carried out but this does not materially change the situation as will be discussed later in this section.

comparisons exhibits a maximum lod score $Z_{max} \geq 3$. Clearly, this overall ("genome-wide") type I error must be higher than the ("locus-specific") type I error associated with testing for linkage with a single marker.

It may be of interest to review the ways in which linkage analysts have tackled the multiple testing problem, particularly with respect to mapping complex traits (Ott, 1997a). In the early days of linkage analysis, very few genetic markers existed so that there did not seem a need to consider a multiple testing problem. For mendelian traits, with an increasing number of markers becoming available in the 1980s, it was recognized that eliminating portions of the genome from consideration increases the prior probability of linkage for the remainder of the genome. As demonstrated in previous versions of this book, these two effects (multiple tests, increased prior probability of linkage) approximately cancel each other so that the critical lod score of 3 still appeared valid for genome-wide linkage testing. For complex traits, however, there did not seem to be an a priori justification for assuming presence of detectable disease loci because part of the justification for genomic screening was that a successful linkage analysis would be statistical proof for the existence of disease genes. Thus, without an increased prior probability of linkage, there was no reason for not increasing the critical lod score with multiple marker testing, and critical lod scores much higher than 3 for complex traits were discussed.

Today, human geneticists somewhat disagree on how to handle genome-wide significance levels. One view is that genome screens should be carried out sensibly, that is, only for traits that are highly likely to involve genes. Arguments involving prior and posterior probabilities of linkage then lead to the conclusion that a critical lod score of 3 is still appropriate (Morton, 1998). On the other hand, and this is my favored view, it is of interest to know the probability of a false positive result, that is, a significant result *without there being linkage.* This is the quantity (the type I error) that should be controlled by a corresponding critical lod score. Thus, linkage is never invoked in these arguments and it is immaterial whether genes for mendelian or complex traits are searched for. Clarification of this situation is one of the important contributions of Lander and Botstein (1989) and Lander and Kruglyak (1995) (see next few paragraphs). Of course, as outlined in Section 4.4, some consideration of the low prior probability of linkage is important in linkage analysis: The rate of false-positive results should be much lower than the rate of true positive results.

Independent Tests. Consider first the situation that the various comparisons are independent of each other, for example, that a disease is tested for linkage versus a set of g markers that are unlinked with each other. Then, at least approximately, the g test results are mutually independent. Overall, success will be claimed when at least one of the comparisons, disease versus each marker, shows a significant result. Let α_1 be the probability that any one comparison shows a significant result by chance alone (i.e., in the absence of linkage). Then, the probability that at least one of the g independent tests shows a significant result by chance is

$$\alpha_g = 1 - (1 - \alpha_1)^g. \tag{4.13}$$

For small values of α_1, one has $\alpha_g \approx g\alpha_1$, that is, the overall significance level is approximately equal to g times the significance level in individual tests. If a fixed overall significance level α_g is desired, then the significance level for individual tests must be adjusted downwards:

$$\alpha_1 = 1 - (1 - \alpha_g)^{1/g}, \tag{4.14}$$

which is obtained by solving (4.13) for α_1. Approximately, for small values of α, $\alpha_1 \approx \alpha_g/g$. These adjustments are known as Bonferroni corrections (Elston and Johnston, 1994). For example, assume that $g = 100$ comparisons should be carried out and the overall significance level should be no greater than $\alpha_g = 0.05$. Each individual comparison must then be tested at a much smaller significance level, which is obtained from (4.14) as $\alpha_1 = 0.0005$.

An important application is multiple marker testing in genome screens. The relevant question is: How frequently will a linkage statistic exceed a specified threshold by chance in a human whole genome scan? In other words, for a given locus-specific threshold and associated pointwise p-value, p, what is the genome-wide significance level, p_G, if significance is claimed when the threshold is exceeded at any one of the marker loci investigated? For a sparse map containing m marker loci, results for different markers are essentially independent so that $p_G = 1 - (1 - p)^m \approx mp$. Clearly, for a given pointwise significance level, the genome-wide rate of false positive results increases with the number of markers tested. Conversely, to maintain a fixed genome-wide significance level of $p_G = 0.05$, say, the pointwise significance level must be decreased (made more stringent) with the number of markers tested. Asymptotically, in lod score analysis, a critical lod score limit of Z_c is equivalent to $\chi^2 = 4.6 \times Z_c$ so that the corresponding one-sided significance level may be obtained from the chi-square distribution (e.g., with the aid of the CHIPROB computer program; see Section 9.5). As mentioned above, for an overall type I error of $p_G = 0.05$ and $m = 100$ independent marker tests, the pointwise significance level must be equal to $p = 0.0005$. This value corresponds to $\chi^2 = 10.84$ and $Z_c = 2.35$ (this theoretically predicted value is below 3 but, for reasons of low prior probability of linkage, Z_c should be kept at a minimum level of 3). With an increasing number of markers tested, the critical lod score limit should increase and may eventually exceed 3.

Dependent Tests. With dense maps, tests for linkage to different markers are no longer independent. Based on mathematical theory, Lander and Kruglyak (1995) explored the pointwise critical lod scores required for an overall, genome-wide significance level of 0.05. The results depend somewhat on the number of markers tested and on the analysis technique applied, because different linkage analysis methods lead to different correlations of results for neighboring markers. In the limit for very dense maps (marker spacing ≤ 0.1 cM), the appropriate critical lod score limits (pointwise p-values) are 3.3 (0.000049) for lod score analysis and 3.6 (0.000022) for affected sib pair analysis (Lander and Kruglyak, 1995). Table 4.3 shows such critical lod scores and corresponding p-values for affected sib pair analysis. For example, for a 5-cM map, the pointwise p-value is 0.000088, corresponding to a lod score limit of slightly over 3. Previously, based on computer simulation of an oligogenic threshold trait and a critical lod score of 4, Suarez et al. (1994) calculated a genome-wide (106 unlinked markers) significance level slightly exceeding 0.05. Sawcer et al. (1997) estimated the empirical genome-wide p-value in ASP families analyzed for multiple sclerosis by nonparametric methods. These authors found that a critical lod score threshold of 3.2 corresponded to a genome-wide false-positive rate of 0.05. This limit is not much higher than the limit of 3.0 originally proposed by Morton (1955). For further discussion of this issue, see Morton (1998).

The last column in Table 4.3 shows genome-wide p-values computed under the assumption that test results for different markers are inde-

Table 4.3. Critical Lod Score for a Genome-Wide Significance Level of 0.05 and Given Marker Spacing in Affected Sib Pair Analysis

Marker Spacing	Critical Lod Score	Pointwise Significance Level	Genome-Wide Bonferroni Significance Level
10 cM	2.88	0.000136	0.046
5 cM	3.06	0.000088	0.059
2 cM	3.24	0.000057	0.093
1 cM	3.35	0.000044	0.139
0.1 cM	3.63	0.000022	0.557

Source: Based on Lander and Kruglyak, 1995.

pendent. For low-density maps, there is good agreement between these Bonferroni significance levels and the correct value of 0.05 (Lander and Kruglyak, 1995), but the former keep increasing as maps become denser. The limiting map spacing is approximately 8 cM between adjacent markers; for sparser maps, test results for different markers appear independent of each other (by virtue of the agreement of the Bonferroni-corrected *p*-values with 0.05).

Genome screens are not the only instance for which multiple testing considerations are relevant. At least one other area is worth noting: In linkage analyses of complex traits, because the genetically relevant disease definition is unknown, researchers typically try different diagnostic schemes and carry out an analysis under each diagnostic scheme. Although results from this type of multiple testing do not seem to be independent of each other, as an approximation, a particular form of Bonferroni correction has been proposed as follows (Kidd and Ott, 1984): If m diagnostic schemes are tried and the significance level in each test is α, then the overall significance level is approximately equal to $m\alpha$. Applying (4.10) to this overall significance level then reads $m\alpha \leq 10^{-Z}$ or $\alpha \leq 10^{[-Z+\log(g)]}$, where Z is the critical lod score if only a single diagnostic scheme were used. To preserve the overall significance level corresponding to Z in a single comparison, one would thus have to raise the lod score limit to

$$Z_c = Z + \log_{10}(m). \tag{4.15}$$

For example, with $Z = 3.3$ and 5 diagnostic schemes, the critical lod score should be raised to 4.0.

The various forms of multiple testing may all be taken into account by properly finding the empirical significance level, that is, the probability of finding a chance result as strong or stronger than the one found in the real analysis. Such overall probabilities are best approximated by computer simulation under no linkage (SIMULATE program; see Section 9.7).

4.8. The Likelihood for Family Data

As introduced in Section 4.3, the lod score is a suitably scaled and transformed likelihood, where the likelihood is defined as the probability of the family data when given values for the unknown parameters are assumed (thus far, only one parameter—the recombination fraction—has been considered). In the examples discussed earlier in this chapter, likelihoods are calculated in an ad hoc manner. Here, pedigree likelihoods are discussed more formally. By way of introduction, the likelihood formulation due to Elston and Stewart (1971) is presented first.

Consider a human pedigree of size m and let x_i denote the phenotype of the ith pedigree member, where x_i refers to the phenotype at one or multiple loci. The likelihood, being the probability of the observations, is then $L = P(x_1, x_2, \ldots, x_m)$. In classical statistical analysis, observations generally are mutually independent so that $L = \Pi P(x_i)$. However, pedigree data are nonindependent, so such a simple representation of the likelihood is not possible. In most cases, however, they are conditionally independent, given genotypes: $P(x_1, x_2, \ldots, x_m | g_1, g_2, \ldots, g_m) = \Pi P(x_i|g_i)$. In other words, an individual's phenotype depends only on his or her genotype. The unconditional likelihood may then be written

$$L = P(x) = \Sigma_g\, P(x, g) = \Sigma_g\, P(x \mid g)\, P(g), \tag{4.16}$$

where $x = (x_1, \ldots, x_m)$ is the array of phenotypes, $g = (g_1, \ldots, g_m)$ is an array of genotypes, and the sum is taken over all sets of genotype assignments to family members (for details, see Section 9.2 on the Elston–Stewart algorithm). The total number of these sets can be large. With only 2 alleles at each of the two loci, there are $H = 4$ haplotypes so that potentially each individual has $H(H + 1)/2 = 10$ genotypes (see Section 1.1). With m family members, there are thus 10^m different sets of genotype arrays. For example, all individuals may have genotype A_1/A_1, or individual 1 has genotype A_1/A_2 and the other individuals have genotypes A_1/A_1, and so on. Not all of these genotype arrays must be considered as many of them are incompatible with mendelian laws. In addition, an individual's phenotype may preclude some of his or her genotypes. For example, in each of the pedigrees on the right side of Figures 4.1 and 4.2, the genotypes in all but one individual are known, and in the single individual with an equivocal genotype, there are just two possibilities. Therefore, the total number of genotypes compatible with the mendelian laws and the phenotypes is just two in each of these two families.

The above representation of pedigree likelihoods is due to Elston and Stewart (1971), who also introduced a recursive way of evaluating it so that likelihood calculations in large pedigrees became possible (see Chapter 9). This so-called *Elston–Stewart* algorithm works by mathematically "peeling" one sibship after another from the pedigree, starting at the bottom (youngest generation) and moving upwards through the pedigree (for details, see Section 9.2). Extensions of this algorithm allow for the presence of pedigree loops and permit pedigree traversing (peeling) in various directions (Thompson, 1986). Such a modified Elston–Stewart algorithm has been implemented in the LINKAGE programs and allows for the simultaneous consideration of multiple loci.

For the Elston–Stewart algorithm and its extensions, computational effort increases linearly with the number of pedigree members (founders) but exponentially with the number of marker loci included in the analysis. Thus, potentially very large pedigrees may be analyzed by this algorithm with relatively little effort. For the Lander–Green (1987) algorithm, on the other hand, computational effort increases exponentially with pedigree size but only linearly with the number of loci. These are the two basic algorithms for likelihood calculation currently known. Both have been extended in various ways (e.g., Kruglyak et al., 1995; O'Connell and Weeks 1995; Idury and Elston, 1997).

Kruglyak et al. (1996) introduced several improvements to the Hidden Markov Model that underlies the Lander–Green algorithm. While in the Elston–Stewart algorithm, the unobserved (hidden) quantity is the genotype, Kruglyak et al. (1996) condition phenotypes on underlying inheritance vectors, $v = (p_1, m_1, p_2, m_2, \ldots, p_n, m_n)$, where n is the number of nonfounders in the pedigree, and p_i and m_i refer to paternal and maternal meioses, respectively; $p_i = 0$ or 1 depending on whether the grandpaternal or grandmaternal allele was transmitted (in the paternal meiosis), and analogously for m_i (see Section 6.2 in Ott [1991b]). Briefly, parametric and nonparametric linkage analysis can then be based on a scoring function, $S(v, F)$, with F denoting observed phenotypes; for incomplete data (inheritance vectors incompletely known), the expected value of the scoring function is defined as $E(S) = \Sigma \, S(v, F) \, P(v)$, with summation over all possible inheritance vectors. Depending on the type of analysis (parametric or nonparametric), the scoring function takes different analytical forms. For details, see Kruglyak et al. (1996). This approach has been implemented in the GENEHUNTER program.

Most linkage analyses are carried out under assumptions of mendelian inheritance. Some extensions have been proposed and implemented; for example, likelihood calculation under mixed models (single gene acting on a polygenic background). Based on a particular formulation of the likelihood for polygenic data (Ott, 1979a), Bonney (1992) had introduced so-called regressive models in which a polygenic background is approximated by regression of children's phenotypes on those of their parents. However, none of these approaches are in much use for linkage analysis, except perhaps for the method implemented in the PAP program (Hasstedt, 1982).

4.9. Some Special Methods

For linkage analyses between a locus anywhere on a chromosome and a chromosomal variant located around the centromere, the term centromere or centromeric linkage has been used (Bailey, 1961; Ferguson-Smith et al., 1975). Genetically very different from this is *centromere mapping* by means of ovarian teratomas (Ott et al., 1976). In ovarian teratomas, the proportion of second-division segregants, a quite different quantity from the recombination fraction, is estimated. The use of human ovarian teratomas for this type of centromere-related mapping rests on the assumption that these benign tumors originate parthenogenetically from a single germ cell by suppression of the second meiotic division (Linder, Kaiser McCow, and Hecht, 1975). Newer developments of this mapping approach take into account the varied origin of ovarian teratomas (Chakravarti and Slaugenhaupt, 1987; Deka et al., 1990).

Molecular genetics techniques allow the recognition of alleles of suitable genetic marker loci in *individual sperm cells* of a man (see review by Arnheim, Li, and Cui, 1990). This method has the potential to score dozens or even hundreds of meioses in a single individual, and appropriate statistical analysis methods have been developed (Boehnke et al., 1989; Lazzeroni et al., 1994). Analysis of single sperm may also be achieved using regular linkage programs. One way of doing this would be to define an artificial mate of the man, whose sperm has been investigated, where that mate is taken to be homozygous at each marker locus. Each sperm is then treated as a child of the man and his mate.

4.10. Problems

Problem 4.1. In the analysis of the pedigree shown in Figure 4.1, recombination events were counted based on the children in the last generation only. Shouldn't one include in the analysis the offspring of the grandparents?

Problem 4.2. In the example family with a phase-unknown parent presented in Section 4.3 (right side of Figure 4.2), the estimate of θ obtained assuming the more plausible phase is the same as the maximum likelihood estimate. Convince yourself that this is not generally the case. Consider the same mating as the one shown on the right side of Figure 4.2 but assume different offspring such that, for parental phase I, there are k recombinants out of n opportunities for recombination. For each of the two cases, (1) $k = 1, n = 5$, and (2) $k = 1, n = 4$, derive the estimates of θ (1) by assuming phase I to be known, and (2) by maximizing the lod score for unknown phase.

Problem 4.3. For the example covered at the end of Section 4.5, compute the power for the two test strategies, (1) H_0 versus H_1, and (2) H_0 versus H_2. Evaluate the power for the case $\theta = \theta_m = \theta_f = 0.01$. You need not derive any new formulas; you may simply manipulate the equations given in the text.

Problem 4.4. For $n = 20$ informative meioses in phase-known double backcross families, calculate (1) the empirical significance level (Section 4.6), and (2) its upper bound (equation 4.10) associated with $k = 1, 2, 3, 4$, and 5 observed recombinants. Convince yourself that the significance level stays below its upper bound.

Problem 4.5. Assume that, in a linkage analysis between a disease and a marker, a lod score of -7.16 was observed at $\theta = 0$. How do you interpret this result?

5.

The Informativeness of Family Data

This chapter is of a somewhat technical nature and introduces the concept of informativeness for linkage. It requires some familiarity with calculus and may be skipped by the less mathematically minded reader, with the exception of the last section on number of individuals required for linkage analysis, which is of general interest. This chapter provides detailed instructions, for example, on how to calculate offspring genotype probabilities and measures of informativeness. The reader who wants to carry out serious statistical work should find useful guidance in it. An interpretation of differences between expected lod scores and Fisher's expected information is given at the end of Section 5.6.

The discussion of mating types in this chapter is rather general and explores informativeness of family data based only on mating types and relationships among family members. The more complicated problem of calculating expected lod scores conditional on observed phenotypes at one locus is covered in Section 9.7.

5.1. Measures of Informativeness

The "usefulness" of a genetic marker for linkage analysis is generally measured by its heterozygosity (see Section 2.2). The higher this value, the more informative a family pedigree will be for linkage between a trait and this marker. In this sense, heterozygosity may be viewed as a measure of marker informativeness: It is the probability of being heterozygous expected under Hardy-Weinberg equilibrium. Below, informativeness is discussed in a broader context.

Observed Informativeness. Amount of data collected and pedigree structures generally determine how well one is able to discriminate between different hypotheses (e.g., linkage versus no linkage) or estimate

84

parameters (e.g., the recombination fraction). In statistical genetics, for a given set of observations on family data, two measures of informativeness are in general use: (1) the maximum of the lod score, and (2) Fisher's (1925) statistical *information*.

The maximum lod score was introduced in Section 4.3 and measures the evidence for linkage versus absence of linkage. By definition, it is equal to zero for $\hat{\theta} = \frac{1}{2}$. When recombination events can be counted, k being the number of recombinants in n meioses, the maximum lod score is given by equation (4.11).

Fisher's (estimated) information measures the precision with which the recombination fraction is estimated in a given set of family data. It does so by assessing how fast the log likelihood (or lod score) curve falls off from its peak at $\hat{\theta}$, that is, by determining curvature. The degree of curvature is defined as the negative of the second derivative of the natural log likelihood, evaluated at $\hat{\theta}$:

$$\hat{I}(\hat{\theta}) = -d^2 \ln L(\hat{\theta})/d\hat{\theta}^2, \tag{5.1}$$

where $\hat{I}(\hat{\theta})$ is called the estimated total amount of information. Note that $\hat{\theta}$ must be an *analytical* maximum (the first derivative of the log likelihood must be zero at $\theta = \hat{\theta}$). If an estimate is unbiased, $1/\hat{I}(\hat{\theta})$ is the approximate sample variance of the recombination estimate. For counts of recombination events, the likelihood is proportional to $\theta^k(1 - \theta)^{n-k}$ and evaluation of (5.1) yields $\hat{I}(\hat{\theta}) = n / [\hat{\theta}(1 - \hat{\theta})]$. In statistics, information is a technical term with a specific definition (see Section 5.3). This is why in this book "informativeness" is used for the more general meaning of "information content."

The two measures of informativeness do different things and thus have somewhat different properties. Whereas the maximum lod score refers to the test for linkage, Fisher's information is relevant for the precision of the recombination fraction estimate. Of course, the test for linkage and the precision of the θ estimate are related: the better we can estimate θ, the easier it is to distinguish between linkage and no linkage. In linkage analysis, the testing aspect is generally more relevant than the estimation aspect, and the maximum lod score is generally used as a measure for informativeness as it directly represents the test criterion (the log of the maximized likelihood ratio). In Figure 5.1, the two measures are graphed for counts of recombination events (for convenience, one known recombination event is assumed). Both are highest for $\hat{\theta} = k/n = 0$. The maximum lod score gradually decreases toward $\hat{\theta} = \frac{1}{2}$, at which point it is zero, because that estimate conveys no evidence for linkage. Fisher's estimated information initially decreases much faster than the

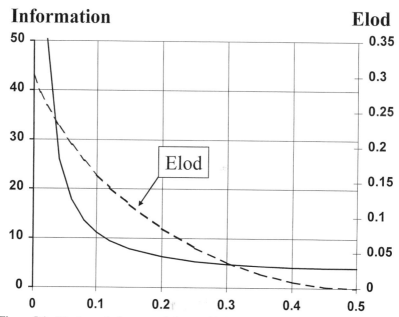

Figure 5.1. Maximum lod score and observed information for an estimated recombination fraction from counts of recombination events (n is set to 1).

maximum lod score (but then levels off faster) and reaches a minimum (>0) at $\hat{\theta} = \frac{1}{2}$. For known recombination events, the lod score curve is not completely flat at $\hat{\theta} = \frac{1}{2}$, which is why the information is positive at $\hat{\theta} = \frac{1}{2}$. Whereas the maximum lod score is zero at $\theta = \frac{1}{2}$ (no informativeness), this is not the case for Fisher's information: There *is* information available for estimation the recombination fraction if it is equal to $\frac{1}{2}$, but this information is much larger for recombination fractions close to zero.

Expected Informativeness. Fisher's information and the lod score may be computed for a set of observed data, as above, or averaged over all possible outcomes for some data or family structures. When averaged, they measure the expected informativeness that a body of data is capable of furnishing, which is discussed in Sections 5.2 and 5.3. These expected measures may be used to assess expected informativeness for detecting linkage or estimation recombination fractions, or to compare informativeness of different bodies of data. As will be outlined below, although the expected lod score is zero at $\theta = \frac{1}{2}$, its limiting value for θ close to $\frac{1}{2}$ may be positive.

A good measure of informativeness is additive over different data sets. Both the expected lod score and Fisher's expected information possess this additivity property. A few nonadditive measures are in current use, which will be discussed in Section 5.2.

5.2. Expected Lod Score and Related Quantities

In comparing different family types or bodies of data, one is interested in the average or expected evidence for linkage that a particular family type is able to provide. One then needs to know all of the possible phenotype constellations for that family type and their probability of occurrence, this probability typically depending on the true value, *r*, of the recombination fraction. The *i*th set of possible phenotypes is associated with the lod score, $Z_i(\theta)$, which is a function of the unknown parameter θ (the recombination fraction). All quantities to be discussed in this section are based on these lod score curves and their probabilities of occurrence. It will be very important to distinguish between the true (but usually unknown) value of the recombination fraction, *r*, and the formal or assumed value, θ, in the estimation of the recombination fraction. A simple example is shown in Figure 5.2: For a family in which three known meioses can be scored, there are four possible outcomes and, thus, four

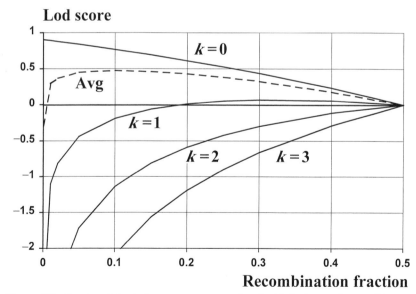

Figure 5.2. Graphs of the lod score curves associated with *k* observed recombinants in *n* = 3 recombination events.

possible lod score curves. The formal parameter, θ, determines the values of the lod score curves while r determines their probabilities of occurrence.

Expected Lod Score. The expected lod score was introduced in a previous edition of this book and has since been proved to be an extremely useful quantity in statistical genetics. For some fixed value of θ, the expectation of the lod score function, also called expected lod score or ELOD, $E[Z(\theta)]$, is the weighted average of the $Z_i(\theta)$'s, with the weights being the probabilities of occurrence of each $Z_i(\theta)$. Usually, only the maximum of the expected lod score curve is called the ELOD. This ELOD is closely related to Shannon's entropy (Shannon and Weaver, 1949) and the Kullback–Leibler information (Kullback and Leibler, 1951; Kullback, 1959). Relations among these quantities were described by Akaike (1985).

For example, when $n = 3$ recombination events can be scored, there are four possible outcomes, $k = 0..3$, where k denotes the number of recombinants. The probability of each outcome is given by the binomial formula, $P(k;r) = \binom{n}{k}r^k(1 - r)^{n-k}$, which depends on the true value r of the recombination fraction. The lod score $Z_k(\theta)$ for the kth outcome is calculated using (3.2). For any given value of θ, the weighted average of the $Z_k(\theta)$ then yields the expected lod score,

$$E[Z(\theta)] = \sum_{k=0}^{n} P(k;r)Z_k(\theta), \tag{5.2}$$

the weights being given by the $P(k;r)$. For $n = 3$, Table 5.1 demonstrates these calculations. The bottom row, in the columns labeled "$Z(\theta)$," shows the resulting expected lod scores. As pointed out in Section 3.3, when the maximum likelihood estimate is consistent, the maximum of the ELOD curve occurs at the value $\theta = r$. In Table 5.1, the maximum of the ELOD curve is equal to 0.480 (at $\theta = r = 0.10$). Graphs of these curves are

Table 5.1. Calculation of Expected Lod Score, $E[Z(\theta)]$, for $n = 3$ Meioses and Expected Z_{max}, under the True Recombination Fraction, $r = 0.1$

		$Z(\theta)$ at $\theta =$				
k	$P(k)$	0.01	0.09	0.10	0.11	Z_{max}
0	0.729	0.890	0.780	0.766	0.751	0.903
1	0.243	−1.106	−0.224	−0.188	−0.157	0.074
2	0.027	−3.101	−1.229	−1.143	−1.065	0
3	0.001	−5.097	−2.234	−2.097	−1.973	0
Average		0.291	0.479	**0.480**	0.479	0.676

Note: k, n, and $P(k)$ are as in Table 3.1, and the average is a weighted mean with $P(k)$ as weights.

shown in Figure 5.2. Each curve depends only on θ and on the phenotypes of the data, not on r. The weighted average of these curves (i.e., the expected lod score function) is also shown. Depending on the true value r of the recombination fraction, the weight attached to each lod score function is different, leading to a different expected lod score. It is only the weighing of the individual lod score functions that depends on r.

For a fixed value of θ, observed lod scores may be added over different families to obtain the total lod score for all families combined (see Section 4.3). Therefore, the expected lod score, $E[Z(\theta)]$, is also additive over families (assuming r fixed). In fact, the ELOD of 0.48 in Table 5.1 could have been obtained simply by just such an addition: Each recombinant occurs with probability r and contributes $\log(2\theta)$ to the lod score, and each nonrecombinant occurs with probability $1 - r$ and contributes $\log(2 - 2\theta)$. At $\theta = r$, the ELOD may be obtained as $E[Z(r)] = n[r\log(2r) + (1 - r)\log(2 - 2r)]$ which, for $n = 3$ and $r = 0.1$, is equal to 0.48, as in Table 5.1. As an application of this additivity property, what number of families of size $n = 3$ meioses are required for the total expected lod score to be at least 3 (assuming $r = 0.10$)? The answer is obtained by calculating $3/0.48 = 6.25$, that is, 7 such families are required.

Maximum of the Expected Lod Score (MELOD). As was pointed out above, consistent estimates of the recombination fraction are characterized by the maximum of the ELOD curve occurring at $\theta = r$. Under some sampling schemes or wrong assumptions on parameter values, the θ estimate may be inconsistent, in which case the maximum of the expected lod score curve is not equal to the ELOD, the value of $E[Z(\theta)]$ at $\theta = r$. The curve's maximum value has been called the MELOD (Terwilliger and Ott, 1994). Later in this book, to determine consistency of an estimate in a particular situation, it will be necessary to calculate analytically at what value of θ the expected lod score has its maximum. This may be done by computing the first derivative, $dE[Z(\theta)]/d\theta$, setting it equal to zero and solving the resulting equation for θ. In these calculations, again, one must be careful to distinguish between θ and r: The derivative is taken only with respect to θ, not r (r is a constant when taking derivatives with respect to θ). For example, when recombinants and nonrecombinants can be counted directly, the expected lod score function per recombination event is given by

$$E[Z(\theta)] = r\log(2\theta) + (1 - r) \log[2(1 - \theta)] = 0.4343[r\ln(2\theta) \\ + (1 - r)\ln(2 - 2\theta)]. \tag{5.3}$$

With this, one calculates $dE/d\theta = 0.4343[2r/(2\theta) - 2(1 - r)/(2 - 2\theta)]$. Setting this equation equal to zero and solving it for θ yields $\theta = r$. After verification that the second derivative at $\theta = r$ is negative, one concludes that $E[Z(r)]$ is a maximum.

Expectation of the Maximum Lod Score (EMLOD). In practice, linkage analysis furnishes the maximum lod score not at $\theta = r$ (as this is unknown) but wherever the maximum occurs in the interval $0 \leq \theta \leq$ ½. Analogously, for each of the possible lod score curves, one may determine its maximum value, $Z_{max}^{(i)}$. The weighted average of these maxima, $E(Z_{max}) = E[max_\theta Z(\theta)] = \Sigma_i P_i Z_{max}^{(i)}$, with P_i being the probability of occurrence of the ith lod score curve, has been called the EMLOD and is often used as a measure of informativeness. For the data in Table 5.1, the maxima of the lod score curves are given in the Z_{max} column. Their weighted average is obtained as 0.676. As Z_{max} is never negative, its distribution is generally expected to be positively skewed. Clearly, ELOD $\leq$ MELOD $\leq$ EMLOD. Because the Z_{max} values are obtained at different θ values, $E(Z_{max})$ is not exactly additive over families (see Problem 5.7).

Power. The three measures discussed so far in this section are averages (expectations) and do not have a direct probabilistic interpretation. However, their densities may be taken to be approximately symmetric so that the median is roughly the same as the mean (this approximation presumably holds best for the ELOD). Thus, the probability that an individual maximum lod score exceeds the ELOD (or MELOD or EMLOD) is approximately equal to 50%. In practice, for a given body of data, one may be interested in the probability, given a true value r of the recombination fraction, that the maximum lod score will exceed some limit, Z_c. This probability (called the power of the linkage test) may again be obtained on the basis of the collection of all possible lod score curves. It is computed by evaluating all possible outcomes of a set of data and their probabilities of occurrence and by determining for each outcome whether the associated Z_{max} (at any θ) reaches or exceeds Z_c. The sum of the probabilities of all those outcomes for which $Z_{max} \geq Z_c$ is the power. For the example data in Table 5.1, $P(Z_{max} \geq 3) = 0$, $P(Z_{max} \geq 0.5) = 0.729$, and $P(Z_{max} \geq 0.05) = 0.972$. This information measure has the advantage that it has a direct intuitive (probabilistic) interpretation that lends itself to prediction of rates of success of linkage analyses. Its disadvantage is that it is not additive over different sets of family data as the maximum of the lod score for each outcome is evaluated at different θ values.

In this section, the ELOD was covered for general types of family data. For pedigrees with a specific observed structure and unknown phenotypes, the ELOD is usually approximated by computer simulation, which is covered in Section 9.7. A special case will be the conditional ELOD given phenotypes already observed at one locus, usually a disease locus. The object is then to determine, before marker typing, what maximum lod score a researcher is likely to find once he or she carries out marker genoyping. For a marker with an assumed number of alleles and genetic distance to the disease locus, the associated maximum lod score will fluctuate around its expected value depending on the possible marker genotypes occurring in each family member and their probabilities of occurrence. If a highly polymorphic marker is assumed, this variability may be small as most parents will be heterozygous for the marker and thus informative for linkage. For a simple mendelian disease, under particularly suitable conditions (full penetrance, no phenocopies, tight linkage between marker and disease loci, no pedigree loops, everybody typed), it is reasonable to consider the *highest* lod score achievable rather than the expected lod score as there will be no variability. In this section, only averages (e.g., of lod scores) were considered and not their variances. Variability of maximum lod scores is discussed in Section 9.7.

5.3. Expected Information and Variance

In Section 5.1, Fisher's estimated total amount of information, $\hat{I}(\hat{\theta})$, was introduced. For example, consider a family with one recombinant and three nonrecombinant offspring. The corresponding log likelihood is given by $\ln[L(\theta)] = \ln\theta + 3\ln(1 - \theta)$ with a maximum at $\hat{\theta} = \frac{1}{4}$. The second derivative is computed as $[\ln(L(\theta))]'' = -1/\theta^2 - 3/(1 - \theta)^2$, so that one obtains $\hat{I}(0.25) = 1/(0.25)^2 + 3/(0.75)^2 = 21.3$. It is customary to use the symbol I for the total information over all observed data, and i for a single observation or a single pedigree (a sampling unit), where the caret identifies *estimated* information.

Whereas the estimated information is evaluated at the MLE of the parameter in question, the *expected information* is computed as a function of the true value r of the recombination fraction. For categorical data falling independently into c different classes (Elandt-Johnson, 1971; Rao, 1973, Section 5g), Fisher's expected information per observation (or per pedigree) is given by

$$i(r) = \sum_{\ell=1}^{c} q_i^2(r)/p_i(r), \tag{5.4}$$

where $q_\ell(r) = dp_\ell(r)/dr$ and $p_\ell(r)$ is the probability of occurrence of the ℓth class. In (5.4), $(dp_\ell/dr)^2/p_\ell$ may be called the contribution of the lth class to the expected information. For example, in counts of recombinant and nonrecombinant offspring, one has $c = 2$ classes, recombinants occurring with probability $p_1 = r$, and nonrecombinants occurring with probability $p_2 = 1 - r$. With $dp_1/dr = 1$ and $dp_2/dr = -1$, equation (5.4) yields

$$i(r) = 1/[r(1 - r)] \tag{5.5}$$

as the expected information per offspring. The total expected information for n such offspring is then equal to $I(r) = n \times i(r)$.

It was mentioned in Section 3.3 that maximum likelihood estimates such as $\hat\theta$ are asymptotically (in large samples) normally distributed and unbiased. Their *asymptotic variance* is equal to the inverse of the expected information. Approximately, then, the standard error of $\hat\theta$ is given by

$$\sigma(\hat\theta) \approx 1/\sqrt{I(r)} = 1/\sqrt{[n\,i(r)]}. \tag{5.6}$$

Equation (5.4) can be extended to the case of several parameters estimated simultaneously (Elandt-Johnson, 1971). Here, only the case of two parameters, r_1 and r_2, is outlined in detail; these parameters are not necessarily recombination fractions. Let $p_\ell = p_\ell(r_1, r_2)$ be the probability of occurrence of the ℓth phenotype class, where this probability is determined by the two parameters. Then, the so-called information matrix is equal to

$$I(r_1, r_2) = ni(r_1, r_2) = n\begin{pmatrix} a & c \\ c & b \end{pmatrix}, \tag{5.7}$$

where $a = \Sigma(\partial p_\ell/\partial r_1)^2/p_\ell$, $b = \Sigma(\partial p_\ell/\partial r_2)^2/p_\ell$, and $c = \Sigma(\partial p_\ell/\partial r_1)(\partial p_\ell/\partial r_2)/p_\ell$, the sums extending from $\ell = 1$ through c. For two parameters estimated simultaneously, the number c of phenotype classes must be equal to three or more. The inverse of $I(r_1, r_2)$ yields the approximate variance–covariance matrix,

$$V(\hat\theta_1, \hat\theta_2) \approx \frac{1}{n(ab - c^2)}\begin{pmatrix} b & -c \\ -c & a \end{pmatrix}, \tag{5.8}$$

where a, b, and c are as in equation (5.7). Then, for example, the approximate variance for the estimate of the first parameter is given by $\sigma^2(\hat\theta_1) = b/[n(ab - c^2)]$. The approximate correlation coefficient between $\hat\theta_1$ and $\hat\theta_2$ (the estimates of r_1 and r_2) is obtained as

$$\rho(\hat\theta_1, \hat\theta_2) \approx -c/\sqrt{(ab)}. \tag{5.9}$$

Approximate *estimated* standard errors and correlation may be calculated when the true parameter values in the equations above are replaced by their estimates. In practice, estimated standard errors are often obtained directly from the curvature of the log likelihood curve or by assuming normality of the estimates; that is, fitting a quadratic curve or surface to the log likelihood at the maximum likelihood estimate(s) (see Chapter 8).

For more than two parameters, the information matrix is easily calculated in analogy to the rules given above but inversion is then no longer straightforward. For given parameter values, a simple approach is to obtain the numerical expression for the information matrix and to invert it with the aid of a computer program. For example, consider the following small program written in SPSS command syntax:

```
matrix.
compute x =
{  0.0490,     -0.0155,    -0.0155;
  -0.0155,      7.8978,     0.6317;
  -0.0155,      0.6317,     7.8978}.
print inv(x).
end matrix.
```

It inverts an information matrix and prints the resulting variance-covariance matrix on screen. For example, the first element of the covariance matrix then represents the variance (here: 20.43) of the first parameter; its standard deviation (standard error) is obtained as the square root of the variance.

5.4. Mating Types

In experimental genetics, matings were given specific names depending on the genotypes of the mates. Consider two parental populations, P_1 and P_2, where individuals in P_1 are all homozygous *AA* at some locus, and individuals in P_2 are homozygous *aa* for another allele at that locus. Crossing $P_1 \times P_2$ leads to a uniform population of all heterozygous *Aa* individuals, the so-called F_1 generation (filial generation no. 1). The mating $F_1 \times F_1$ is called an *intercross,* and their offspring form the F_2 generation (filial generation no. 2). A cross $F_1 \times P_1$ or $F_1 \times P_2$ is called a *backcross* (or *testcross*).

These mating types can be extended to more than one locus. For example, let one of the mates be a double heterozygote, phase known or unknown. If the other mate is doubly homozygous, singly heterozygous, or doubly heterozygous, the mating is called a *double backcross,* a *single backcross,* or a *double intercross,* respectively. In human genetics, these terms are rarely used as they are defined on the basis of only two alleles per locus. Many matings, particularly when highly polymorphic marker loci are used in linkage analyses, involve three or four different alleles per locus. The classical mating type designations then no longer apply.

In subsequent sections, I will calculate how much linkage information per offspring is provided by a mating type. The main purpose is to demonstrate how to carry out such calculations rather than to compile an exhaustive list of mating types. For various classical mating types, their information content has been given by Mather (1936).

The first step in calculating an information measure (ELOD or Fisher's expected information) for a given mating type is to list all possible haplotypes (gametes) each parent can produce. Each pair of haplotypes (one from each parent) will then constitute an offspring genotype. Depending on the polymorphism of the loci involved, some of the offspring genotypes will be indistinguishable and can be collected into a single class. This collapsing of genotypes represents a reduction in genetic variability. Genotype probabilities will generally depend on the true recombination fraction, r, which may be different in male (r_m) and female (r_f) parents. In this chapter, however, r_m and r_f are taken to be equal.

The next step consists of combining into a single class those genotypes leading to the same phenotype, which represents a further reduction of variability. It is these reductions in variability that lead to a loss of information. Different mating types will be seen to lead to a larger or smaller reduction in the number of classes as one proceeds from pairs of haplotypes to genotypes to phenotypes. Offspring phenotype classes and their probabilities of occurrence then determine the amount of information, for example, through equation (5.4). In the subsequent section, this procedure will be demonstrated step by step.

Below, only two loci will be considered at a time. Alleles at one locus will be enumerated alphabetically, A, B, C, and so on, while alleles at the other locus will be numbered from 1 through n.

5.5. Double Intercross with Two Alleles

In this section, according to the general scheme outlined in the previous few paragraphs, detailed instructions are provided for calculating expected information and lod score. Consider a mating *A1/B2* $\times$ *A1/B2* (double intercross) and assume codominant inheritance at each locus. Phase is assumed known so that, for example, allele *A* at the first locus is in coupling with allele *1* at the second locus. To obtain a list of all possible offspring genotypes with their probabilities of occurrence, one must prepare an exhaustive list of the haplotypes (gametes) that each parent can produce, including the probabilities with which they are produced. In this mating, each parent can produce four haplotypes. For example, a haplotype contains the A allele with probability $\frac{1}{2}$. Given that it does, the other allele is a 2 when a recombination takes place, where a recombination occurs with probability r. Therefore, the probability of an $A2$ haplotype occurring is equal to $\frac{1}{2}r$.

In Table 5.2, the haplotypes and their probabilities of formation are given along the borders. To keep this table general, male and female recombination rates are distinguished as r_m and r_f, respectively. In subsequent calculations, however, this distinction will be dropped. Gametes from the two parents combine to form genotypes, each pair of gametes yielding a genotype. The parents are assumed to mate at random with respect to their genotypes. Therefore, offspring genotype probabilities are obtained simply by multiplying the probabilities of the parental haplotypes that make up the offspring genotypes. For example, haplotypes $A1$ from the mother (probability $\frac{1}{2}[1 - r_f]$) and $B1$ from the father (probability $\frac{1}{2}r_m$) combine to form the genotype $A1/B1$. Its probability of occurrence is $\frac{1}{4}r_m(1 - r_f)$. In this mating, both parents produce an identical set of haplotypes; therefore, haplotype $A1$ could come from the father and $B1$ from the mother, which would lead to the same genotype as before. That genotype, $A1/B1$, thus has probability of occurrence $\frac{1}{4}[r_m(1 - r_f) + (1 - r_m)r_f]$, which, for $r = r_m = r_f$, is equal to $\frac{1}{2}r(1 - r)$. Inspection of Table 5.2 reveals that the 16 pairs of parental haplotypes give rise to 10 unique genotypes.

Each genotype gives rise to a phenotype, but some genotypes lead to the same phenotype. The probability of such a phenotype is then simply the sum of the probabilities of its component genotypes. So, based on the list of genotypes, one prepares a list of unique phenotypes because, in linkage analysis, offspring will be distinguishable only through their

Table 5.2. Offspring Genotypes from Mating $A1/B2 \times A1/B2$

Haplotypes from Other Parent		Haplotypes from One Parent			
		$A1$ $\frac{1}{2}(1 - r_m)$	$B2$ $\frac{1}{2}(1 - r_m)$	$A2$ $\frac{1}{2}r_m$	$B1$ $\frac{1}{2}r_m$
$A1$	$\frac{1}{2}(1 - r_f)$	$A1/A1$	$A1/B2$	$A1/A2$	$A1/B1$
$B2$	$\frac{1}{2}(1 - r_f)$	$B2/A1$	$B2/B2$	$B2/A2$	$B2/B1$
$A2$	$\frac{1}{2}r_f$	$A2/A1$	$A2/B2$	$A2/A2$	$A2/B1$
$B1$	$\frac{1}{2}r_f$	$B1/A1$	$B1/B2$	$B1/A2$	$B1/B1$

phenotypes. As can be seen from Table 5.3, the 10 unique genotypes determine nine unique phenotypes.

Many but not all offspring phenotypes reveal unequivocal recombination events in the parents. For example, a BB-11 individual occurs by a recombination in each parent. Also, an AA-12 offspring has received a recombinant haplotype from one parent and a nonrecombinant from the other, but it is unknown which parent passed on which haplotype (if recombination rates were distinguished by the sex of the parents, such uncertainty in the parental origin of the haplotypes would lead to a correlation between the male and female recombination fraction estimates). The most "uncertain" offspring phenotype is AB-12, a double heterozygote with unknown phase, which corresponds to four cells in Table 5.2. It originates either from two recombinant or two nonrecombinant haplotypes.

Probabilities of occurrence of the nine offspring phenotypes are listed in Table 5.3. Each of these nine classes will contribute to the measures of expected informativeness. Classes with equal probability of occurrence lead to the same lod score and contribution to expected information. Thus, they may be combined into one class. This leads to four phenotype classes, each with a different probability of occurrence, as shown in Table 5.4.

Table 5.4 may be used to calculate observed lod scores, expected information, and expected lod scores as follows: If some linkage data consist of the data type considered here (phase-known double intercross matings) and n_ℓ is the number of offspring in the lth class, the total observed lod score for these data is simply equal to $\Sigma n_\ell Z_\ell(\hat{\theta})$.

Table 5.3. Phenotypes of Offspring from Mating $A1/B2 \times A1/B2$, with Associated Probabilities p_i of Occurrence

i	Phenotype	p_i
1	AA-11	$\frac{1}{4}(1 - r)^2$
2	AA-12	$\frac{1}{2}r(1 - r)$
3	AB-12	$\frac{1}{2}[r^2 + (1 - r)^2]$
4	AB-22	$\frac{1}{2}r(1 - r)$
5	AA-22	$\frac{1}{4}r^2$
6	AB-22	$\frac{1}{2}r(1 - r)$
7	BB-11	$\frac{1}{4}r^2$
8	BB-12	$\frac{1}{2}r(1 - r)$
9	BB-22	$\frac{1}{4}(1 - r)^2$
Total		1

Table 5.4. Offspring Phenotypes with Equal Probabilities Combined into One Class Each, Mating $A1/B2 \times A1/B2$ ($q = dp/dr$)

ℓ	i^a	p_ℓ	q_ℓ	$Z_\ell(\theta)$
1	$1 + 9$	$\frac{1}{2}(1 - r)^2$	$r - 1$	$\log[4(1 - \theta)^2]$
2	$2 + 4 + 6 + 8$	$2r(1 - r)$	$2(1 - 2r)$	$\log[4\theta(1 - \theta)]$
3	$5 + 7$	$\frac{1}{2}r^2$	r	$\log(4\theta^2)$
4	3	$\frac{1}{2}[r^2 + (1 - r)^2]$	$2r - 1$	$\log[2\theta^2 + 2(1 - \theta)^2]$
Total		1	0	

^{a} Refers to the index i used in Table 5.3.

Fisher's expected information per offspring is obtained from Table 5.4 using (5.4). One finds

$$i(r) = \frac{2}{r(1 - r)} - \frac{4r(1 - r)}{r^2 + (1 - r)^2} - 2. \tag{5.10}$$

The general shape of the graph of $i(r)$ looks very much like the estimated information curve in Figure 5.1 : It is positive at $r = \frac{1}{2}$ and tends to infinity as r approaches 0. For small values of r, (5.10) is approximately equal to $2/r$, that is, twice as large as the corresponding value for the phase-known double backcross mating (see Section 5.7), the reason being that in this mating type both parents are informative for linkage and the "equivocal" offspring type ($\ell = 4$ in Table 5.4) becomes "unequivocal" for $r = 0$.

Expected lod scores are calculated from Table 5.4 in analogy to equation (5.2) as

$$E_r[Z(\theta)] = \Sigma p_\ell(r) \, Z_\ell(0). \tag{5.11}$$

The result is a function of the formal parameter θ, while the shape of the function depends on the true value r of the recombination fraction. As outlined at the end of Section 3.3, the maximum of the expected lod score, the ELOD, must occur at $\theta = r$. Substituting r for θ in equation (5.11), one obtains the ELOD per offspring in the data type considered here as

$$E[Z(r)] = (1 - r^2)\log[2(1 - r)] + r(2 - r)\log(2r) \\ + \frac{1}{2}[r^2 + (1 - r)^2]\log[2r^2 + 2(1 - r)^2]. \tag{5.12}$$

For any given true value r of the recombination fraction, the ELOD (5.12) provides a measure for the average linkage information per offspring in phase-known double intercross matings. It is zero at $r = \frac{1}{2}$ and rises to its maximum of 0.45 at $r = 0$. To obtain, for example, an expected lod score of 3 or more, assuming tight linkage, one needs to investigate seven ($3/0.45 = 6.67$) offspring from matings $A1/B2 \times A1/B2$. With tight linkage, in contrast to the situation with the expected information, the ELOD for this family type is only 50% higher than that for the phase-known double backcross mating (see Section 5.7). Thus, for the same amount of "linkage information content," one requires 50% more offspring of phase-known double backcross matings than of double intercross matings.

5.6. Double Intercross with More Than Two Alleles

The phase-known double intercross of the previous section was used as a model mating to introduce the calculation of expected information and ELOD. That mating is also relatively common in gene mapping, particularly in the CEPH reference families (Dausset et al., 1990), where parental phase is often known owing to grandparental genotypes. However, parents may share more than two alleles at a marker. Thus, in this section, the two-allele mating type is extended to a type involving more polymorphic markers and, consequently, an increase in expected information and ELOD.

Consider two very polymorphic genetic markers such that, with high probability, four different alleles segregate in a family at each marker locus. Specifically, consider the phase-known mating *A1/B2 × C3/D4*. Going through the same steps as in the previous section shows that all of the 16 offspring genotypes are distinct. Because parental origin of each allele is unequivocally known, all of the phases in the offspring are known (each offspring is a double heterozygote). Inspection of the 16 phenotypes (genotypes in this case) reveals that only three different phenotype probabilities occur, $\frac{1}{4}(1 - r)^2$, $\frac{1}{4}r(1 - r)$, and $\frac{1}{4}r^2$. Combining phenotypes with equal probabilities into one class each leads to three class probabilities of $(1 - r)^2$, $2r(1 - r)$, and r^2. These are binomial probabilities corresponding to counts of $k = 0, 1$, or 2 recombinants in $n = 2$ recombination events as each offspring may be scored for one recombination event in each parent.

Offspring from the mating *A1/B2 × C3/D4* are maximally informative in that each exhibits two known recombination events. According to equation (5.5), Fisher's expected information for two recombination counts is equal to $2/[r(1 - r)]$, and the corresponding ELOD is obtained from equation (5.3) as $2r\log(2r) + 2(1 - r)\log[2(1 - r)]$. The expected information (5.10) and the ELOD (5.12) obtained above for the mating *A1/B2 × A1/B2* are smaller than those obtained here, the differences being entirely due to an increase in the degree of marker polymorphism. The ratio of the ELOD for the 4-allele case over that for the 2-allele case is shown in Figure 5.3 (upper curve). Also shown is the analogous ratio of the expected information (lower curve). For example, at a recombination fraction of $r = 0$ between the two loci, the ELOD equals $E[Z(0)] = 0.601$ in the 4-allele case and 0.451 in the 2-allele case, leading to a ratio of 1.33. On the other hand, the expected information tends to infinity in both cases as $r \to 0$, but in the limit the corresponding ratio is 1.

The ELOD measures informativeness for detecting linkage, whereas the expected information is a measure for the precision of the recombination fraction estimate, the latter being important in gene mapping given that linkage is established. Thus, for linkage detection, under tight linkage, families with highly polymorphic markers are more powerful than those segregating less polymorphic markers: For the mating types considered here, 100 offspring in the 4-allele case yield an ELOD as high as do $100 \times 0.601/0.451 = 133$ offspring in the 2-allele case. On the other hand, under tight linkage, the precision of the recombination fraction estimate (expected information) is essentially the same for four or two alleles. With looser linkage, as r approaches ½, offspring in the 4-allele case tend to be twice as informative as those in the 2-allele case, both for linkage detection and for estimation of the recombination fraction; then, only half as many offspring of 4-allele matings as of 2-allele matings are needed on average. At $r = $ ½, the ratio of ELODs is undefined 0/0, but the limiting value for $r \to$ ½ is as shown in Figure 5.3.

A particular type of phase-unknown mating of two doubly heterozygous individuals is represented by parents of children affected with a recessive disease, when linkage to a highly polymorphic marker is

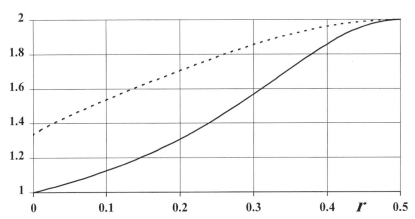

Figure 5.3. Ratios of ELOD (dashed line) and expected information (solid line) for mating *A1/B2* × *C3/D4* over those for mating *A1/B2* × *A1/B2*.

investigated. Calculations of the ELOD, conditional on number of affected and unaffected offspring, will be presented at the end of Section 11.3.

5.7. Phase-Known Double Backcross

The phase-known double backcross mating, $A1/B2 \times A1/A1$, has already been referred to at various places in this book. It allows a direct estimate of the recombination fraction, $\hat{\theta} = k/n$, where k is the number of recombinants among the n offspring. Fisher's expected information is given in equation (5.5). The ELOD per offspring is obtained from equation (5.3) as $E[Z(r)] = r\log(2r) + (1 - r)\log[2(1 - r)]$. At $r = 0$, because $0^0 = 1$ and $\log(1) = 0$, one finds $E[Z(0)] = \log(2) = 0.30$. The phase-known double backcross often serves as a standard against which informativeness of other mating types is compared, for each offspring is equivalent to one recombination event.

For this mating, as well as for all other matings with known parental genotypes (including known phase), n families with 1 offspring each provide the same information as, for example, $n/2$ families with 2 offspring each or as 1 family with n offspring. This simple relationship no longer holds when parental genotypes are not unambiguously known, as will be seen in subsequent sections.

5.8. Phase-Unknown Double Backcross with Two Offspring

As was pointed out in Section 4.1, one needs at least three generations of individuals to be able to unequivocally count recombinants and nonrecombinants. Two-generation families also yield information on linkage but not in a direct way (see y statistics, Section 4.1). A typical such family is the phase-unknown double backcross—a mating between a double heterozygote and a double homozygote. Specifically, assume that the possible genotypes of the double heterozygote are $A1/B2$ (I) and $A2/B1$ (II), where I and II identify the two phases. The other parent is taken to have genotype $A1/A1$.

For a single offspring, the probability of an observed phenotype (the likelihood) is calculated as demonstrated below. Consider, for example, an offspring with phenotype $x = A1/A1$. One can easily calculate the probability of occurrence of x once the phase is known. Therefore, one must condition on the phases and compute offspring probabilities as $P(x) = P(x|\text{I})P(\text{I}) + P(x|\text{II})P(\text{II})$, which, in this case, yields $\frac{1}{2}(1 - r) \times \frac{1}{2} + \frac{1}{2}r \times \frac{1}{2} = \frac{1}{4}$, where r is the true recombination fraction and, according to population genetics, the phases occur with probabilities of ½ each (assuming linkage equilibrium; see Section 11.4). Because $P(x)$ does not depend on r for this offspring type, the lod score associated with such an observation is zero. Carrying out these calculations for each possible offspring genotype shows that none of them is informative for linkage. Consequently, the phase-unknown double backcross with a single offspring is not useful for linkage analysis. It was previously mentioned that a parent must be doubly heterozygous to be potentially informative for linkage. This condition is thus seen to be necessary but not sufficient.

Consider now two offspring from the mating type assumed above, for example, both offspring with phenotypes $x_1 = x_2 = A1/A1$. The likelihood for these two observations is given by $P(x_1, x_2) = P(x_1, x_2|I)P(I) + P(x_1, x_2|II)P(II)$. For given phase, the two observations are conditionally independent so that one obtains $P(x_1, x_2) = \frac{1}{4}(1 - r)^2 \times \frac{1}{2} + \frac{1}{4}r^2 \times \frac{1}{2} = [(1 - r)^2 + r^2]/8$, which is denoted here by f_1. Similarly, for $x_1 = A1/A1$ and $x_2 = A2/A1$, one obtains $P(x_1, x_2) = \frac{1}{4}r(1 - r) = f_2$. When these calculations are carried through for all possible pairs of offspring genotypes, it turns out that each has either probability f_1 or f_2, which is shown in Table 5.5. As outlined in Section 5.5, one may collapse equal genotype probabilities into a single class so that one is left with a table of two rows and two columns (Table 5.6). The first row and column each correspond to an offspring who is a nonrecombinant given phase I—call this a type 1 phenotype. The second row and column correspond to a recombinant given phase I—call this a type 2 phenotype. The result is shown in Table 5.6. For example, the table entry in the first row and first column is simply the sum of the corresponding uncollapsed four terms, $4f_1 = \frac{1}{2}[(1 - r)^2 + r^2]$. The margins reflect the result obtained in the previous paragraph, namely, that a single offspring is uninformative for linkage.

Table 5.6 demonstrates the important general fact that offspring genotypes are not mutually independent when parental genotypes are equivocal.

Table 5.5. Joint Genotype Probabilities of Two Offspring from a Mating [A1/B2 or A2/B1] × A1/A1, $f_1 = [(1 - r)^2 + r^2]/8$, $f_2 = r(1 - r)/4$

	Child 2			
Child 1	A1/A1	B2/A1	A2/A1	B1/A1
A1/A1	f_1	f_1	f_2	f_2
B2/A1	f_1	f_1	f_2	f_2
A2/A1	f_2	f_2	f_1	f_1
B1/A1	f_2	f_2	f_1	f_1

Table 5.6. Joint Offspring Genotype Probabilities from a Phase-Unknown Double Backcross Mating (Table 5.5 Collapsed)

	Child 2		
Child 1	Type 1	Type 2	Total
Type 1	$[(1 - r)^2 + r^2]/2$	$r(1 - r)$	½
Type 2	$r(1 - r)$	$[(1 - r)^2 + r^2]/2$	½
Total	½	½	1

In this case, nonindependence is demonstrated, for example, by $P(x_1 =$ type 1, $x_2 =$ type 2) $\neq P(x_1 =$ type 1) $P(x_2 =$ type 2), or $\frac{1}{2}[(1 - r)^2 + r^2] \neq \frac{1}{2} \times \frac{1}{2}$, where x_1 and x_2 are phenotypes of child 1 and child 2, respectively. The correlation coefficient for Table 5.6 is calculated as $\rho = (1 - 2r)^2$. The quantity $1 - 2r$ is known as the *linkage parameter*. Correlation between the offspring genotypes is zero only when there is absence of linkage, $r = \frac{1}{2}$; otherwise, it is positive. This is, of course, the basis for the sib pair method referred to in Section 4.7 and Chapter 13.

The list of joint genotypes of offspring pairs in Table 5.6 shows that only two probabilities occur (binomial situation) so that, again, genotypes with equal probabilities may be combined into a single class. Phase-unknown double backcross families thus occur in two classes with class probabilities of $p = 2r(1 - r)$ and $1 - p = r^2 + (1 - r)^2$. Class 1 with frequency p corresponds to offspring of unequal type (one offspring is type 1, the other is type 2), whereas class 2 with frequency $1 - p$ corresponds to offspring with equal type (both offspring are type 1 or both are type 2), these class frequencies being independent of the population allele frequencies as long as the two loci are in linkage equilibrium (see Section 11.4). If they are not, the two phases in the informative parent are not equally frequent and their frequency depends on the allele frequencies.

Knowing the offspring phenotype (genotype) distribution allows calculation of expected information and ELOD per unit of observation, which is, in this case, a pair of offspring. The relevant quantities are shown in Table 5.7 and lead to an expected information of

$$i(r) = \frac{2}{r(1 - r)} \frac{(1 - 2r)^2}{[1 - 2r(1 - r)]}. \tag{5.13}$$

In the limit of no recombination, two offspring from the phase-unknown double backcross carry the same amount of information as two offspring from a phase-known double backcross. Thus, at $r = 0$, not knowing the

Table 5.7. Phenotype Classes of Pairs of Offspring from a Phase-Unknown Double Backcross Mating

Phenotype	ℓ	p_ℓ	q_ℓ	$z_\ell(\theta)$
Type unequal	1	$2r(1-r)$	$2(1-2r)$	$\log[4\theta\,(1-\theta)]$
Type equal	2	$r^2 + (1-r)^2$	$-2(1-2r)$	$\log[2\theta^2 + 2(1-\theta)^2]$
Total		1	0	

phase does not lead to a loss of precision of the θ estimate. It does so, however, as r increases. At $r = \frac{1}{2}$, in contrast to the phase-known double backcross, there is even no information left for estimating r; that is, the expected lod score curve is completely flat at $r = \frac{1}{2}$. The ELOD is calculated as $\sum_\ell p_\ell(r) Z_\ell(\theta)$, which, when evaluated at $\theta = r$, leads to

$$E[Z(r)] = 2r(1-r)\log[4r(1-r)]$$
$$+[r^2 + (1-r)^2]\log[2r^2 + 2(1-r)^2]. \quad (5.14)$$

For $r = 0$, note that $0^0 = 1$ so that the first term is equal to zero. One then obtains $E[Z(0)] = \log(2) = 0.30$, which is only half as much as the ELOD for *two* offspring from a phase-known double backcross. This result has been interpreted to mean that, for detecting linkage, one loses one offspring because of not knowing the phase. But one generally loses even more than that. Consider the ratio R of the ELOD for two offspring from a phase-known mating over the ELOD for two offspring from a phase-unknown mating. At $r = 0$ we have $R = 2$ but, with increasing recombination fraction, R increases until it becomes infinite in the limit as $r \to \frac{1}{2}$. For example, at $r = 0.1, 0.2,$ and 0.3, one obtains $R = 3.32,$ $5.82,$ and 12.80, respectively.

Although the recombination fraction is generally estimated by maximizing the lod score, for a number n of phase-unknown double backcross families with two offspring each, a direct estimation is possible. Let k denote the number of class 1 families (offspring are of unequal type), where each such family occurs with probability $p = 2r(1-r)$. Because the maximum likelihood estimate of p is equal to k/n, solving for r leads to the following estimate of the recombination fraction:

$$\hat{\theta} = \begin{cases} \frac{1}{2}[1 - \sqrt{1 - 2k/n}] & \text{if } k < \frac{1}{2}n \\ \frac{1}{2} & \text{if } k \geq \frac{1}{2}n. \end{cases} \quad (5.15)$$

From (5.13), the approximate standard error of $\hat{\theta}$ is obtained as $1/[n \times i(r)]$ when r is known, and an estimated approximate standard error is obtained by substituting $\hat{\theta}$ for r.

5.9. Phase-Unknown Double Backcross with More Than Two Offspring

If parental genotypes are equivocal (e.g., phase-unknown), then offspring genotypes are statistically dependent (see previous section) so that the number of offspring per family is relevant in likelihood calculations. Let m denote the number of offspring of a phase-unknown double backcross mating and n the number of such families. Offspring phenotypes are of two kinds: Type 1 is a nonrecombinant under one of the parental phases (phase I, say) but a recombinant under the other, and for type 2 the situation is reversed. Given phase I, a type 1 offspring occurs with probability r and a type 2 offspring with probability $1 - r$, with r being the true recombination fraction. The conditional probability that i type 1 individuals out of m offspring are observed is thus $P(i|I) = \binom{m}{i}r^i(1 - r)^{m-i}$ for phase I and $P(i|II) = \binom{m}{i}(1 - r)^i r^{m-i}$ for phase II. The unconditional probability of i type 1 individuals is then $P(i) = \frac{1}{2}[P(i|I) + P(i|II)]$, $i = 0 \ldots m$. Now, for any i, $P(i)$ is equal to $P(m - i)$ so that two such probabilities each can be combined into one class (for $i = m - i$, only a single probability exists). Thus, the resulting class probabilities are $P(i) + P(m - i) = \binom{m}{i}[r^i(1 - r)^{m-i} + r^{m-i}(1 - r)^i]$ for $i \neq m - i$, while $P(i) - \binom{m}{i}r^i (1 - r)^{m-i}$ for $i = m - i$. The number of distinct classes for a phase-unknown double backcross family is given by

$$c = \begin{cases} \frac{1}{2}(m + 1) & \text{if } m \text{ is odd} \\ 1 + \frac{1}{2}m & \text{if } m \text{ is even.} \end{cases} \tag{5.16}$$

Each family falls into one of these c classes. When $c > 2$, the probability distribution of m such families is multinomial.

The simplest case, $m = 2$, is binomial and was covered in the previous section. The case of $m = 3$ offspring each (see Section 4.5) again leads to $c = 2$ classes: A family of class 1 consists of three offspring who are either all recombinants or all nonrecombinants, with the corresponding probability of occurrence being $p = 3r(1 - r)$. The other family class occurs with probability $1 - p = r^3 + (1 - r)^3$. From this, the expected information per family is derived as

$$i(r) = \frac{3}{r(1 - r)} \frac{(1 - 2r)^2}{[1 - 3r(1 - r)]}. \tag{5.17}$$

Lod scores corresponding to the two family classes are $Z_1(\theta) = \log[4\theta(1 - \theta)]$ and $Z_2(\theta) = \log[4\theta^3 + 4(1 - \theta)^3]$, from which the ELOD may be obtained.

For $m > 3$, formal derivation of expected information and ELOD becomes cumbersome. For a phase-unknown family with m offspring, the ELOD at $r = 0$ turns out to be equal to $(m - 1)\log(2)$, which is the same as the ELOD for a phase-known family with $m - 1$ offspring. Therefore, as noted in the previous section, one tends with tight linkage to "lose" one offspring for not knowing the phase, but the loss is relatively larger at larger values of the recombination fraction. At $r = 0$, this "loss" of one offspring may be explained heuristically as follows: In the absence of recombination, the phenotype of the first offspring reveals parental phase so that effectively phase is known for subsequent offspring. If recombination occurs ($r > 0$), phase is not completely revealed so that, even after knowing the first offspring, information from the other offspring is not as good as in a phase-known situation.

The observed lod score for a phase-unknown double backcross family with k type 1 individuals among m offspring is given by

$$Z(\theta) = (m - 1)\log(2) + \log[\theta^k(1 - \theta)^{m-k} + (1 - \theta)^k\theta^{m-k}]. \qquad (5.18)$$

Figure 5.4 shows a comparison of observed lod scores with the same values of $k = 1$ and $m = 7$ for a phase-known (equation 3.2) and a phase-unknown family (equation 5.18). The graphs are given for the whole range of values, $0 \leq \theta \leq 1$. Apart from the higher lod score for the phase-known family, a major difference between the two curves is that, in the phase-known case, the lod score has only one peak whereas in the phase-unknown case, it has two. The estimates are practically the same, $\hat{\theta} = 0.14$. In linkage analysis, lod scores are generally calculated only for the range $0 \leq \theta \leq \frac{1}{2}$. However, when a large pedigree with many

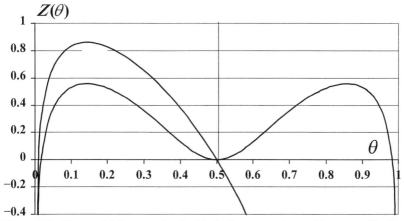

Figure 5.4. Observed lod scores for double backcross matings with seven offspring each (phase known: One recombinant; phase unknown: One type 1 individual).

different matings is analyzed or when several families are combined, inspecting the combined lod score at θ values higher than $\frac{1}{2}$ shows whether the data contain a sizeable proportion of phase-unknown matings. When the maximum at $\theta > \frac{1}{2}$ is close to the maximum at $\theta < \frac{1}{2}$, little phase-known information is present. In addition, when the maximum of the lod score is much higher for $\theta > \frac{1}{2}$ than for $\theta < \frac{1}{2}$, this warrants scrutiny for possible errors in the data; it is for this reason that the ILINK computer program of the LINKAGE package (see Section 8.3) computes estimates of $\theta > \frac{1}{2}$.

In equation (5.18), the two terms in the logarithm correspond to the two parental phases, whose unconditional (population) probabilities were assumed to be equal to $\frac{1}{2}$ each. Because of unknown phase, it was said above that counting recombinants and nonrecombinants among the offspring was not possible. In many cases, however, the conditional proba-bility of phase I, say, given the observations, is so close to 0 or 1 that phase may essentially be assumed to be known. Applying Bayes theorem, this conditional probability is calculated as $P(\text{phase I}|F) = P(F|\text{phase I}) P(\text{phase I}) / P(F)$, where F stands for the observations, $P(F)$ is the pedigree likelihood, and $P(\text{phase I}) = \frac{1}{2}$. Thus, one obtains

$$
\begin{aligned}
P(\text{phase I}|F) &= \frac{\theta^k(1 - \theta)^{m-k}}{\theta^k(1-\theta)^{m-k} + \theta^{m-k}(1 - \theta)^k} \\
&= \frac{1}{1 + [\theta|(1 - \theta)]^{m-2k}}.
\end{aligned}
\tag{5.19}
$$

Clearly, with small θ or k, it takes only a small number of offspring for the phase to have probability close to 1.

5.10. Conditional ELODs: Maximum or Average Lod Score?

Thus far, the ELOD and other measures of informativeness were considered conditional only on pedigree structure but not on any observed phenotype. In this section, the important case of conditional ELODs, given phenotypes at one locus, is briefly discussed. In practice, the most relevant situation is that phenotypes at a disease locus are known, whereas marker phenotypes have not yet been observed and it is desired to predict lod scores before marker typing, assuming that a marker with certain properties (linked with disease locus, polymorphic) will be found. Calcula-tions for this situation are much more involved and results are usually approximated by computer simulation. This section demonstrates a numer-ical approach that is applicable to small pedigrees. A simple solution, practiced by many researchers, is to find the maximum lod score possible for given observed disease phenotypes. It will be shown below that this technique is generally unsatisfactory.

Consider the small pedigree shown in Figure 5.5. Of the two parents, the mother is affected with an autosomal dominant disease, and so is one of the four children; the remaining three children are unaffected. What (maximum) lod score can we expect from this family? The reasoning generally invoked is as follows: "In a genome screen, it will always be possible to find a highly polymorphic marker closely linked with the disease. Therefore, we should take as our measure of informativeness the maximum lod score or, equivalently, that lod score (at $\theta = 0$) obtained under the assumption of no recombinants. In this family, for example, the genotype of child II-3 will reveal the phase in the mother so that the remaining three children will furnish three nonrecombinations, each providing a lod score contribution of $2 \times \log(2)$. Thus, the maximum lod score is equal to 0.903." Indeed, with tight linkage ($\theta = 0$), full penetrance for genetic cases, no occurrence of phenocopies, disease allele frequency essentially zero, marker 100% polymorphic, and everybody available for genotyping, this is the only lod score possible. The problem is, however, that this line of reasoning is also applied to situations of incomplete penetrance even though, in that case, multiple lod scores can be obtained yet only the maximum is taken into account. Below, an example is outlined that demonstrates the fallacy of this procedure: It is shown that even with no recombinations and complete marker heterozygosity, various maximum lod scores are possible that may be quite different from the overall maximum lod score.

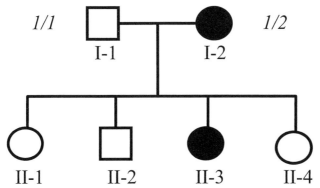

Figure 5.5. Artificial small family with a dominant disease to show maximum possible lod score.

For given or assumed marker characteristics, disease phenotypes, and true value, r, of the recombination fraction, calculating conditional lod scores is complicated because of the many possibilities that one must keep track of. This is discussed in more detail in Section 9.7; see also the description in Boehnke (1986). For small pedigrees, when it is feasible to enumerate all possible marker genotypes, a *numerical approach* is suitable and furnishes exact results. For example, for the small family with observed disease phenotypes in Figure 5.5, assume known marker genotypes for the parents so that the affected parent is always heterozygous, *2/3*, that is, informative for linkage; the unaffected parent is not informative as the disease is dominant and rare, so he may as well have known marker genotype, *1/1*. Further assume absence of phenocopies but incomplete penetrance of 0.90 for genetic cases, and complete linkage, $r = 0$. Each of the four offspring potentially has one of two marker genotypes, *1/2* or *1/3*. Thus, there is a total of $2^4 = 16$ possible marker genotype configurations, which are listed in Table 5.8. Each of these configurations furnishes a maximum lod score. Consider using a linkage program to determine these lod scores. For example, each of the 16 configurations may be represented as a family for which lod scores are calculated by the MLINK program for assumed values of $\theta = 0$, 0.01, 0.02, and so on. Table 5.8 shows the resulting maximum lod scores, Z_{max},

Table 5.8. List of 16 Possible Offspring Genotypes for Pedigree in Figure 5.5, Associated Maximum Lod Scores and Probabilities of Occurrence for Penetrance of 90%

| Case | Genotype of | | | | Z_{max} | $\hat{\theta}$ | $L(\theta = 0) \times 10^9$ |
	II-1	II-2	II-3	II-4			
1	½	½	½	½	0	.50	.016
2	½	⅓	½	½	0	.50	.162
3	⅓	½	½	½	0	.50	.162
4	⅓	⅓	½	½	.004	.33	1.620
5	½	⅓	⅓	½	.799	0	16.195
6	½	⅓	⅓	½	.004	.33	1.620
7	⅓	½	⅓	½	.004	.33	1.620
8	⅓	⅓	⅓	½	0	.50	.162
9	½	½	½	⅓	0	.50	.162
10	½	⅓	½	⅓	.004	.33	1.620
11	⅓	½	½	⅓	.004	.33	1.620
12	⅓	⅓	½	⅓	.779	0	16.195
13	½	⅓	⅓	⅓	.004	.33	1.620
14	½	⅓	⅓	⅓	0	.50	.162
15	⅓	½	⅓	⅓	0	.50	.162
16	⅓	⅓	⅓	⅓	0	.50	.016

and estimates of the recombination fraction, $\hat{\theta}$, at which $Z_{\max}$ occurs. Now, we must figure out the conditional probability of occurrence of each of the 16 marker genotype configurations. Because the pedigree likelihood is proportional to the probability of observing the data, all we need to do is to look up likelihood values furnished by the MLINK program, and this should be done for calculations done under $\theta = 0$ because we assumed a true recombination fraction of zero. The program furnishes log likelihoods; Table 5.9 shows the corresponding likelihoods obtained by taking antilogs of the log likelihoods. To compute proper probabilities, we proceed as follows.

Only three values of $Z_{\max}$ occur among the 16 possible genotype configurations. They are listed in Table 5.9. For each value of $Z_{\max}$, the sum of the corresponding likelihoods is also shown. These sums are converted to probabilities by dividing them by their sum, 43.114. Thus, $Z_{\max}$ values of 0, 0.004, and 0.779 occur with respective conditional probabilities of 0.02, 0.23, and 0.75. As mentioned above, many researchers tend to argue that eventually a fully polymorphic marker that is tightly linked with the disease locus will be found, which is certainly plausible. However, our example shows that this does not guarantee that the maximum possible lod score will be observed. In the case considered here, the marker is fully informative and linkage is complete, yet incomplete penetrance allows for the occurrence of several lod scores. The maximum possible lod score of 0.779 occurs only with probability 75%. That is, even under these ideal conditions, there is a probability of 25% that marker genotypes will be such that the maximum lod score observed is lower than the maximum possible lod score. It is easy to see how this may occur. For example, offspring II-3 may have genotype *1/2*. As there are no phenocopies and no recombinations, the *2* allele in the mother must be in coupling with the disease allele. If one or more of the unaffected offspring also received a *2* allele and, thus, a disease allele, they must be nonpenetrant disease gene carriers, in which case absence of linkage may be more plausible than linkage.

Table 5.9. Maximum Lod Scores and Their Probabilities of Occurrence with Penetrance of 90% for Pedigree in Figure 5.5

$Z_{\max}$	$\Sigma L(\theta = 0)$	Probability
0	1.004	0.02
0.004	9.720	0.23
0.779	32.390	0.75
Sum	43.114	1

Rather than considering the maximum possible lod score, it is more meaningful, for example, to look at the probability that the maximum lod score exceed 3, or the average maximum lod score (called EMLOD). For our contrived example with three possible outcomes of Z_{max}, the EMLOD is given by $0 \times 0.02 + 0.004 \times 0.23 + 0.779 \times 0.75 = 0.585$, which is quite a bit smaller than 0.779.

The case shown here is simple yet realistic. More realistic situations, with a larger number of possible maximum lod scores, occur in collections of pedigrees. For example, for two pedigrees such as the one shown in Figure 9.3, the maximum possible lod score is approximately 3.12 yet the average is only 1.03 (see Section 9.7). Often, after marker genotypes have been obtained, researchers compare their observed maximum lod score with the maximum possible lod score in their families (the latter is approximately furnished by computer simulation; see Section 9.7). I have heard researchers say, "for our families, the maximum possible lod score is 3.7 and we are approaching this value." For the example data in Figure 5.5, researchers should expect to find the maximum possible lod score only in 75% of all cases. If researchers consistently find the maximum possible lod score and never any values much lower than the maximum, this is unexpected statistically and may be due to a selection bias.

5.11. Number of Observations Required to Detect Linkage

In planning a linkage analysis, an important question is how many individuals or families one reasonably needs to establish linkage or to localize a disease locus on a map of markers. The answer will depend on various factors influencing informativeness such as penetrance, heterogeneity, and so forth, and is discussed in Section 12.2. A more specific approach is to numerically determine the conditional expected lod score for a given set of families with given phenotypes. It is usually carried out by computer simulation and is discussed in Section 9.7. In this section, the focus is on the number of offspring required for linkage and its dependency on mating types.

As a starting point, consider known recombination events (offspring of phase-known double backcross matings). One may now ask what number, n, of these are required such that with high probability, ϕ (power), one will find a significant linkage ($Z_{max} \geq Z_0$) when the true recombination fraction is equal to r. The result may be obtained from the following approximate formula (Elandt-Johnson, 1971, equation 13.69 modified):

$$n \approx [1.073\sqrt{Z_c} + x_\phi \sqrt{r(1 - r)}]^2/(r - \frac{1}{2})^2, \tag{5.20}$$

where x_ϕ is the normal deviate associated with an upper tail probability ϕ; for example, $x_\phi = 0.84$ for a power of 80% and $x_\phi = 1.28$ for a power of 90%. Table 5.10 presents some numbers calculated using equation (5.20). To detect a recombination fraction of 5% or smaller using the customary criterion, $Z_c = 3$, roughly 20 recombination events are required.

Depending on the informativeness associated with different mating types, a large number of families with small informativeness will be required for the same total information content as is furnished by a small number of families with high informativeness. Consider two family types with respective ELODs of E_1 and E_2 per family. Assume that n_1 families of type 1 have been collected. The total ELOD for the type 1 families is thus equal to n_1E_1. How many families of type 2 are required such that their total ELOD is the same as that furnished by the type 1 families? For an equal total ELOD from families of type 2, the equation $n_1E_1 = n_2E_2$ must hold so that the number of families of type 2 is obtained as

$$n_2 = R\,n_1, \; R = E_1/E_2. \tag{5.21}$$

In later chapters, the ratio R will be calculated for various factors reducing informativeness. At the end of this book (Section 11.10), such results will serve as a quick guide for deciding how many families are required in a given linkage study.

As a simple example, consider the following expected lod scores at $r = 0$: $\log(2) = 0.301$ for one known recombination event or for two offspring from a phase-unknown double backcross; $2 \times \log(2)$ for three offspring from a phase-unknown double backcross; and $5 \times \log(2)$ for 6 offspring from a phase-unknown double backcross. Take $n_1 = 16$ as the number of known recombination events needed for a linkage analysis (Table 5.8). How many phase-unknown families with three offspring each are required for the same ELOD as the 16 known

Table 5.10. Number of Known Recombination Events Required to Find $Z_{max} \geq Z_0$ with Power ϕ, Given True Recombination Fraction r

Z_0	ϕ	True Recombination Fraction					
		0.01	0.05	0.10	0.20	0.30	0.40
2	0.80	11	14	20	38	91	373
	0.90	11	16	23	46	111	461
3	0.80	16	21	28	54	126	516
	0.90	16	22	31	62	150	618

recombination events? With $E_1 = \log(2)$ and $E_2 = 2 \times \log(2)$, one finds $n_2 = (E_1/E_2)n_1 = \frac{1}{2} \times 16 = 8$ families.

In planning a linkage analysis one may ask what is more informative, a large number of small families or a small number of large families? An answer to this question depends on several factors such as problems of genetic heterogeneity. In terms of ELODs, when phase-unknown double backcross matings are considered, results of the previous paragraph show that a small number of large families is better. Consider a total number of 6 offspring from a varying number of families of different sizes: (1) two offspring each in three families, (2) three each in two families, and (3) all six offspring in a single family. The corresponding total ELODs for these three cases are (1) $3 \times \log(2)$, (2) $4 \times \log(2)$, and (3) $5 \times \log(2)$.

5.12. Problems

Problem 5.1 Show formally that a mating in which no parent is a double heterozygote is not informative for linkage. Assume the mating $A1/B1 \times C1/C2$ and proceed in analogy to Table 5.2. List all possible offspring genotypes.

Problem 5.2. In Table 5.4, the first three phenotype classes identify known recombination events, whereas the fourth class represents ambiguous cases. Researchers sometimes analyze data by simply omitting the latter. Using probabilities and lod scores given in the table, determine whether and to what extent discarding this information introduces an asymptotic bias in the recombination fraction estimate. *Hint*: Set the first derivative with respect to θ of the expected lod score function equal to zero and solve the resulting equation for θ as a function of r; this will yield the value of θ at which the expected lod score function has its maximum. Make sure that the conditional probabilities used sum to 1.

Problem 5.3. Show that a pair of offspring from a phase-unknown double backcross mating carries the same amount of expected information (equation 5.13) as one offspring from the double intercross mating $A1/B2 \times A2/B1$ (codominant inheritance at each locus). *Hint*: Show that, for both cases, the same number of phenotype classes and the same class probabilities occur.

Problem 5.4. Assume two trait loci with alleles T and t at locus 1 and alleles D and d at locus 2. Both traits follow a strictly dominant mode of inheritance, $T > t$ and $D > d$. For a phase-known mating $Td/tD \times Td/tD$, derive Fisher's expected information, $i(r)$, and the ELOD, $E[Z(r)]$, and evaluate these quantities numerically for a range of values, $0 \le r \le \frac{1}{2}$.

Problem 5.5. Compute the ELOD at recombination fraction r for the mating $A1/B2 \times A?/A?$. The second parent is untyped at the second locus, which has alleles *1* and *2* with the respective population gene frequencies p and $1 - p$.

Problem 5.6. Consider two parents and n children, all individuals being doubly heterozygous (*1/2, 1/2*), that is, each has genotype *1/2* at each of two loci (phase unknown). Is this family informative for linkage? *Hint*: Derive the likelihood ratio $L(\theta)/L(\frac{1}{2})$ and check whether it is different from 0 for $\theta < \frac{1}{2}$. What is the likelihood ratio at $\theta = 0$?

Problem 5.7. Verify in an example that the ELOD, $E[Z(r)]$, is additive over families but the expected maximum lod score, $E(Z_{max})$, is not (Section 5.2). *Hint*: Use the data of Table 5.1 for a phase-known double backcross family of size 3, carry out analogous calculations for two families of size 3 (which are the same as for one family of size 6), and compare the results. It is easiest to obtain $P(k)$ with the BINOM program, and $Z(0.10)$ and Z_{max} with the EQUIV program.

6.

Multipoint Linkage Analysis

Traditionally in human genetics, linkage analysis has been carried out as a sequence of pairwise (two-point) comparisons between a trait locus and each of a number of marker loci. For each comparison, trait versus ith marker, or marker versus marker, lod scores are computed and combined over families and investigators. With today's dense linkage maps, simultaneous analysis of several linked loci (multipoint analysis) is the rule. In practice, at least as a first step, two-point lod scores are still computed and reported in most studies.

In connection with disease loci, "multipoint analysis" may refer to two conceptionally different things. In *parametric* multipoint analysis, which is the topic of this chapter, linkage relationships between a mendelian disease gene (known or assumed mode of inheritance) and maps of markers are investigated. In *nonparametric* multipoint analysis, mode of inheritance of the disease does not enter calculations and the term "multipoint" refers only to marker loci (see Chapter 13). For complex traits, as outlined in Chapter 15, two-point analysis is more appropriate than (parametric) multipoint analysis (but nonparametric multipoint analysis is quite appropriate).

Some theoretical aspects of multipoint analysis may be found in Bailey (1961). In human genetics, early approaches to multipoint analysis include those of Renwick and Bolling (1971), Cook et al. (1974), and Meyers et al. (1975, 1976). A few multipoint analyses in classical genetics will be quoted below (e.g., Fisher, 1922b).

This chapter addresses theoretical and practical aspects of parametric multipoint analysis. Most of the material covered refers to marker loci, but it applies equally well to mendelian disease loci. Particular aspects of linkage analysis for disease loci are addressed in Chapters 12 (mendelian traits) and 15 (complex traits). Although some examples are provided below, specific computational problems are deferred until Chapter 9. The first section of this chapter introduces notation and terminology required

114

for the joint analysis of several loci. Basic principles of multipoint analysis are addressed in Sections 6.2 and 6.3; they are somewhat theoretical and of interest mostly to students of statistical genetics. Sections 6.4 and 6.5 introduce interference, and later sections are devoted to several practical aspects of multipoint analysis.

6.1. Notation and Terminology

With many loci, linkage analysis is quantitatively as well as qualitatively different from two-point analysis. For one thing, the order of loci now matters. Also, the number of parameters, haplotypes, and genotypes increases drastically with the number of loci considered. This section introduces notation and terms required in subsequent sections. If some of this seems too abstract, it may be best to skip this portion of the text and consult it only when required. Examples will be provided in subsequent sections.

As pointed out in Section 1.2, the total number of different haplotypes or gametes with respect to a number of loci is given by the product of the numbers of alleles at these loci, $H = \Pi n_i$. For example, presence of 3 alleles at each of 5 loci defines $H = 3^5 = 243$ haplotypes. For any individual, the total number of different multilocus genotypes (pairs of haplotypes) is equal to $H(H + 1)/2$. With $H = 243$, one has 29,646 possible genotypes. The sheer size of this figure gives an impression of the computational problems that may be involved in the calculation of the likelihood (equation 4.16). Calculation of genotype probabilities will be demonstrated in Section 6.2.

Thus far a fixed order of loci has been assumed. As will be seen below, genotype probabilities are generally different for different locus orders. It is thus important to consider the number, n_0, of different possible orders. It is simply equal to the total number of permutations divided by 2, because two orders are considered the same if one is just the mirror image of the other, for example 1-2-4-3 and 3-4-2-1. Therefore,

$$n_0 = \frac{n!}{2} = \frac{n(n-1)(n-2) \ldots (3)(2)(1)}{2}. \tag{6.1}$$

For example, $n = 3$ loci can occur in $n_0 = 3$ possible orders, and $n = 5$ loci in 60 orders. For large n, it may not be easy to enumerate all possible orders. A systematic method of listing these orders (Johnson, 1963) is implemented in the PERMUTE program (this is important for programmers; linkage analysts rarely have a need for this method).

Table 6.1. Numbering System for Loci and Map Segments

Locus number	*1*	*2*	*3*	. . .		*n* − 1		*n*
Interval number	0	1	2	3		. . .	*n* − 1		*n*

A set of n loci defines $n - 1$ intervals between adjacent loci. When the lengths of these intervals are known, this collection of loci is called a *map* (sometimes an ordered set of loci, without knowledge of map distances, is also called a map). If, in addition, an interval is defined to the left of the leftmost locus and one to the right of the rightmost locus, $n + 1$ intervals are distinguished, which may be numbered as shown in Table 6.1. The ith interval is denoted by I_i.

In two-point linkage analysis, support for linkage is customarily expressed in terms of the lod score, which is the logarithm of the likelihood ratio, L_1/L_0, with L_1 being the likelihood under linkage and L_0 referring to absence of linkage. With multiple loci, depending on the hypotheses considered, multiple ways of expressing support have been defined (Keats et al., 1991); some of these terms, however, are rarely used in practice. Three measures of statistical support are distinguished, each based on $\log_{10}(L_1/L_2)$, with L_1 and L_2 being defined below for specific support measures. *Global support* indicates the evidence that a locus belongs to a map of loci. It is calculated by taking L_1 as the maximum likelihood when the locus is inserted in the map and L_2 as the likelihood when the locus is not on the map. "Definite" linkage of the locus with the map is said to be established when global support is 3 or more. *Interval support* measures the evidence that a locus is in a particular interval of the map, where L_1 is the maximum likelihood with the locus being in that interval and L_2 is the highest likelihood obtained by placing the marker in any other interval. To express *support for a given order*, L_1 is taken as the maximum likelihood of the best supported order and L_2 is the maximum likelihood for the given order.

Loci with interval support of at least 3 are termed *framework loci*, and a map composed entirely of such loci is called a *framework map* (Keats et al., 1991). A map is called *comprehensive* if it aims to include all syntenic loci (no support requirements for a comprehensive map).

In addition to the three types of multilocus support mentioned above, a fourth type has customarily been used to designate the overall evidence that a set of loci form a linkage group. It is obtained as the maximum likelihood L_1 under the best supported order divided by the likelihood L_0 assuming all loci are unlinked,

$$\log(L_1/L_0) = \log[L(\theta_{12}, \ldots, \theta_{n-1,n}) / L(\frac{1}{2}, \frac{1}{2}, \ldots, \frac{1}{2})], \quad (6.2)$$

where θ_{ij} is the recombination fraction between loci i and j. The support defined by equation (6.2) has been called *generalized lod score;* it measures the overall evidence that a set of loci forms a linkage group.

The four types of support considered above are all single numbers, obtained by maximizing likelihoods over portions of the genome. In analogy to the two-point situation, support for the various positions, x, of a single locus relative to a map of loci can be expressed as a *map-specific multipoint lod score*, $Z(x) = \log[L(x)/L(\infty)]$, where x is any map position of the locus in question on the fixed marker map, and the infinite location, $x = \infty$, indicates that the single locus is off the map ($\theta = \frac{1}{2}$ between the single locus and any of the marker loci on the map). For example, if x specifies the location of a locus in interval 0 of the marker map and θ_{ij} denotes the recombination fraction between loci i and j, this map-specific multipoint lod score is given by

$$Z(\theta_{01}, \theta_{12}, \theta_{23}, \ldots, \theta_{n-1,n})$$
$$= \log[L(\theta_{01}, \theta_{12}, \ldots, \theta_{n-1,n}) / L(\frac{1}{2}, \theta_{12}, \ldots, \theta_{n-1,n})]. \quad (6.3)$$

Another transformation of the likelihood ratio $L(x)/L(\infty)$ is the *location score*, $S(x) = 2 \times \ln[L(x)/L(\infty)]$ (Lathrop et al., 1984). It is a simple multiple of the lod score; that is, $S(x) = 2 \times \ln(10) \times Z(x) = 4.6 \times Z(x)$. Obviously, it would not be meaningful to make use of generalized lod scores when mapping a new locus to a known map of markers. The generalized lod score would not represent the evidence for the relation between the new locus and the map of markers; the relation among the latter is known from other sources.

For calculations outlined later in this chapter, it is important to distinguish between joint and marginal recombination probabilities. When gametes are produced by a parent, in each interval a recombination either does or does not occur. For example, on the right side of Figure 6.1, a

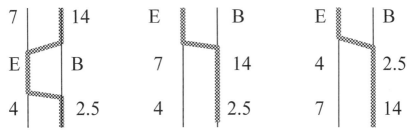

Figure 6.1. Crossover events leading to the haplotype received by individual 3.5 in Figure 6.2 for different locus orders.

recombination occurs in interval 1 (top) but none occurs in interval 2. The probability, which specifies for each interval whether a recombination has occurred or not, is called an *n-fold recombination fraction* (Risch and Lange, 1979), a multilocus, or *joint recombination probability*. Its notation may be formalized as follows: For n loci, consider an array $\varepsilon = (\varepsilon_1, \varepsilon_2, \ldots, \varepsilon_{n-1})$, in which $\varepsilon_i = 1$ if a recombination occurs in interval I_i and $\varepsilon_i = 0$ for no recombination in I_i. The joint recombination probability is then conveniently written as $G(\varepsilon)$. For example, with four loci, the fact that a recombination occurs in intervals I_1 and I_2 but not in I_3 is denoted by $\varepsilon = (1, 1, 0)$ and its probability of occurrence is $G[(1,1,0)]$ or simply g_{110}. As there are two possibilities in each of the $n - 1$ intervals, the possible number of arrays ε and thus of joint recombination probabilities is equal to 2^{n-1}. Joint recombination events are mutually exclusive, and the sum of the probabilities $G(\varepsilon)$ over all ε is equal to 1.

On a gamete received from a parent, a recombination between two loci is said to have occurred when the two alleles at these loci (one at each locus) originated in different grandparents. The probability of occurrence of such a recombination is just the regular two-point *recombination fraction*. It is a *marginal recombination probability* and is given by the joint recombination probabilities in the intervals between the two loci. For example, in Table 6.2, the g_{ij} are joint and the $\theta_{k\ell}$ are marginal recombination probabilities. In general, a gamete received from a parent consists of a sequence of segments, where grandparental origin of alleles alternates from one segment to the next. In other words, one segment contains loci whose alleles were received from one grandparent, the next segment contains loci whose alleles originated in the other grandparent, and so on. The boundary between two segments is given by a recombination breakpoint.

6.2. Three-Point Analysis with Known Phase

This and the next two sections cover the theoretically important case of the joint analysis of three loci. In human linkage analysis, the material

Table 6.2. Joint Recombination Probabilities (g_{ij}) and Two-Point Recombination Fractions (θ) for Recombination (R) and Nonrecombination (NR) among Loci A, B, and C

	Loci B and C		
Loci A and B	R	NR	Total
R	g_{11}	g_{10}	θ_{AB}
NR	g_{01}	g_{00}	$1 - \theta_{AB}$
Total	θ_{BC}	$1 - \theta_{BC}$	1

presented here is not so much of practical usefulness as it facilitates an understanding of the basic principles in multipoint linkage analysis.

The basic data type for three-point linkage analysis consists of the *n* offspring from phase-known matings in which one parent is triply heterozygous and the other is triply homozygous (a triple backcross). This mating is written as *ABC/abc* × *abc/abc*, with alleles *A* and *a* at locus *A*, *B* and *b* at locus *B*, and alleles *C* and *c* at locus *C*. In Section 1.2, a recombination between two loci was introduced as that process in a parental meiosis leading to the occurrence of two alleles (one at each locus) from different grandparents in the same haplotype of a child (see Figure 1.1). As one has only two maternal or two paternal grandparents, any offspring cannot be recombinant for each of the three locus pairs, *AB, BC,* and *AC*. Rather, for example, a recombination for *AB* and *BC* implies nonrecombination for *AC*. On the other hand, no individual can be recombinant for only one pair of loci and not for any other; for example, recombination for *AB* and nonrecombination for *BC* implies recombination for *AC*. All of this is based entirely on the definition of recombination and holds irrespective of the particular order of loci.

For any number of loci, if haplotypes can be recognized in offspring, one may, for example, indicate grandmaternal origin of an allele by *0* and grandpaternal origin by *1*. A haplotype is then characterized by a string of *0*'s and *1*'s, where a change from *0* to *1* or *1* to *0* identifies the occurrence of a recombination between the two corresponding loci (for examples, see White et al., 1985, Table 2).

With respect to joint recombination events for *AB* and *BC*, assuming locus order *A-B-C*, four classes of offspring are distinguished. The corresponding probabilities of occurrence are listed in Table 6.2. Double recombinants with recombination for *AB* and *BC* occur with probability g_{11}. Single recombinants with a recombination for loci *AB* but none for *BC* have probability g_{10}). Single recombinants with a recombination for *BC* but none for *AB* have probability g_{01}. Finally, nonrecombinants occur with probability g_{00}. Because $\Sigma\Sigma g_{ij} = 1$, there are three independent parameters, say, g_{11}, g_{10}, and g_{01}. The maximum likelihood estimates of the multinomial parameters g_{ij} are simply the corresponding observed proportions of offspring, $\hat{g}_{ij} = n_{ij} / n$.

As a simple example, consider Figure 6.2, which shows the most likely genotypes for three X-chromosomal marker loci in part of family 21 of Musarella et al. (1989). Let *A, B,* and *C* stand for the loci *DXS85*, *DXS255*, and *DXS14*, respectively. Following gametes from parents to the children, one finds $n_{00} = 6$ cases of nonrecombinant haplotypes; $n_{10} = 1$ haplotype (received by individual 2.7) is recombinant for *AB* and nonrecombinant for *BC*, and $n_{11} = 1$ haplotype (received by individual

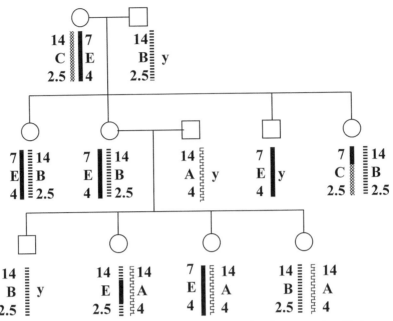

Figure 6.2. Portion of family 21 showing segregation of haplotypes at three X-chromosomal marker loci. (Based on Musarella et al., 1989, Figure 7.)

3.5) is recombinant for both AB and BC. No case of a single recombinant between B and C ($n_{01} = 0$) is observed in this small family segment. The total number of haplotypes counted is $n = 8$.

Recombination fractions are obtained from the joint recombination probabilities as follows: The probability of a recombination between loci A and B, irrespective of what happens between B and C, is $\theta_{AB} = g_{11} + g_{10}$ (Table 6.2). Analogously, $\theta_{BC} = g_{11} + g_{01}$. Finally, a recombination between loci A and C occurs when there is recombination between A and B and none between B and C, *or* a recombination between B and C and none between A and B; thus, the probability of this happening is given by $\theta_{AC} = g_{01} + g_{10}$. For example, the data of the previous paragraph give estimates $\hat{\theta}_{AB} = (1 + 1)/8 = \frac{1}{4}$, $\hat{\theta}_{BC} = \frac{1}{8}$, and $\hat{\theta}_{AC} = \frac{1}{8}$.

The relations leading from the g_{ij}'s to the θ's are easily inverted to yield joint recombination probabilities in terms of two-point recombination fractions, where the indicated restrictions ensure that the joint probabilities g_{ij} are nonnegative:

$$g_{11} = \frac{1}{2}(\theta_{AB} + \theta_{BC} - \theta_{AC}), \qquad\qquad \theta_{AC} \le \theta_{AB} + \theta_{BC} \qquad (6.4a)$$
$$g_{10} = \frac{1}{2}(\theta_{AB} - \theta_{BC} + \theta_{AC}), \qquad\qquad \theta_{BC} \le \theta_{AB} + \theta_{AC} \qquad (6.4b)$$

$$g_{01} = \tfrac{1}{2}(-\theta_{AB} + \theta_{BC} + \theta_{AC}), \qquad\qquad \theta_{AB} \le \theta_{BC} + \theta_{AC} \qquad (6.4c)$$

$$g_{00} = 1 - g_{11} - g_{10} - g_{01} = 1 - \tfrac{1}{2}(\theta_{AB} + \theta_{BC} + \theta_{AC}) \qquad (6.4d)$$

With the g's defined as in Table 6.2, equations (6.4a–d) do not depend on locus order (but see the locus-specific inequalities [6.9]). In practice, one usually works with yet another set of parameters involving the coefficient of coincidence, which will be introduced in Section 6.4.

The log likelihood for three-point observations is given by

$$\ln L(g_{11}, g_{10}, g_{01}) = \sum_i \sum_j n_{ij} \log(g_{ij}). \qquad (6.5)$$

When all two-point recombination fractions involving the three loci are equal to $\tfrac{1}{2}$, the g_{ij}'s become $\tfrac{1}{4}$ each. A generalized lod score may thus be obtained from (6.5) as

$$Z(g_{11}, g_{10}, g_{01}) = \sum_i \sum_j n_{ij} \log(4g_{ij}). \qquad (6.6)$$

For example, with the data from Figure 6.2, $n_{00} = 6$, $n_{01} = 0$, $n_{10} = n_{11} = 1$, one finds $Z = 6 \times \log(4g_{00}) + \log(4g_{10}) + \log(4g_{11})$. At the maximum likelihood estimates, $\hat{g} = n_{ij}/n$, the maximum of the generalized lod score for the given observations is obtained as 2.26.

In human genetics, three-point data rarely occur as counts of haplotypes from phase-known double backcross matings. In many matings, only one of the two intervals is informative. For example, in Figure 6.2, individual 2.7 is homozygous at marker *DXS14* and thus uninformative for recombination events between loci *DXS255* and *DXS14*. Her sons (not shown; she had no daughters) contribute information only for the recombination fraction θ_{BC} but not for joint recombination probabilities at both intervals. Therefore, the likelihood for the data shown in Figure 6.2 plus the data contributed by the sons of individual 2.7 cannot be represented in the simple form of (6.5) or (6.6).

When, in a collection of families, each family is informative for the recombination fraction between two markers only, then the total lod score is simply the sum of the two-point lod scores,

$$Z(\theta_{AB}, \theta_{BC}, \theta_{AC}) = Z(\theta_{AB}) + Z(\theta_{BC}) + Z(\theta_{AC}). \qquad (6.7)$$

A formula analogous to (6.7) applies to more than three loci. As a first step, linkage data are often analyzed in pairwise comparisons. However, the overall log likelihood cannot generally be represented as a sum of two-point log likelihoods as in equation (6.7) because of sample nonindependence of $\hat{\theta}_{AB}$ $\hat{\theta}_{BC}$, $\hat{\theta}_{AC}$. Some approximate analysis approaches are based on combinations of two-point lod scores (see Section 6.7).

In several respects, three-point (and generally multipoint) analysis yields more information than does two-point analysis (Fisher, 1954). As shown by Thompson (1984), "three-way data provide very much more information, particularly with regard to the problem of ordering the loci"; where individuals informative for all three loci are observed, information is lost (or overestimated) by summarizing the data in pairwise form. Assuming absence of interference, Lathrop et al. (1985) calculated the relative efficiency of three-locus versus two-locus estimates of recombination rates. They found that three-point data can be over five times as efficient, thus requiring less than one-fifth the number of observations than two-point data for the same precision of the estimates. Some 10 to 15 years ago, there were heated debates on this matter; however, nobody doubts today that multipoint analysis has its clear advantages.

6.3. Phase-Unknown Triple Backcross with Two Offspring

As will be seen below, for many multilocus problems, explicit solutions are unavailable; they can be found analytically only for special cases such as phase-unknown triple backcross matings with two offspring each, which will be covered in this section. Results will not be of much practical value but they give insight into several important theoretical aspects, for example, why maximum likelihood estimates in linkage analysis generally are biased. Readers less interested in theory may skip this section.

Consider three loci with two alleles each, where alleles are designated as *A, a; B, b;* and *C, c* at loci *A, B,* and *C,* respectively. Assume a triply homozygous parent, *abc/abc,* and a triply heterozygous parent (*A/a, B/b, C/c*). In the latter, four phases are possible: (I) *ABC/abc,* (II) *ABc/abC,* (III) *AbC/aBc,* and (IV) *Abc/aBC.* Under regular conditions (linkage equilibrium, see Chapter 11), each of these phases occurs with probability ¼. While the triply homozygous parent produces only one kind of haplotype, *abc,* potentially eight different haplotypes originate from the heterozygous parent, which are listed in Table 6.3 along with their conditional probabilities of occurrence given parental phase. For example, under phase I, with no recombination in interval *1* but a recombination in interval *2,* that is, with probability g_{01} (Table 6.2), either an *ABc* or an *abC* haplotype occurs. The probability for each of these two possibilities is ½ so that, under phase I, the haplotype *ABc* is produced with probability ½g_{01}, as is the haplotype *abC.*

Assuming dominance at each locus, haplotype symbols in Table 6.3 may be interpreted as offspring phenotype symbols. The figures in Table 6.3 then give the conditional probabilities with which offspring phenotypes occur. Now, in analogy to the phase-unknown double backcross (see

Table 6.3. Conditional Haplotype Probabilities Given Phase, Produced by a Triply Heterozygous Parent (*A/a, B/b, C/c*)

		Phase			
i	Haplotype	I	II	III	IV
1	*ABC*	$\frac{1}{2}g_{00}$	$\frac{1}{2}g_{01}$	$\frac{1}{2}g_{11}$	$\frac{1}{2}g_{10}$
2	*ABc*	$\frac{1}{2}g_{01}$	$\frac{1}{2}g_{00}$	$\frac{1}{2}g_{10}$	$\frac{1}{2}g_{11}$
3	*AbC*	$\frac{1}{2}g_{11}$	$\frac{1}{2}g_{10}$	$\frac{1}{2}g_{00}$	$\frac{1}{2}g_{01}$
4	*Abc*	$\frac{1}{2}g_{10}$	$\frac{1}{2}g_{11}$	$\frac{1}{2}g_{01}$	$\frac{1}{2}g_{00}$
5	*aBC*	$\frac{1}{2}g_{10}$	$\frac{1}{2}g_{11}$	$\frac{1}{2}g_{01}$	$\frac{1}{2}g_{00}$
6	*aBc*	$\frac{1}{2}g_{11}$	$\frac{1}{2}g_{10}$	$\frac{1}{2}g_{00}$	$\frac{1}{2}g_{01}$
7	*abC*	$\frac{1}{2}g_{01}$	$\frac{1}{2}g_{00}$	$\frac{1}{2}g_{10}$	$\frac{1}{2}g_{11}$
8	*abc*	$\frac{1}{2}g_{00}$	$\frac{1}{2}g_{01}$	$\frac{1}{2}g_{11}$	$\frac{1}{2}g_{10}$
Total		1	1	1	1

Section 5.8), assume two offspring in each family. Their joint probabilities of occurrence are computed as in the following example: Assume phenotype ABC (genotype *ABC/abc, i* = 1 in Table 6.3) for child 1 and phenotype AbC (genotype *AbC/abc, i* = 3) for child 2. Given phase I, the joint probability of occurrence of these two phenotypes is $(\frac{1}{2}g_{00}) \times (\frac{1}{2}g_{11})$; under phase II, it is $(\frac{1}{2}g_{01}) \times (\frac{1}{2}g_{10})$, and so on. The unconditional probability for the phenotype ABC in child 1 and AbC in child 2, is then calculated as $\frac{1}{4}(\frac{1}{2}g_{00})(\frac{1}{2}g_{11}) + \frac{1}{4}(\frac{1}{2}g_{01})(\frac{1}{2}g_{10}) + \ldots = (g_{11}g_{00} + g_{10}g_{01})/$ 8. Disregarding the order of the two offspring, their joint probability of occurrence is given by $\frac{1}{4}(g_{11}g_{00} + g_{10}g_{01})$. In this manner, the probabilities for all $8 \times 9/2 = 36$ possible pairs of phenotypes are calculated. It then turns out that, among the 36 probabilities, only four different values occur so that phenotypes with the same probabilities may be combined into a single class (see Section 5.8). Offspring phenotypes with the same probabilities are listed in Table 6.4, along with the probabilities p_k of the

Table 6.4. Offspring Phenotype Classes in Phase-Unknown Triple Backcross Families with Two Offspring

k	*ij*	P_k
1	11, 22, 33, 44, 55, 66, 77, 88, 45, 36, 27, 18	$g_{11}^2 + g_{10}^2 + g_{01}^2 + g_{00}^2$
2	12, 34, 35, 17, 46, 28, 56, 78	$2(g_{11}g_{10} + g_{01}g_{00})$
3	23, 14, 15, 26, 37, 48, 67, 58	$2(g_{11}g_{01} + g_{10}g_{00})$
4	13, 24, 25, 16, 47, 38, 57, 68	$2(g_{11}g_{00} + g_{10}g_{01})$
Total		1

Note: i and *j* refer to the numbering of haplotypes in Table 6.3, interpreted here as phenotypes. Cases *i* > *j* are not listed.

resulting phenotype classes. The lod score associated with the kth phenotype class is given by $\log(4p_k)$, because $g_{ij} = \frac{1}{4}$ under absence of linkage.

As there are four offspring phenotype classes in Table 6.4, their probabilities are determined by three independent parameters (degrees of freedom), say, p_1, p_2, and p_3 (class frequencies). Their maximum likelihood estimates are given by the multinomial proportions, $\hat{p}_k$, that is, the proportions of families with offspring phenotype class k. The p_k depend on the joint recombination probabilities, g_{ij}, or, equivalently, on the recombination fractions θ_{AB}, θ_{BC}, and θ_{AC}. Because the number of the latter parameters is also equal to 3, their MLEs can simply be obtained as functions of the $\hat{p}_k$ (Weir, 1996). The equations for p_k in Table 6.4 are easily solved, for example, by writing $p_3 + p_4 = 2(g_{11}g_{01} + g_{10}g_{00} + g_{11}g_{00} + g_{10}g_{01}) = 2(g_{11} + g_{10})(g_{01} + g_{00}) = 2\theta_{AB}(1 - \theta_{AB})$. Solving this quadratic leads to

$$\hat{\theta}_{AB} = \begin{cases} \frac{1}{2} - \frac{1}{2}\sqrt{1 - 2(\hat{p}_3 + \hat{p}_4)} & \text{if } \hat{p}_3 + \hat{p}_3 < \frac{1}{2} \\ \frac{1}{2} & \text{otherwise.} \end{cases} \tag{6.8}$$

In an analogous manner, $\hat{\theta}_{BC}$ is determined by $\hat{p}_2 + \hat{p}_4$, and $\hat{\theta}_{AC}$ by $\hat{p}_2 + \hat{p}_3$.

The multinomial proportions $\hat{p}_k$ are known to be unbiased estimates of the class probabilities p_k, that is, $E(\hat{p}_k) = p_k$. However, nonlinear functions of MLEs such as the recombination fractions (6.8) are generally biased. This suggests that, in essentially all cases of practical importance, recombination estimates are biased, but this bias tends to disappear as the number of observations increases because MLEs are generally consistent (see Section 3.3).

The ranges of the estimates (6.8) are restricted by the inequalities in equations (6.4a–c), which do not depend on locus order. For a given order of the loci, *A-B-C,* one usually requires an additional restriction, namely that θ_{AC} be at least as large as either of θ_{AB} and θ_{BC},

$$\theta_{AC} \geq \theta_{AB} \text{ and } \theta_{AC} \geq \theta_{BC}. \tag{6.9}$$

This imposes limits on the ranges of the p_i so that often the θ_{ij} cannot be estimated directly using equation (6.8). For example, $\hat{p}_1 = 0.45$, $\hat{p}_2 = 0.10$, $\hat{p}_3 = 0.15$, and $\hat{p}_4 = 0.30$ lead to $\hat{\theta}_{AB} = 0.342$, $\hat{\theta}_{BC} = 0.276$, and $\hat{\theta}_{AC} = 0.146$. Such estimates are inadmissible, and the recombination fractions have to be estimated by numerical maximization of the likelihood under the restrictions (6.9) (for an example, see Section 6.7).

6.4. Interference in the Three-Point Cross

In many species, a frequent observation is that in different intervals between genes on a chromosome, recombinations do not occur independently of each other. This non-independence is called *interference.* For three loci in the order *A-B-C,* the frequency of double recombinations (a recombination in each of the two intervals) has been denoted by g_{11} (see Table 6.2). Under independence, a double recombination occurs with probability $\theta_{AB}\theta_{BC}$ where θ_{ij} is the recombination fraction between loci i and j. In genetics, the deviation from independence is measured by the *coefficient of coincidence* (Muller, 1916),

$$\gamma = g_{11}/(\theta_{AB}\theta_{BC}) = \tfrac{1}{2}(\theta_{AB} + \theta_{BC} - \theta_{AC})/(\theta_{AB}\theta_{BC}), \tag{6.10}$$

and interference is defined as $I = 1 - \gamma$ (Strickberger, 1985). Thus, interference is absent ($I = 0$) for $\gamma = 1$, negative ($I < 0$) for $\gamma > 1$, and positive ($I > 0$) for $\gamma < 1$.

It is often more convenient to work with γ rather than with θ_{AC}. From (6.10), one obtains

$$\theta_{AC} = \theta_{AB} + \theta_{BC} - 2\gamma\,\theta_{AB}\theta_{BC}. \tag{6.11}$$

Replacing θ_{AC} in (6.4a–d) by the right side of (6.11) leads to the new parameterization,

$$g_{11} = \gamma\,\theta_{AB}\theta_{BC} \tag{6.12a}$$
$$g_{10} = \theta_{AB}(1 - \gamma\,\theta_{BC}) \tag{6.12b}$$
$$g_{01} = \theta_{BC}(1 - \gamma\,\theta_{AB}) \tag{6.12c}$$
$$g_{00} = 1 - \theta_{AB} - \theta_{BC} + \gamma\,\theta_{AB}\theta_{BC}. \tag{6.12d}$$

In some organisms, the recombination fraction across two intervals is larger than the sum of the recombination fractions in the two intervals, $\theta_{AC} > \theta_{AB} + \theta_{BC}$. This phenomenon is referred to as *map expansion* (Holliday, 1964); human geneticists sometimes use this term with different meanings. However, in a three-point cross this cannot occur as it would require a negative value for g_{11}.

In three-point analysis, the requirement that probabilities assume values between 0 and 1 and recombination fractions be between 0 and $\tfrac{1}{2}$ puts limits on the possible range of γ in equation (6.10). Assume fixed values of θ_{AB} and θ_{BC}. Then the lower limit of γ is attained when no double recombinants occur, $g_{11} = 0$, in which case $\gamma = 0$. In addition, one must have $\theta_{AC} \le \tfrac{1}{2}$ so that, using (6.11), one obtains $\gamma \ge (\theta_{AB} + \theta_{BC} - \tfrac{1}{2})/(2\theta_{AB}\theta_{BC})$. Therefore, the lower limit of γ is given by $\gamma \ge \max[0, (\theta_{AB} + \theta_{BC} - \tfrac{1}{2})/(2\theta_{AB}\theta_{BC})]$. From the right side of equation (6.10), one can see that the upper limit of γ is given by the requirements that $\theta_{AC} = (g_{10} + g_{01}) \le \tfrac{1}{2}$ and that each of g_{10} and g_{01} be nonnegative, which leads to an upper limit for γ of $1/\theta_{AB}$ or $1/\theta_{BC}$, whichever is smaller. Put together, these limits read

$$\max[0, (\theta_{AB} + \theta_{BC} - \tfrac{1}{2})/(2\theta_{AB}\theta_{BC})] \leq \gamma \leq \min(1/\theta_{AB}, 1/\theta_{BC}). \quad (6.13)$$

In some organisms, for tightly linked loci (sum of the recombination fractions in two intervals of 1% or less), instances of high negative interference are observed, and multiply recombinant gametes are common. This phenomenon is related to gene conversion rather than multiple recombinations occurring within a short distance (Strickberger, 1985). In most species, however, interference seems to be positive ($I > 0$, $\gamma < 1$) so that one usually assumes $\gamma \leq 1$ and takes "interference" to mean "positive interference." Also, complete interference is usually taken to mean $\gamma = 0$. The limitation to nonnegative interference sharpens the restrictions (6.9) on θ_{AC}. With $\gamma \leq 1$, rearranging (6.10) leads to

$$\theta_{AB} + \theta_{BC} - 2\theta_{AB}\theta_{BC} \leq \theta_{AC} \leq \min(\theta_{AB} + \theta_{BC}, \tfrac{1}{2}). \quad (6.14)$$

For small distances and under the assumption of complete interference, map distances are equal to recombination fractions (Morgan map function) so that, for three loci A-B-C, the recombination fraction between loci A and C is simply the sum, $\theta_{AC} = \theta_{AB} + \theta_{BC}$. For other cases, θ_{AC} may be obtained via the map functions. This may be done with the MAPFUN program by calculating map distances, x_1 and x_2 from θ_{AB} and θ_{BC}, adding them, and converting their sum back into a recombination fraction. For some of the map functions, explicit *addition formulas* can be obtained. Based on (6.11), setting $\gamma = 1$ leads to the Haldane addition formula, $\theta_{AC} = \theta_{AB} + \theta_{BC} - 2\theta_{AB}\theta_{BC}$. For the Kosambi map function, the coefficient of coincidence is given by

$$\gamma = 2\theta_{AC} = 2(\theta_{AB} + \theta_{BC})/(1 + 4\theta_{AB}\theta_{BC}) \quad (6.15)$$

(Bailey, 1961). Dividing (6.15) by 2 leads to the Kosambi addition formula,

$$\theta_{AC} = (\theta_{AB} + \theta_{BC})/(1 + 4\theta_{AB}\theta_{BC}). \quad (6.16)$$

Estimates of the coincidence coefficient γ are obtained when the recombination fractions in (6.10) are replaced by their estimates. However, estimates of γ have a large standard error (Elandt-Johnson, 1971) so that distinguishing $\gamma < 1$ from $\gamma = 1$ (absence of interference) can be difficult, which is demonstrated as follows: Consider three ordered loci A-B-C and a phase-known triple backcross mating with n offspring (see Section 6.2). Thus, there are four offspring phenotype classes with probabilities of occurrence given by (6.12a–d). Based on these, a 3×3 information matrix with respect to parameters γ, θ_{AB}, and θ_{BC} may be obtained as described in Section 5.3 (the 3×3 information matrix at the end of Section 5.3 corresponds to our parameter values $\gamma = 0.55$, $\theta_{AB} = 0.15$, and $\theta_{BC} = 0.15$). For simplicity, assume the same recombination rates in the two intervals, $\theta = \theta_{AB} = \theta_{BC}$. Then, offspring classes identified by equations (6.12b) and (6.12c) have the same probabilities of occurrence and may be pooled into one class. From the resulting three probabilities, the 2×2 information matrix with respect to parameters γ and θ may be set up according to the rules given in Section 5.3; it furnishes the same results for γ as would be obtained with the three-parameter approach for $\theta_{AB} = \theta_{BC}$. For selected values of γ and θ, Table 6.5 shows standard errors for the estimates of the coincidence coefficient per observation, which are seen to be large. The values of γ listed in Table 6.5 are those predicted by the Kosambi formula, but calculations were made without assuming a map function. Also given in Table 6.5 are approximate numbers n of offspring (meioses) required to detect a deviation from $\gamma = 1$. They were calculated by

$$n = (1.64\sigma_0 + 0.84\sigma_1)^2/(\gamma - 1)^2 \tag{6.17}$$

(adapted from Elandt-Johnson, 1971, p. 380), where $\sigma_0 = \sigma(\hat{\gamma}; \gamma = 1, n = 1)$ is the standard error of the γ estimate when γ is equal to 1 and recombination fractions are as given in the table, $\sigma_1 = \sigma(\hat{\gamma}; \gamma < 1, n = 1)$ is the standard error for values of γ and θ as given in the table, and constants 0.84 and 1.64 were chosen for a power of 80% at a significance level of 5%, respectively. Results indicate that testing for the presence of interference is most powerful for moderate values of $\theta \approx 0.15$. Even though a power of 80% represents a rather mild requirement for a statistical test, over 800 meioses are required to detect interference, which makes it difficult to establish significant positive interference in generally available data sets. The role of interference for ordering loci will be discussed in Section 6.6.

As outlined in Section 1.5, map functions $\theta = M(x)$ relate map distance x between two loci to the recombination fraction θ between them. One way of obtaining such map functions is to apply Haldane's method

Table 6.5. Asymptotic Standard Error of Coincidence Coefficient Estimates and Number n of Meioses Required for Detecting Positive Interference

γ	θ	$\sigma(\hat{\gamma}; \gamma < 1, n = 1)$	$\sigma(\hat{\gamma}; \gamma = 1, n = 1)$	n
0.04	0.01	19.99	99.01	34,826
0.20	0.05	8.85	19.00	2,327
0.38	0.10	5.92	9.00	1,013
0.55	0.15	4.52	5.67	847
0.69	0.20	3.56	4.00	949
0.88	0.30	2.28	2.33	2,285

(see Karlin, 1984, for an overview). For three ordered loci, *1-2-3*, assume map distance x and recombination fraction θ between loci *1* and *2*, and map distance Δx between loci *2* and *3*. Letting Δx go to zero, Haldane (1919) obtained the *marginal coincidence coefficient*,

$$\gamma_0 = (1 - d\theta/dx)/(2\theta), \tag{6.18}$$

where $d\theta/dx = M'(x)$ is the first derivative (the slope) of the map function, and γ_0 is viewed as a function of θ [or of x when $M(x)$ is substituted for θ]. Rearranging terms in (6.18) leads to the differential equation,

$$d\theta/dx = 1 - 2\theta\,\gamma_0. \tag{6.19}$$

Solving (6.19) under specific assumptions on γ_0 leads to various well-known map functions. For the map functions of Haldane (equation 1.2), Morgan (1.1), Kosambi (1.3), Carter and Falconer (1.4), and Felsenstein (1.6), the respective marginal coincidence coefficients are given by $\gamma_0 = 1, 0, 2\theta, (2\theta)^3$, and $K - 2\theta(K - 1)$. Kosambi interference, for example, tends to be complete ($\gamma_0 = 0$) as θ tends toward zero and increases linearly with θ until it is equal to 1 at $\theta = \frac{1}{2}$.

The marginal coincidence coefficient (6.18) is often used as a convenient measure to characterize map functions regarding their interference properties. For a given θ, it is proportional to minus the slope $M'(x)$ on the map function; that is, a larger slope indicates stronger marginal interference. However, as pointed out by Risch and Lange (1979), marginal coincidence does not necessarily give an accurate picture of coincidence as defined by (6.10) for two map lengths. Marginal coincidence may even be less than 1 with coincidence exceeding 1.

6.5. Crossover Distributions and Testing for Interference

In the human genome, interference has a positional and a numerical aspect. *Positional interference* refers to the fact that crossovers do not tend to occur in close proximity of each other, whereas *numerical interference* is reflected in the distribution of crossovers, that is, the numbers of chromosomes carrying 0, 1, 2, and so on, crossovers. Interference in the three-point cross, discussed in the previous section, covers both these aspects of interference (Ott, 1997b). Because testing for interference in the three-point cross is difficult owing to the required large number of observations, several authors have resorted to whole-chromosome approaches hoping that the increase in observations on additional marker loci will increase power, which is the topic of this section. Most of the material refers to numerical interference, with a few comments on positional interference. Interference in map functions will be discussed first, followed by newer results on testing for interference through crossover distributions.

Multilocus-Feasible Map Functions. Because estimates of the coincidence coefficient from three-point data are quite imprecise (Table 6.5), another avenue is sometimes taken to estimate interference. It makes use of the fact that map functions incorporate different levels of interference and allow the joint consideration of more than three loci. Particularly the Rao map function (see Section 1.5) has been fitted to observed data by varying its parameter p. Using linkage data for loci on chromosome 3 of *Drosophila,* Lalouel (1977) found an estimate for p of 0.56, which suggests interference operating approximately at the Kosambi level. He also reported suggestive evidence of nonuniformity of interference along the chromosome. Pascoe and Morton (1987) investigated data for the X chromosome of *Drosophila* and estimated p at 0.33, corresponding to an interference level between that predicted by the Kosambi and Carter–Falconer map functions.

As discussed in Sections 6.1 and 6.2, a joint recombination probability (gamete probability) refers to presence or absence of a recombination in each of the intervals on a map. On the other hand, the recombination fraction is the probability of a recombination occurring in an interval irrespective of what happens in other intervals. This concept may be generalized to a quantity called recombination value, which is the probability that a recombination occurs in a region of the genome consisting of multiple, but not necessarily contiguous intervals. There is a one-to-one relationship between recombination values and gamete probabilities (Karlin and Liberman, 1978), which allows the prediction of all gamete probabilities based on a given map function (Liberman and Karlin, 1984). It turns out that most classical map functions fail to furnish valid gamete probabilities for more than three loci (Bailey, 1961). Liberman and Karlin (1984) defined a map function as *multilocus-feasible* when it yields proper joint recombination probabilities; that is, gamete probabilities ranging from 0 through 1. They showed that a map function $\theta = M(x)$ is multilocus-feasible when

$$(-1)^k M^{(k)}(x) \leq 0, \quad k = 1, 2, \ldots, \tag{6.20}$$

for all $x \geq 0$, that is, when all even-numbered derivatives, $M^{(2k)}(x) = d^{2k}M(x)/dx^{2k}$, are nonnegative and all odd-numbered derivatives are less than or equal to zero. For example, the Kosambi, Carter–Falconer, and Rao map functions are not multilocus-feasible for more than three loci. However, it has been argued that multilocus-feasible map functions are not generally realistic (Evans et al., 1993)—for one thing, such map functions only refer to numerical interference and disregard positional aspects of interference.

Historically, many map functions have been derived based on specific assumptions on the functional form of the marginal coincidence coefficient (equation 6.18). Based on the concept of multilocus-feasibility, Karlin and Liberman (1978) and Risch and Lange (1979) presented a general class of map functions in which the nonrandomness of crossovers is in the numbers of crossovers that occur, not in their locations. The results of these authors may be summarized as follows: Let c_k denote the probability of occurrence of k crossovers. Then, $m = \Sigma_k kc_k$ is the mean number of crossovers. Let $f(s) = \Sigma c_k s^k$ be the probability generating function (Feller, 1968) of any distribution c_k of the number of crossovers. An associated map function may then be constructed as

$$\theta = M(x) = \frac{1}{2}[1 - f(1 - 2x/m)]. \tag{6.21}$$

As an application of (6.21), take the binomial distribution, $c_k = \binom{N}{k}p^k q^{N-k}$, $q = 1 - p$, which was also considered by Liberman and Karlin (1984). Its probability generating function is given by $f(s) = (ps + q)^N$, and its mean is $m = Np$. If $f(s)$ is evaluated at $s = 1 - 2x/m$ and inserted in (6.21), one obtains the map function (1.8). It introduces interference by restricting the number of crossovers, whose upper limit is given by the mapping parameter, N. Map distances are restricted to the interval $0 \leq x \leq N/2$, that is, total map length is $L = N/2$. For $N = 1$, the binomial map function coincides with the Morgan map function. The limiting marginal interference for small x is obtained as $\lim(c_0)_x \to_0 = (N - 1)/N$.

Weeks et al. (1993) incorporated interference into a linkage program through multilocus-feasible map functions. When applied to six loci from the CEPH consortium map of chromosome 10, their program found significant evidence in favor of positive interference as modeled by the Sturt map function. In simulation studies, multilocus-feasible map functions appeared relatively powerful for the detection of interference (Weeks et al., 1994).

Other Methods of Allowing for Interference in Multilocus Analysis. An interesting ad hoc approach was taken by Pascoe and Morton (1987). These authors assumed absence of more than three crossovers and postulated that a crossover divides the chromosome into two segments between which there is no interference. This permits writing down the joint recombination probabilities for the different gamete classes.

Goldgar and Fain (1988) proposed a chiasma-based model for joint recombination probabilities, which includes the relative positions of the different crossovers. The model contained an interference parameter that makes closely spaced crossovers unlikely. A maximum of three crossovers was permitted. Application of this model to X-chromosome data of *Drosophila* resulted in a better fit than that achieved by other methods. For map distances up to about $x = 50$ cM, the graph of Goldgar and Fain's (1988) map function (full model) exhibits stronger marginal interference than that of the Rao map function and, for larger x, it exhibits smaller marginal interference. It has been suggested that restrictions in the numeric distribution of chiasmata is of greater significance for models of multilocus recombination than restrictions in locations of multiple chiasmata (Goldgar, Fain, and Kimberling, 1989).

Zhao et al. (1990) developed a method for jointly estimating recombination fractions and interference coefficients in multilocus linkage analysis. It is based on a multiplicative model and maximum-likelihood estimation of recombination fractions and interference coefficients. When applied to seven-locus data from *Drosophila*, the method detected pairwise and higher-order interference.

The chi-square model for the occurrence of crossovers along a chromosome, first proposed in the 1940s without a biological basis, has been reintroduced for modeling certain aspects of the crossover process (Zhao et al., 1995). Interference based on this model has been incorporated into pedigree analysis (Lin and Speed, 1996). However, discussion of these models for crossover formation are beyond the scope of this book.

Chiasma and Crossover Distributions. Some of the whole-chromosome approaches have involved crossover counts (numerical interference), which is discussed in the following few paragraphs. Several fallacies in these approaches seem to have gone unnoticed and are pointed out below. In particular, it has been assumed that under absence of interference, crossover distributions should follow the Poisson frequency law, which could be tested on the basis of the number of crossovers observed on a given chromosome.

In this context, the basic phenomenon on a chromosome is the chiasma. The frequency distribution of chiasmata associated with a particular chromosome may be estimated, for example, by the proportion of chromosomes showing 0, 1, 2, etc., chiasmata (remember that chiasmata may be observed under the microscope). An assumption often made is that under absence of interference, the number, c, of chiasmata, must follow the Poisson frequency law, that is,

$$P(c) = \lambda^c e^{-\lambda}/c!, \ c = 0, 1, 2, \ldots, \tag{6.22}$$

where $P(c)$ denotes the probability that in a meiosis exactly c chiasmata occur on a given chromosome. The parameter λ in equation (6.22) is the mean of $P(c)$ and its variance.

Observing chiasmata under the microscope appears to be somewhat unreliable. With a dense map of fully informative (100% polymorphic) markers, it is far easier to genetically observe crossovers than to count chiasmata. Thus, we need to know the distribution of crossovers resulting from a distribution of chiasmata. As outlined in Section 1.3, assuming absence of *chromatid* interference, each chiasma leads to a crossover with probability ½ (Mather, 1938). Thus, with a given fixed number, c, of chiasmata on a chromosome, the frequency distribution of crossovers is Binomial $(c, ½)$,

$$P(k|c) = \binom{c}{k}(½)^c, \text{ if } k \leq c, \tag{6.23}$$

and $P(k|c) = 0$ if $k > c$. From this, elementary probability calculus leads to the unconditional frequency distribution of crossovers (Ott, 1996) as

$$P(k) = \sum_{c=0}^{\infty} P(k|c)P(c). \tag{6.24}$$

Equation (6.24) applies to any distribution, $P(c)$. In particular, if $P(c)$ is Poisson as given by equation (6.22), $P(k)$ can be shown to also follow the Poisson frequency law, but with parameter $\lambda/2$ rather than λ as in (6.22). Thus, it seems easy enough to investigate haplotypes for a given chromosome and classify them as to how many crossovers each haplotype shows. However, there are two problems with this simple approach.

The first problem refers to the transformation (6.24) from $P(c)$ to $P(k)$. The matrix $P(k|c)$ is of full rank, that is, the transformation (6.23) is $1:1$—each $P(c)$ leads to a unique $P(k)$ and vice versa. An algorithm for the inverse transformation of (6.24) may be found in Ott (1996). Also, it is biologically intuitive that any chiasma distribution $P(c)$ must lead to a valid crossover distribution $P(k)$, that is, one must have $0 \leq P(k) \leq 1$ for all k. However, the reverse is not necessarily true. It is easy to come up with values for $P(k)$ that lead to some values of $P(c) > 1$ or $P(c) < 0$. For example, consider the crossover distribution $P(k = 0) = 0.2$, $P(k = 1) = 0.5$, and $P(k = 2) = 0.3$. Calculations outlined in Ott (1996) lead to the chiasma distribution $P(c = 0) = 0$, $P(c = 1) = -0.2$, and $P(c = 2) = 1.2$, which clearly is invalid. Therefore, the associated crossover distribution $P(k)$ must be called invalid on biological grounds as it cannot have arisen from any known chiasma distribution. Consequently, estimates of crossover distributions based on frequency counts of crossovers in haplotypes cannot be taken at face value unless they conform to a valid chiasma distribution. In other words, a crossover distribution must be estimated under the restriction that its associated chiasma distribution be valid, and this restriction tends to lower the evidence for interference. The relevant calculations to do that have been implemented in a computer program, CROSSOVR, which is available at URL ftp://linkage.rockefel ler.edu/software/utilities/. Instructions for using the program are given at URL http://linkage.rockefeller.edu/ott/linkutil.htm.

The second problem referred to above is based on the biological observation that in each meiosis at least one chiasma occurs. Thus, the Poisson distribution (6.22) is not a realistic representation for the frequencies with which chiasmata occur. In a previous analysis (Ott, 1996), the requirement of an obligatory chiasma was modeled as a truncated Poisson distribution for which the class $P(c = 0)$ is never observed. However, as pointed out by Dr. Pak Sham (personal communication, 1996), a more realistic model is that of a shifted Poisson distribution: the number of chiasmata is equal to $c + 1$ with c following a Poisson distribution, $c = 0, 1, \ldots$. Under this assumption, the frequency distribution for crossovers is obtained as

$$P(k) = \tfrac{1}{2} \frac{(\lambda + k)\, \lambda^k}{\lambda\, k! e^\lambda}; \; k = 0, 1, 2 \ldots; \gamma > 0 \qquad (6.25)$$

(Ott et al., 1998). It is this form of $P(k)$ that is incorporated in the current version of the CROSSOVR program.

Distribution of Distances between Adjacent Crossovers. Methods discussed in the previous few paragraphs all relied on detecting *numerical* interference. A method designed to assess *positional* interference has been proposed by Weber et al. (1993). It focuses on chromosomes with exactly two crossovers and tests whether the observed distance between them agrees with what would be expected under no interference. In that case, the distribution (histogram) of their absolute distances, d_c, from each other should follow a straight line with maximum height at $d_c=0$ and sloping down to zero at $d_c =$ chromosome length (Weber et al., 1993). One could then form classes of d_c values and compare in a chi-square test observed numbers of chromosomes falling into the different classes with the numbers expected under no interference.

Effects of Incomplete Marker Polymorphism. Thus far it has been assumed that crossovers may be observed in small intervals on maps of fully polymorphic markers. However, realistic maps consist of markers with high but not perfect heterozygosity. For example, consider three markers where the middle marker has heterozygosity of 75%. Crossovers may be observed to fall into intervals 1 or 2. However, because of incomplete heterozygosity, in 25% of all cases a parent will be homozygous for the middle marker. Thus, if two crossovers occurred, one in each interval, then no crossover will be seen (this is a rare case), and if one crossover took place it is unknown in which interval it occurred. In this situation, crossovers should be modeled as occurring on an underlying perfect yet unobservable map, with inferences being drawn on the basis of imperfect marker maps (Ott et al., 1998).

6.6. Three-Point Locus Ordering

In previous sections, three-point and multipoint analysis were considered under the tacit assumption that locus order was given. In this and the next two sections, problems of locus ordering are discussed. Below, the focus is on ordering three loci as this case shows particularly nicely the salient features of locus ordering.

In principle, order of three loci *ABC* is determined by the magnitude of the (true) recombination fractions θ_{AB}, θ_{BC}, and θ_{AC}, where θ_{ij} is the two-point recombination fraction between loci i and j. The largest of these indicates which of the three loci are farthest apart, as spelled out by inequalities (6.9) for the order *ABC*. Another order, for example, *ACB*, is determined by inequalities analogous to those of (6.9), that is, $\theta_{AB} \geq \theta_{AC}$ and $\theta_{AB} \geq \theta_{BC}$. A geometric interpretation of the different restrictions among the recombination fractions imposed by gene order is as follows: Consider a three-dimensional space with coordinates θ_{AB}, θ_{BC}, and θ_{AC}. With $0 \leq \theta_{ij} \leq \frac{1}{2}$, the three coordinates span a cube with sides of length $\frac{1}{2}$ each. In this cube, the three orders of the loci *A, B,* and *C* represent three non-overlapping regions as defined by the inequalities mentioned above. Note that these regions are not subspaces in the statistical sense, rather they are all of the same dimensionality as the sample space (cube).

Based on estimates $\hat{\theta}_{AB}, \hat{\theta}_{BC}$, and $\hat{\theta}_{AC}$, the largest of these values, say, $\hat{\theta}_{BC}$, determines order by specifying that the flanking loci are *B* and *C*. This estimated order may not correspond to the true, unknown order. By chance, $\hat{\theta}_{BC}$ may have turned out largest, while in fact the true value of θ_{BC} might not be largest. It is thus useful to consider the plausibility of different locus orders, that is, to evaluate the maximum likelihood or the lod score under each gene order and compare these maxima with each other.

Different locus orders imply different interpretations of the observations. For example, consider the three loci *A = DXS85, B = DXS255,* and $C = DXS14$ in Figure 6.2. For the order ABC, individual 3.5 was seen to be a double recombinant. For different assumed locus orders, however, Figure 6.1 shows that the same individual is only a single recombinant. Relationships among the three orders may be formalized as outlined below.

As an artificial example, consider $n = 20$ offspring from a phase-known triple backcross mating. Assume that 17 offspring are nonrecombinants. Among the three recombinant offspring, let $n_{AB} = 1$ offspring be recombinant for AB, $n_{BC} = 2$ offspring recombinant for BC, and $n_{AC} = 3$ offspring recombinant for AC. The sum of these numbers exceeds three because a recombinant individual must be recombinant for two of the three possible relations (see second paragraph in Section 6.2). Depending on the order of the three loci, these numbers of recombinants fall into different classes of gametes (Table 6.2) received by the offspring. For a given order, let R_1 be the number of offspring recombinant for the first interval, irrespective of whether they are recombinant or not in the second interval. R_2 is the number of offspring recombinant in the second interval, while R_3 is the number of offspring recombinant over both intervals, that is, with recombination for the two flanking loci. Then, in analogy to equations (6.4a–c), numbers of gametes in the different classes are given by

$$k_{11} = \tfrac{1}{2}(R_1 + R_2 - R_3), \tag{6.26a}$$
$$k_{10} = R_1 - k_{11}, \tag{6.26b}$$
$$k_{01} = R_2 - k_{11}, \tag{6.26c}$$
$$k_{00} = n - k_{11} - k_{10} - k_{01}, \tag{6.26d}$$

where k_{11} is the number of doubly recombinant (in intervals 1 and 2) gametes, k_{10} those with recombination in interval 1 and nonrecombination in interval 2, k_{01} those with nonrecombination in interval 1 and recombination in interval 2, and k_{00} is the number of nonrecombinant gametes.

Table 6.6 shows the results of our example for the three locus orders

Table 6.6. Offspring Numbers from Phase-Known Triple Backcross Matings Interpreted under Three Locus Orders

	Order *ABC*			Order *BAC*			Order *BCA*		
	R_2	N_2	Σ	R_2	N_2	Σ	R_2	N_2	Σ
R_1	0	1	1	1	0	1	2	0	2
N_1	2	17	19	2	17	19	1	17	18
Σ	2	18	20	3	17	20	3	17	20

Note: R_i = recombination in interval i, N_i = nonrecombination in interval i.

(the layout of each of the 2 × 2 tables is as in Table 6.2). For example, under order *BAC*, interval 1 refers to the chromosomal region between loci *B* and *A* (so, we have $R_1 = 1$), and interval 2 refers to region $AC (R_2 = 3)$. The number of recombinants between flanking loci (*B* and *C*) is $R_3 = 2$. Thus, equation (6.26a) tells us that under order *BAC* our artificial sample data contain $k_{11} = 1$ doubly recombinant offspring. In this manner, the table for order *BAC* is completed and the other two tables set up. Depending on locus order, in our data, there are either 0, 1, or 2 double recombinants.

The next task is to calculate log likelihoods under each of the three locus orders. This amounts to estimating the probabilities g_{ij} with which observations in each of the four cells of a given 2 × 2 table in Table 6.6 occur. It is instructive to consider two possible ways of estimating the *g*'s even though only the second one is generally applied. One approach is to directly estimate the four gamete class frequencies, g_{ij}, subject to the restriction that the coefficient of coincidence (6.10) be between zero and one, $0 \le \gamma \le 1$ (6.14). The multinomial class frequencies are estimated simply as $\hat{g}_{ij} = k_{ij}/n$. Under locus order *ABC*, one obtains $\hat{g}_{11} = 0$, $\hat{g}_{10} = \frac{1}{20} = 0.05$, $\hat{g}_{01} = 0.10$, and $\hat{\theta}_{00} = 0.85$. The estimated coefficient of coincidence is $\hat{\gamma} = 0$. The maximum of the generalized lod score (6.6) for order *ABC* is thus obtained as $Z = 1 \times \log(4 \times 0.05) + \ldots + 17 \times \log(4 \times 0.85) = 7.540$ (the zero class contributes nothing to this sum). For order *BAC*, the unrestricted estimate of the coefficient of coincidence is $(\frac{1}{20}) / [(\frac{1}{20}) \times (\frac{3}{20})] = \frac{20}{3}$, which exceeds the upper limit of 1. Thus, on $0 \le \gamma \le 1$, the estimate is $\hat{\gamma} = 1$, implying independence of recombination in the two intervals. Consequently, the gamete class frequencies are given by the products of the marginal frequencies, that is, by equations (6.12a–d) with $\gamma = 1$. Thus, under locus order *BAC*, the frequency of doubly recombinant gametes is estimated as $\hat{g}_{11} = 1 \times (\frac{1}{20}) \times (\frac{3}{20}) = 0.0075$, $\hat{g}_{10} = 0.0425$, $\hat{g}_{01} = 0.1425$, and $\hat{g}_{00} = 0.8075$. With these estimates, the lod score (6.6) is obtained as 6.645. Formally, the drop in lod score from 7.540 is due to restricting $\hat{\gamma}$. Finally, under the order *BCA*, one again finds $\hat{\gamma} = 1$, and the lod score is obtained as 5.546.

Because estimates of the coincidence coefficient tend to be very inaccurate (see Section 6.4), another approach is more common. Rather than estimating γ, one either assumes an appropriate value, most often $\gamma = 1$, or a certain level of interference predicted by a map function. Each of these will be done here. For the three loci considered here, define the map distance x_{AB} as a vector from *A* to *B* such that x_{AB} is positive for locus order *AB* and negative for order *BA*. Analogously, define x_{BC} as a map distance vector from *B* to *C*. Then, $x_{AC} = x_{AB} + x_{BC}$ is the map distance from loci A to C. For locus order ABC, x_{AB} and x_{BC} are both positive. For BAC, x_{AB} is negative but smaller in absolute value than x_{BC}, and for BCA, $-x_{AB} > x_{BC}$. The three locus orders may thus be represented as regions of a plane with coordinate axes x_{AB} and x_{BC}, as shown in Figure 6.3. The graph of the lod score, $Z(x_{AB}, x_{BC})$, then forms a mountainous surface above the plane.

In Table 6.6, observations for different locus orders were presented in 2×2 tables, where rows correspond to recombination and nonrecombination in the first interval and columns analogously correspond to the second interval. For our calculations of lod scores $Z(x_{AB}, x_{BC})$, it is more convenient to refer to a fixed 2×2 table, in which rows correspond to the interval AB and columns correspond to BC, irrespective of locus order. So, our assumed observations are $n_{11} = 0$, $n_{10} = 1$, $n_{01} = 2$, and $n_{00} = 17$, that is, observations in the four cells are the same for the different orders, but their interpretation changes with order. In the graph for different locus orders (Figure 6.3), a given point (x_{AB}, x_{BC}) determines order of the three loci as well as absolute map distances among them. For instance, $x_{AB} = -0.32$ and $x_{BC} = 0.12$ imply order BCA. Using a particular map function, one then translates absolute map distances ($|x_{AB}| = 0.32$, $x_{BC} = 0.12$, $|x_{AC}| = 0.20$) into recombination fractions. For the map distances given here, the Kosambi function furnishes $\theta_{AB} = 0.2824$, $\theta_{BC} = 0.1177$, and $\theta_{AC} = 0.1900$ (may be done with the MAPFUN program). Based on these recombination fractions, using equations (6.4a–d), one obtains the following gamete probabilities: $g_{11} = 0.10505$, $g_{10} = 0.17735$, $g_{01} = 0.01265$,

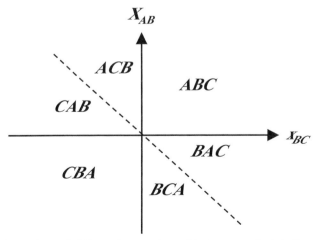

Figure 6.3. Regions of different locus orders with three gene loci A, B, and C. $x =$ map distance.

and $g_{00} = 0.70495$, corresponding to offspring numbers $n_{11} = 0$, $n_{10} = 1$, $n_{01} = 2$, and $n_{00} = 17$. Notice that under the current order, *BCA*, it is the $n_{01} = 2$ gametes that are the double recombinants. The lod score at the assumed point $(x_{AB}, x_{BC}) = (-0.32, 0.12)$ is then calculated by equation (6.6) as $Z = 0 + 1 \times \log(4 \times 0.17735) + 2 \times \log(4 \times 0.01265) + 17 \times \log(4 \times 0.70495) = 4.91$.

Based on the Kosambi map function, Table 6.7 presents calculations of the previous paragraph for a grid of x_{AB} and x_{BC} values. The lod score appears as a mountainous surface with three hills separated by two crevices, each dipping down to $-\infty$. The hills correspond to the three locus orders (Figure 6.3), and the top of each hill defines estimates of x_{AB} and x_{BC} under the given locus order. These estimates, accurate to two decimal places, are given on the right side of Table 6.8, which also lists analogous results for other map functions. Under each map function, the best locus order is *ABC*. With increasing interference, the difference in maximum lod score between the best and second best locus order also increases, the major reason being that different locus orders predict different numbers of double recombinants and these become less likely with increased interference. Hence, map functions with stronger interference permit better discrimination between locus orders. In the limit for complete interference (binomial map function with at most $N = 1$ crossover, or Sturt map function with map length $L = \frac{1}{2}$), the maximum lod score is 7.540 under locus order *ABC*. Any other order has zero likelihood as it requires more than one crossover between the flanking loci.

Essentially all currently available human genetic maps have been

Table 6.7. Lod Scores Z (x_{AB}, x_{BC}) under Kosambi Interference for the Observations in Table 6.6

x_{AB}	Map Distance, x_{BC}					
	0.05	0.10	0.15	0.20	0.25	0.30
0.10	7.22	7.38	7.29	7.09	6.84	6.57
0.05	7.35	7.53	7.44	7.25	7.01	6.75
0.01	6.98	7.17	7.10	6.92	6.69	6.43
0.00	$-\infty$	$-\infty$	$-\infty$	$-\infty$	$-\infty$	$-\infty$
−0.01	4.46	5.41	5.74	5.83	5.80	5.70
−0.05	$-\infty$	5.35	6.00	6.21	6.24	6.17
−0.10	3.34	$-\infty$	5.39	5.98	6.15	6.14
−0.15	4.17	3.86	$-\infty$	5.25	5.79	5.93
−0.20	4.50	4.57	4.01	$-\infty$	5.02	5.53
−0.25	4.61	4.83	4.65	4.00	$-\infty$	4.74
−0.30	4.60	4.89	4.86	4.58	3.89	$-\infty$
−0.40	4.42	4.76	4.83	4.77	4.60	4.26

Table 6.8. Maximum Lod Scores and Estimates of Absolute Map Distances x_1 and x_2 in the Two Intervals for Different Orders of Three Loci *A*, *B*, and *C* and for Different Map Functions (Observations as in Table 6.6)

Order	Haldane			Binomial ($N = 2$)			Kosambi		
	x_1	x_2	Z	x_1	x_2	Z	x_1	x_2	Z
A B C	.05	.11	7.493	.05	.11	7.515	.05	.10	7.527
B A C	.05	.18	6.645	.05	.16	6.382	.06	.18	6.247
B C A	.11	.18	5.546	.11	.17	5.022	.12	.20	4.912

obtained under the assumption of no interference. Justification for this approach has been given by Speed et al. (1992) who showed that ordering loci under no interference will consistently estimate the true order even when there is interference.

Statistical tests for declaring one locus order "significantly" better than another cannot be carried out through customary likelihood ratio tests because locus orders correspond to different regions of the same parameter space. One avenue might be to test for goodness of fit of different orders with the observations. All of those locus orders with good fit of the observations would then form a confidence space of locus orders. Although such tests have been developed for certain simple data types (Lathrop et al., 1987; Ott and Lathrop, 1987a), they have not been extended to more general situations. However, these analytical tests reveal the following important properties of the locus ordering problem: Power for ordering loci is very small for closely linked loci and reaches an optimum value at recombination rates of about 20% between loci (Bishop, 1985; Ott and Lathrop, 1987a). Thus, to establish order among closely spaced markers a rather high number of observations is required. In practice, one locus order is considered better than another if the difference in associated lod scores exceeds the threshold of 3 ("maps with 1000 : 1 odds").

6.7. Mapping under Complete Interference

In many applications, it is reasonable to assume occurrence of at most one crossover in a local map, which is equivalent to complete interference (the term "crossover" is often used although "recombination" would be more exact). Ordering loci may then be carried out in a simplified manner (Fain et al., 1989). For example, consider a set of ordered loci, *A-B-C-D-E-F*, and a multiple phase-known backcross mating, *ABCDEF/ abcdef × abcdef/abcdef*. Assume that an offspring receives a recombinant haplotype such as *ABCdef*, in which a crossover (recombination) has occurred between loci C and D. Looking at pairs of loci only, one recognizes that any haplotype to the left of the crossover point (AB, AC, and BC) is nonrecombinant, and the same is true for haplotypes involving pairs of loci to the right of the crossover (*de*, *df*, and *ef*). However, any locus on the left side of the crossover is recombinant with any locus on the right side of the crossover. Hence, the point of crossover divides the loci into two distinct groups. For unknown locus order, the argument may now be reversed. If a crossover has occurred, pairwise nonrecombinant loci form a group of (unordered) loci, which must be separated by the crossover from any other locus. A single crossover permits division of the loci into two separated groups. Another crossover at a different location will introduce a new point of separation such that three ordered groups of loci are present, with the loci in each group still unordered. Eventually, when a crossover has occurred in each interval, the order of all loci has been unequivocally established.

This method of mapping is also being used to place disease loci on a map of known markers. For example, the breast cancer locus, *BRCA1*, was partially fine-mapped in this manner (Easton et al., 1993). Another example is quoted in Section 1.4.

Complete interference allows a simple quantification of the number of observations required for ordering loci. To confirm order among three closely linked loci, as pointed out above, occurrence of at least one crossover in each of the two intervals is required. Let M_1 and M_2 be two markers at a distance r from each other. Consider a new marker, M_0, located between M_1 and M_2, at a distance x from M_1 (toward M_2). To detect that M_0 is indeed between M_1 and M_2, one must make the following two observations:

- A recombination (at least one) between M_1 and M_0 that places M_0 toward M_2 of M_1.
- A recombination (at least one) between M_0 and M_2 that places M_0 toward M_1 of M_2.

Due to interference, these recombinations will not occur in the same meiosis, that is, they represent independent events. The probability that the above two conditions occur in n meioses is given by

$$P(x) = [1 - (1 - x)^n][1 - (1 - \{r - x\})^n].$$

For small x and $(r - x)$, this simplifies to

$$P(x) \approx [nx][n(r - x)] = n^2 x(r - x).$$

Thus far, these probabilities are conditional on a fixed position x of M_0. Assume now that M_0 can be at any position between M_1 and M_2 with equal probability. That is, x is a uniformly distributed random variable with density $1/r$ between 0 and r. With the approximate expression for $P(x)$ above, one finds the unconditional probability for detecting M_0 as

$$P = \int_0^r n^2 x(r-x) \frac{1}{r} dx = \frac{n^2 r^2}{6}.$$

This may be solved for

$$n = \frac{\sqrt{6P}}{r}$$

which is the number of fully informative meioses required to localize M_0 between M_1 and M_2 with power P.

With incomplete marker polymorphism, this number is likely to increase. Let h be the heterozygosity of markers M_1 and M_2, and h_0 be the heterozygosity of M_0. For a recombination to be seen in intervals (M_1, M_0) or (M_0, M_2), both markers delimiting the intervals must be heterozygous, which occurs with probability hh_0, independently in each interval. This leads to $P = h^2 h_0^2 n^2 r^2/6$ or

$$n = \frac{\sqrt{6P}}{hh_0 r}. \tag{6.27}$$

For example, assume marker heterozygosities of $h = h_0 = 0.80$. To localize a new marker into a 5 cM-wide interval with power $P = 0.90$ requires $n = 73$ meioses. If the new marker has heterozygosity $h_0 = 0.30$, which is fairly typical of a single nucleotide polymorphism, the number of meioses is increased to $n = 194$. Of course, these calculations assume absence of errors. In practice, pedigree errors (undetected laboratory errors, nonpaternities, etc.) run at a rate of close to 1% so that it becomes almost academic to consider positioning a disease locus into a very small interval by genetic mapping.

Once loci are confidently ordered, recombination fractions in the different intervals must be estimated. For the remainder of this section, a particular example of such estimation under complete interference will be considered. This material is mostly of importance to statistical geneticists and may be skipped by readers with more general interests in linkage analysis. The example in question refers to three loci in *Drosophila*, which had been analyzed by Fisher (1922b) on the basis of pairwise counts of recombinants and nonrecombinants. (A thorough maximum likelihood analysis of these and additional loci was described by Smith [1989].) The three ordered loci are *scute* (locus A), *beaded* (locus B), and *rough* (locus C), with observed two-point recombination fraction estimates of $\hat{\theta}_{AB} =$

4/279 [recombinants / (recombinants + nonrecombinants)] = 0.0143, $\hat{\theta}_{BC} = 11/455 = 0.0242$, and $\hat{\theta}_{AC} = 453/6388 = 0.0709$. The estimated recombination rate between the flanking loci is seen to be larger than the sum of those in the two intervals between these loci. The coefficient of coincidence is thus estimated to be zero (complete interference). Below, as an example of the EM algorithm, iterative maximum likelihood estimation of the recombination fractions is demonstrated.

Consider the layout of Table 6.2 and assume absence of double recombinants, $g_{11} = 0$. Then, gamete frequency g_{10} is equal to θ_{AB}, and $g_{01} = \theta_{BC}$, where θ_{AB} and θ_{BC} are the recombination rates to be estimated, while $\theta_{AB} + \theta_{BC} = \theta_{AC}$ under complete interference. In addition to being a recombination rate, θ_{AB} is also the frequency of (multipoint) gametes recombinant for AB and nonrecombinant for BC, and θ_{BC} is the frequency of gametes recombinant for BC and nonrecombinant for AB. The frequency of nonrecombinant gametes is then given by $1 - \theta_{AB} - \theta_{BC}$. The number of observations is $n = 7122$, which is taken to be the total number of gametes in Table 6.9 (probabilities analogous to those in Table 6.2). Let k_{ij} be the number of recombinants and s_{ij} the number of nonrecombinants for each pair of loci. Thus, $k_{AB} = 4$, $s_{AB} = 275$, $k_{BC} = 11$, $s_{BC} = 444$, $k_{AC} = 453$, and $s_{AC} = 5935$. The object is now to count gametes by dividing up the two-point numbers of recombinants and nonrecombinants into the various gamete classes. In the EM algorithm, although one wants to *estimate* the proportions of gametes, θ_{AB} and θ_{BC}, they are initially assumed to be known as having some "starting value." For our data, this procedure is outlined as follows.

What is the number, $\theta_{AB}n$, of gametes recombinant for AB and nonrecombinant for BC (upper right-hand cell in Table 6.9)? First, this number must comprise all of the $k_{AB} = 4$ recombinants for AB, because these

Table 6.9. Counts of Gametes Recombinant (R) and Nonrecombinant (NR) for Loci AB and BC

AB	Loci BC	
	R	NR
R	0	$4 + \dfrac{444\theta_{BC}}{1 - \theta_{BC}} + \dfrac{453\theta_{AB}}{\theta_{AB} + \theta_{BC}}$
NR	$11 + \dfrac{275\theta_{BC}}{1 - \theta_{AB}} + \dfrac{453\theta_{BC}}{\theta_{AB} + \theta_{BC}}$	$\dfrac{275\,(1 - \theta_{AB} - \theta_{BC})}{1 - \theta_{AB}} + \dfrac{444\,(1 - \theta_{AB} - \theta_{BC})}{1 - \theta_{BC}} + 5935$

contribute only to the first row of Table 6.9, whereas double recombinants for *AB* and *BC* are lacking. Next, the $s_{BC} = 444$ nonrecombinants for *BC* are distributed over the two cells of the second column in Table 6.9. The upper and lower cell probabilities are θ_{AB} and $1 - \theta_{AB} - \theta_{BC}$ (their sum is $1 - \theta_{BC}$), respectively, so that the respective relative cell probabilities are $\theta_{AB}/(1 - \theta_{BC})$ and $(1 - \theta_{AB} - \theta_{BC})/(1 - \theta_{BC})$. Consequently, $444 \times \theta_{AB}/(1 - \theta_{BC})$ of the $s_{BC} = 444$ nonrecombinants for *BC* are expected to fall into the upper cell and thus contribute toward our number $\theta_{AB}n$ of gametes. The last type of observation to be considered here are the $k_{AC} = 453$ recombinants for *AC,* which must be distributed over the diagonal of Table 6.9. Of these, a proportion $\theta_{AB}/(\theta_{AB} + \theta_{BC})$ contributes toward our gametes in the upper right cell, that is, the number of these recombinants to be counted as gametes recombinant for *AB* and nonrecombinant for *BC* is equal to $453 \times \theta_{AB}/(\theta_{AB} + \theta_{BC})$. Hence, the desired number of gametes recombinant for *AB* and nonrecombinant for *BC* amounts to $\theta_{AB}n = 4 + 444 \times \theta_{AB}/(1 - \theta_{BC}) + 453 \times \theta_{AB}/(\theta_{AB} + \theta_{BC})$.

The number, $\theta_{BC}n$, of gametes recombinant for *BC* and nonrecombinant for *AB* is determined in an analogous manner. That number certainly comprises all of the $k_{BC} = 11$ recombinants for *BC*. Next, the $s_{AB} = 275$ nonrecombinants for *AB* are distributed over the second row of Table 6.9, $275 \times \theta_{BC}/(1 - \theta_{AB})$ of which fall into the left cell and are counted toward our number of gametes recombinant for *BC* and nonrecombinant for *AB*. Finally, the $k_{AC} = 453$ recombinants for *AC*, distributed over the diagonal of Table 6.9, contribute toward our gametes with a number of $453 \times \theta_{BC}/(\theta_{AB} + \theta_{BC})$, the remainder having been counted as the other gamete type above.

These results are summarized in Table 6.9. For information purposes, the number of nonrecombinant gametes is also given, which includes all of the $s_{AC} = 5935$ nonrecombinants for *AC* (sum of upper left and lower right cells). The two proportions of gametes are now estimated by dividing their number (upper right cell of Table 6.9 for θ_{AB}, lower left cell for θ_{BC}) by the total number of gametes ($n = 7122$),

$$\theta_{AB} = [4 + 444 \times \theta_{AB}/(1 - \theta_{BC}) \\ + 453 \times \theta_{AB}/(\theta_{AB} + \theta_{BC})]/7122, \tag{6.28a}$$

$$\theta_{BC} = [11 + 275 \times \theta_{BC}/(1 - \theta_{AB}) \\ + 453 \times \theta_{BC}/(\theta_{AB} + \theta_{BC})]/7122. \tag{6.28b}$$

Equations (6.28) are analogous to expressions for gene counting (Smith, 1957) and contain the quantities to be estimated on both sides of the equations. Estimates are obtained iteratively by inserting initial values for the parameters in the right side, solving the equations, inserting the results as updated estimates on the right side, solving the equations again, and so on. Suitable initial values for θ_{AB} and θ_{BC} are their pairwise estimates, 0.014 and 0.024, respectively, but final results turn out to be independent of initial values as long as these range between 0 and ½. After a large enough number of iterations, the values converge to the multipoint estimates, $\hat{\theta}_{AB} = 0.0326$ and $\hat{\theta}_{BC} = 0.0367$. As one can see, these are quite different from the corresponding two-point estimates. The multipoint recombination fraction estimate between the flanking loci is then $\hat{\theta}_{AB} + \hat{\theta}_{BC} = 0.0693$, which agrees fairly well with the corresponding two-point estimate of 0.0709, as this (two-point) relation is based on a much larger number of observations than the other two pairwise recombination fraction estimates.

Incidentally, gene counting equations other than (6.28) may be derived for the same data. The ones shown below are obtained on the basis of the log likelihood of the (two-point) observations, which is $4 \times \log(\theta_{AB}) + 275 \times \log(1 - \theta_{AB}) + 11 \times \log(\theta_{BC}) + 444 \times \log(1 - \theta_{BC}) + 453 \times \log(\theta_{AB} + \theta_{BC}) + 5935 \times \log(1 - \theta_{AB} - \theta_{BC})$. Taking partial derivatives with respect to θ_{AB} and θ_{BC}, setting these equal to zero, and solving the resulting equations as if they were obtained from multinomial data leads to the counting equations,

$$\theta_{AB} = \frac{e_1}{e_1 + 275 + 5935(1 - \theta_{AB})/(1 - \theta_{AB} - \theta_{BC})}, \qquad (6.29a)$$

$$\theta_{BC} = \frac{e_2}{e_2 + 444 + 5935(1 - \theta_{BC})/(1 - \theta_{AB} - \theta_{BC})}, \qquad (6.29b)$$

where $e_1 = 4 + 453\theta_{AB}/(\theta_{AB} + \theta_{BC})$ and $e_2 = 11 + 453\theta_{BC}/(\theta_{AB} + \theta_{BC})$. Equations (6.29) differ from (6.28). Depending on the starting values, one or the other pair of equations leads more rapidly to the results at a predetermined accuracy, but both lead to the same final estimates, $\hat{\theta}_{AB} = 0.0326$ and $\hat{\theta}_{BC} = 0.0367$.

This gene counting approach to estimating multipoint recombination rates is suitable for relatively uncomplicated situations and large numbers of offspring. For human family data, using one of the multipoint computer programs will generally be much more practical.

6.8. Map Construction and Gene Localization

Map construction for marker maps is generally based on a subset of the CEPH families (Dausset et al., 1990). Disease loci, on the other hand, are generally mapped based on families specifically collected because they contain affected individuals. In this section, methods for ordering loci are discussed, which includes localizing a new locus, a disease, or a marker locus, on an existing marker map. On a chromosome, consider a set of n loci. In principle, to estimate locus order amounts to evaluating the maximum likelihood for each order. For each assumed order, interval lengths (recombination fractions) must be estimated, which leads to the maximum likelihood under the given order. With n loci, $n!/2$ such orders must be evaluated. For example, $n = 10$ loci correspond to $n!/2 = 1,814,400$ locus orders. If analysis of each order takes only 1 second (it might take more than that), evaluating all orders requires 21 days of uninterrupted computation. Thus, in practice, several other approaches have been proposed (see Weeks, 1991 for an overview).

A well-known method is to choose that locus order as the best which requires the smallest number of recombinations in a given set of data. For loci with full penetrance, this method has indeed been shown to be equivalent to maximum likelihood ordering (Thompson, 1984). To the untrained geneticist, this method might seem to suggest that recombination is something bad that ought not to happen. One should consider, however, that it is the occurrence of recombinations that allows us to order loci. Recombinations are thus essential for gene mapping and one should not try to explain away recombinations in one's data as this biases the resulting estimates of recombination fractions and map distances.

In practice, most methods of map construction work in a step-wise manner by starting with a small number of loci and gradually adding loci. Thus, the first step in the ordering of a set of loci is to carry out conventional two-point linkage analysis for each locus pair. For n loci, this will result in $\frac{1}{2}n(n-1)$ estimates of θ with associated maximum lod scores. Various map construction algorithms [e.g., the one implemented in the MAP-MAKER program (Lander et al., 1987)] and the method employed in the construction of the Généthon maps, then proceed somewhat differently. A possible route would be to select that locus pair with the highest maximum lod score and a map distance not smaller than 10 or 20 cM. Then, each marker is tried in turn for its fit onto this map, and the best fitting marker (see next paragraph) is retained at its estimated map position. In this manner, one marker after another is added to the map.

To add a new marker (or a disease locus) to an existing marker map amounts to estimating its position, x, on the map, where, for example, the first locus on the map is at position $x = 0$. One may then proceed in one of two ways. A simple approach is to keep the existing marker map fixed, that is, interval lengths are not varied, while the new marker is "walked" along the map in small steps. At each position, x, the multipoint lod score or location score, $Z(x)$, is calculated (e.g., with the LINKMAP program). The estimated map position is then given by the maximum lod score, $Z(\hat{x})$. A generally more efficient approach is to drop the new locus into one interval after another. For example, consider markers *A, B, C,* and *D*, with *N* being the new locus. If the latter is assumed to be in interval 1, locus order is *A-N-B-C-D*. The maximum lod score associated with *N* being in interval 1 is then obtained as follows. Let L_1 be the likelihood maximized over the four interval lengths in *A-N-B-C-D*. L_2 is the likelihood maximized over the three interval lengths in *A-B-C-D* (in calculations of L_2, for numerical reasons, locus *N* is retained on the map but with a recombination fraction of 50% relative to each marker). The maximum lod score for *N* being in interval 1 is then given by $\log(L_1/L_2)$. This approach treats existing marker intervals as nuisance parameters and generally works better than the other approach mentioned, but it requires a much higher computational effort. The number of *df* associated with the test statistic $\log(L_1/L_2)$ is equal to 1.

The existence of dense ordered marker maps demonstrates that these approaches have worked quite well in practice. Of course, none of them guarantee that the maximum likelihood order will be found. Once a map has been constructed, various consistency checks are carried out. For example, the CRI-MAP program has a ''flips'' option by which the order of a pair of adjacent markers is reversed, and this is done for each pair of adjacent markers in turn. Presumably, any disturbance such as a ''flip'' will decrease the maximum lod score, or else the map is updated to what is found to be a better map.

To localize a disease locus on a dense map of markers, it may not be necessary to estimate the map position of the disease locus precisely, at least not initially. One may simply assume that the disease is located in the middle of one of the intervals and estimate the interval containing the disease locus. This is the basis of Lander and Botstein's (1986a) *interval mapping,* which these authors showed to be more powerful than using unmapped markers.

With heterogeneous traits (several disease loci exist but only one segregates in a given family), one usually estimates the proportion α of families in which the trait gene is linked with the marker map (with $1 - \alpha$ being the proportion of families in which the trait locus is elsewhere), and the map position x of the trait on the map. An extension of the interval mapping approach to heterogeneous traits (*simultaneous search;* Lander and Botstein, 1986a) consists of simultaneously finding the various disease loci on the gene map, which is more powerful than searching for one disease locus at a time. One of the HOMOG programs may be used for this purpose (see Ott et al., 1990a, for an example). A detailed treatment of genetic heterogeneity is given in Chapter 10.

As is well known, in most genomic regions, sex-specific differences in map distances exist. For accurate marker mapping, these differences must be allowed for although in the initial steps of map building, male and female recombination fractions are often taken to be the same. This topic will be taken up in detail in Section 10.1.

In disease gene mapping, calculating multipoint lod scores is often prohibitively slow if the number of marker loci exceeds 3 or 4. For this reason, several methods have been developed that approximate likelihoods by computer simulation rather than compute them exactly (Lange and Matthysse, 1989; Irwin et al., 1994; Lin, 1996; Heath, 1997, 1998).

It is interesting to note that in a genome-wide multipoint analysis, true and false lod score peaks have somewhat different characteristics: True peaks tend to be wider than false peaks (Terwilliger et al., 1997). This phenomenon is related to the fact that among affected individuals, shared haplotypes at the disease locus extend over a wider region than among unaffected individuals. This was first pointed out by Weber and Stephenson (1993, 1994) and greatly extended by Houwen et al. (1994). Statistically, this is an example of length-biased sampling (Armitage and Berry, 1987; Karlin and Taylor, 1975). However, the value of this phenomenon in parametric linkage mapping may be rather limited.

For mapping purposes, one would expect that a low-density map of highly polymorphic markers may have similar ''value'' for gene mapping as a high-density map of markers with low polymorphisms. Relationships between the two types of maps were investigated analytically by Terwilliger et al. (1992) and in computer simulations by Kruglyak (1997).

Generally, for map distances between markers, it is only point estimates that are obtained, and not interval estimates. Computer programs such as ILINK provide both point estimates and associated sampling variances, but the latter are not usually calculated. It is of interest to have an idea of the number of meioses required to estimate the length of a map interval with a given precision. Accuracy of an estimate may be measured by its coefficient of variation, $C = \sigma/r$, where r = recombination fraction (interval length) and σ = standard deviation of the estimate, $\hat{\theta}$, of r. For a number n of phase-known meioses, $\hat{\theta}$ is just the proportion of meioses resulting in a recombination (binomial situation). Its mean is $E(\hat{\theta}) = r$, with variance $V(\hat{\theta}) = r(1 - r)/n$ and $\sigma = \sqrt{V(\hat{\theta})}$. Thus, the coefficient of variation is given by $\sigma/r = \sqrt{[(1 - r)/(nr)]}$. If one requires that it be smaller than some constant, $\sqrt{[(1 - r)/(nr)]} \leq c$, this translates into a minimum number of meioses of

$$n \geq (1 - r)/(rc^2). \qquad (6.30)$$

For example, if the coefficient of variation should be no larger than 0.20, which is a reasonable and not too stringent value, for an interval with recombination fraction $r = 0.05$, a minimum of $n = 475$ meioses are required. For $r = 0.20$, one obtains $n = 100$. If one equates estimates with true values, writing $\sigma = Cr$, the expected confidence interval around some recombination fraction is given by $r \pm 2s = r \pm 2Cr = r[1 \pm 2C]$. With $C = 0.20$, this yields a confidence interval of $(0.6r, 1.4r)$. For example, one finds $(0.3, 0.7)$ for $r = 0.05$, and $(0.12, 0.28)$ for $r = 0.20$. Thus, even for such rather wide confidence intervals, the number of meioses required is quite large. This demonstrates that generally map lengths tend to be estimated with low precision.

6.9. Map Integration

In addition to genetic maps discussed in this book, other maps have been constructed, most notably radiation hybrid maps (see Section 2.5). Although these maps all refer to ''the same thing'' (ordered human loci, or their constituents, DNA sequences), they are characterized by different metrics. If one map in one area contains little information while another map is highly informative in that area, a combination of the two maps is expected to represent a major improvement over each single map. This motivates the study of *map integration*. Because of the different metrics and other differences between maps, map integration is not straightforward (Weissenbach and Bentolila, 1996). Below, a likelihood approach to map integration is outlined. The analysis types presented are intended to give the user a flavor of what is involved in map integration. For a more detailed study, relevant references should be consulted. Here, the focus is on integrating genetic and radiation hybrid maps, but the approach applies also to other projects of map integration.

Genetic maps are based on recombination frequencies between polymorphic genetic markers. The resulting maps consist of points (marker loci) along a chromosome, with intermarker distances being provided in terms of genetic distance. Genetic distance is defined as the expected number of crossover points (on a gamete) in an interval. For short intervals, it is essentially identical to recombination fraction between the endpoints of the interval. Thus, a set of $n + 1$ marker loci define n genetic lengths, d_i, $i = 1, \ldots, n$. In *radiation hybrid maps*, the expected number of chromosome breaks in an interval is taken as the physical length, x_i, of that interval, where an interval is defined as the piece of chromosome between two adjacent loci.

In terms of statistical analysis, both maps share the property that the underlying quantity defining length cannot generally be observed directly but must be estimated indirectly by maximum likelihood techniques. Computer programs are available that provide likelihoods relative to the parameters of interest. Assume, for the moment, that the same markers are considered in a genetic and radiation hybrid map. Then, $L(d_1, d_2, \ldots, d_n)$ is the likelihood for the genetic map, where d_i is the map length (in Morgans) of the ith interval. Similarly, $L(x_1, x_2, \ldots, x_n)$ is the likelihood for the radiation hybrid map, where x_i is the map length (in Rays) in the ith interval. Because these two maps are statistically independent, the total likelihood for both, genetic and physical data, is simply $L(d_1, \ldots, d_n, x_1, \ldots, x_n) = L(d_1, \ldots, d_n) L(x_1, \ldots, x_n)$, or the product of the two individual likelihoods. Joint estimates of all parameters are given by maximizing the total likelihood over all parameters. Clearly, if these parameters are allowed to vary freely, nothing is gained by maximizing the joint likelihood over maximizing individual likelihoods and multiplying them.

Presumably, there is some regularity in the relationship between the d_i and x_i for the various intervals. The most basic common denominator between the two maps is that locus order is constrained to be the same in the two maps. If estimates of genetic and radiation hybrid maps individually define different locus orders, then the requirement of a common order represents a restriction on interval lengths. In this case, the total likelihood will generally be different from the product of individual likelihoods (under different locus orders). Thus, this first-level map integration amounts to estimating locus order on the basis of genetic and physical likelihoods. If genetic and physical loci are not the same, then there will be, for example, an interval on the genetic map that contains several physical loci. While the length of this interval is estimated based on both genetic and physical data, the distances among physical markers within that interval are estimated based only on the physical likelihood (except that the physical length of the interval tends to be influenced by genetic data).

Another level of map integration is achieved by postulating additional relationships between the d_i and x_i parameters. Consider the ratio, $R_i = d_i/x_i$, and reparametrize so that the variables $\{d_i, x_i\}$ are replaced by $\{d_i, R_i\}$. If the d_i and x_i are estimated independently of each other ($2n$ parameters), this is equivalent to estimating a separate value of R_i in each interval and the reparametrization has no effect. However, the R_i may not fluctuate wildly from one interval to the next but may be constant or show a trend along a chromosome, as does, for many chromosomes, the analogous ratio between male and female recombination fractions (see Section 10.1).

In the simplest case, there is a constant proportionality, $R = R_i = R_j$, in all intervals. If so, the number of parameters to be estimated reduces from $2n$ to only $n + 1$.

Collins et al. (1996) presented an approach to map integration and implemented it in a computer program. Experience shows that the resulting maps are highly reliable.

6.10. Problems

Problem 6.1. Show that the Kosambi map function is not multilocus-feasible, using the fact that $d\theta/dx = 1 - 4\theta^2$. To disprove multilocus feasibility, it suffices to show that (6.20) is violated for any value of x, where $x = 0$ is a convenient choice.

Problem 6.2. What steps would you have to carry out to determine the map length (independent of any mapping function) of a particular chromosome?

Problem 6.3. For three ordered loci A-B-C, assume recombination fractions in the two intervals of 0.05 and 0.08. What is the recombination fraction between loci A and C as predicted by the Haldane and Kosambi map functions?

Problem 6.4. For the recombination fractions of Problem 6.3, what is the coefficient of interference predicted by the binomial map function with parameter $N = 2$?

Problem 6.5. For a given chromosome, assume half of all meioses show one chiasma and half show two chiasmata. (1) For this chromosome, what is the average number of crossovers expected to be observed in gametes (haplotypes)? (2) With what frequencies will gametes with 0, 1, and so on crossovers occur?

7.

Penetrance

One of the problems that make linkage analysis complicated (and interesting) is that crossovers take place on the genotypic level while observations occur on the phenotypic level, and phenotypes often do not fully exhibit underlying genotypes. The concept of penetrance establishes the connection between genotypes and phenotypes and is thus of central importance in linkage analysis. This chapter introduces and discusses penetrance in a predominantly applied manner. In the first three sections, penetrance is assumed to have a fixed value, which helps develop the salient features of incomplete penetrance. The practically important situation of age-dependent penetrance will be discussed in Section 7.5.

7.1. Definitions of Penetrance

Penetrance in the *general sense* or *wide sense* is defined as the conditional probability $P(x|g)$ that an individual with a given genotype g expresses the phenotype x. For example, the zeros and ones in Table 1.1 are penetrances—the probability is 1 that an individual with B/O genotype expresses the B phenotype, and the penetrance is 0 for such an individual to express the A or AB or O phenotype. For certain diseases, penetrance may be less than 1, in which case one speaks of incomplete or reduced penetrance. A given genotype may then lead to one of two or more phenotypes, where unspecified factors are responsible for determining which phenotype is expressed. For example, in insulin-dependent diabetes mellitus, penetrance for the disease has been estimated to be between 2 and 20% (Rotter, 1981).

Penetrance is sometimes used in a *narrow sense* as the probability of being affected (with a disease) given a certain genotype. In other words, penetrance is the phenotype risk given some genotype. Thus, for a simple, fully penetrant recessive disease with disease allele d

and normal allele D, genotype d/d has penetrance 1, and genotypes D/D and D/d have penetrance 0 each. Penetrance in the wide sense coincides with penetrance in the narrow sense when the phenotype is x = "affected". Narrow-sense penetrance refers to diseases and is not generally used in any other context. In this book, both definitions will be used, but it should always be clear from the context which definition applies. The LIPED computer program works with wide-sense penetrance. In the LINKAGE programs, on the other hand, one uses penetrance in the narrow sense by defining a number of so-called liability classes (classes of phenotypes) and specifying in each class, for the different genotypes, the probability of being affected.

If phenotypes are mutually exclusive and exhaustive, the penetrances over all phenotypes for a given genotype sum to 1. In practice, one often works with phenotypes whose definitions "overlap" so that some of the phenotypes are not mutually exclusive. Table 2.4 shows such a case in which, depending on the antigen used for typing for the Lutheran blood group, various phenotypes are distinguished, some of which are not mutually exclusive, for example, the phenotypes $A+B-$ and $A+$.

Most DNA polymorphisms (marker loci) show codominant inheritance so that, in the absence of errors, phenotypes reveal underlying genotypes ($1:1$ correspondence between genotypes and phenotypes). In fact, molecular geneticists tend to refer to genotyping results as "genotypes." Strictly speaking, however, they are phenotypes even though they may unequivocally exhibit underlying genotypes.

Dominant and recessive inheritance are basically distinguished through the penetrance of heterozygotes (Mendel, 1866)—their penetrance is 0 in the recessive case and 1 (with complete penetrance) in the dominant case. For example, consider a dominant disease with disease allele D and normal allele d and assume the penetrances $P(\text{affected}|$ genotype $D/D) = P(\text{affected}|D/d) = f$, and $P(\text{affected}|d/d) = 0$. Hence, $P(\text{unaffected}|D/D) = P(\text{unaffected}|D/d) = 1 - f$ and $P(\text{unaffected}|d/d) = 1$. The phenotype "unknown" is the union of the phenotypes "affected" and "unaffected" (unknown = affected or unaffected) so that it is characterized by a constant penetrance, $P(\text{unknown}|\text{genotype}) = P(\text{affected}|\text{genotype}) + P(\text{unaffected}|\text{genotype}) = 1$, for all genotypes. If penetrance is small, $f \approx 0$, penetrances for unaffected individuals are almost the same, $1 - f \approx 1$, for all genotypes, so that with small penetrance unaffected individuals contribute practically nothing in a linkage analysis. Occasionally, penetrances are purposely chosen to be small to carry out a so-called "affecteds-only" analysis, in which almost all information is derived from affected individuals.

If only susceptible genotypes ever express the disease, an affected phenotype identifies an individual as a carrier of the disease allele (or alleles in the case of a recessive disease). In many diseases, however, *phenocopies* (also called *sporadic cases* or *false positives*) occur. These are individuals who are affected not owing to genetic predisposition (at the locus under study) but due to some unspecified environmental factors or to genes at other locations. Occurrence of phenocopies is modeled by a nonzero penetrance for nonsusceptible genotypes. For example, consider a dominant disease with disease allele D and a normal allele d, with the disease allele having a population frequency of $p = P(D)$. Genotypes D/D, D/d, and d/d may have the respective associated penetrances $f_{DD} = 0.9$, $f_{Dd} = 0.9$, and $f_{dd} = 0.001$, where genotypes D/D and D/d are susceptible and genotype d/d is not susceptible to disease. The population frequency of genetically affected individuals is then equal to $A = p^2 f_{DD} + 2p(1 - p)f_{Dd}$, while the frequency of phenocopies is given by $C = (1 - p)^2 f_{dd}$. The *phenocopy rate*, that is, the proportion of phenocopies among all affected individuals, is equal to $C/(A + C)$. Note that occasionally the term phenocopy rate has been used to denote the penetrance of phenocopies.

If a dominant disease is rare, one has $A \approx 2pf_{Dd}$ and $C \approx (1-2p)f_{dd}$ and the phenocopy rate may be expressed as $(1-2p)/[1 + 2p(R-1)]$, where $R = f_{Dd}/f_{dd}$ is the ratio of penetrances. That is, the actual penetrance values are not relevant, only their ratio matters. This ratio is an important quantity characterizing mendelian inheritance models. It may be taken as a measure for how well a phenotype discriminates among underlying genotypes. There is also an interesting analogy to the following association measure used in epidemiology: Let $P(\text{affected}|G)$ be the proportion of individuals with a risk factor G who are affected with a disease. This proportion may also be interpreted as the risk of contracting the disease given one has the risk factor G. Similarly, $P(\text{affected}|g)$ is the proportion of affecteds among individuals without the risk factor. The risk ratio, $P(\text{affected}|G)/P(\text{affected}|g)$, then measures the effect of the risk factor on disease. If G is taken to mean presence of a disease susceptibility genotype, and g absence of the susceptibility genotype, the penetrance ratio R in linkage analysis is exactly equivalent to the risk ratio in epidemiology (Ott, 1994). For this reason, R is sometimes called risk ratio or relative risk.

7.2. Cost of Incomplete Penetrance

Incomplete penetrance clouds our view of the genotypes—phenotypes no longer unambiguously exhibit underlying genotypes. The consequence of this ambiguity is a loss of information which, for simple situations, may be assessed by computing expected lod scores. A detailed example is worked out below. The reader interested only in results may turn directly to the discussion of Table 7.2 at the end of this section.

Assume a dominant trait with disease allele D and normal allele d and a codominant marker locus with alleles 1 and 2. The penetrance, $f = P(\text{affected}|\text{genotype } D/d)$, at the disease locus is taken to be known and phenocopies are assumed absent. For full penetrance, $f = 1$. Consider a phase-known double backcross mating, $D1/d2 \times d1/d1$. Table 7.1 shows the four possible offspring genotypes, g, with associated probabilities $P(g; r)$ of occurrence, where r is the true recombination fraction between disease locus and marker locus. The recessive genotypes, $d2/d1$ and $d1/d1$, produce only the respective recessive phenotypes, $d21$ and $d11$. Owing to incomplete penetrance, however, the $D1/d1$ genotype expresses the $D11$ phenotype with probability f, and the $d11$ phenotype with probability $1 - f$. Similarly, $D2/d1$ expresses $D21$ and $d21$ with the respective probabilities f and $1 - f$. The unconditional probabilities of occurrence of the offspring phenotypes are computed as $P(x; r) = \Sigma_g P(x|g)P(g; r)$, with $P(x|g) = f$, and are given in the row labeled $P(x)$ of Table 7.1.

The lod score associated with a particular phenotype x is given by $Z_x(\theta) = \log[L(\theta)/L(\frac{1}{2})]$, where $L(\theta) = P(x; \theta)$. The likelihood ratios given in Table 7.1 show that for the dominant phenotypes, which unequivocally exhibit underlying genotypes, the lod scores do not involve the penetrance (this is the basis for the affecteds-only analysis mentioned above). Over all phenotypes possibly occurring in an offspring, the expected lod score is calculated as the weighted average of the lod scores, $\Sigma_x P(x; r)Z_x(\theta)$.

Table 7.1. Offspring Phenotype Probabilities in Phase-Known Double Backcross Families with Incomplete Penetrance, f, at the Disease Locus and True Recombination Fraction, r, between Disease and Marker Loci

		Phenotype x			
Genotype g	$P(g; r)$	$D11$	$d21$	$D21$	$d11$
$D1/d1$	$\frac{1}{2}(1 - r)$	f	0	0	$1 - f$
$d2/d1$	$\frac{1}{2}(1 - r)$	0	1	0	0
$D2/d1$	$\frac{1}{2}r$	0	$1 - f$	f	0
$d1/d1$	$\frac{1}{2}$	0	0	0	1
	$P(x)$	$\frac{1}{2}(1 - r)f$	$\frac{1}{2}(1 - rf)$	$\frac{1}{2}rf$	$\frac{1}{2}(1 - f + rf)$
	$L(\theta)/L(\frac{1}{2})$	$2(1 - \theta)$	$\dfrac{1 - \theta f}{1 - \frac{1}{2}f}$	2θ	$\dfrac{1 - f + \theta f}{1 - \frac{1}{2}f}$

Of interest here is only its maximum (the ELOD), which is attained at $\theta = r$ and is denoted by $E[Z(r; f)]$. The ratio, $R = E[Z(r; f)]/E[Z(r;1)]$, of the expected lod score with incomplete penetrance over that with full penetrance may be taken as a measure of relative informativeness for detecting linkage when the penetrance is f. As an aside, for values of r close to ½, the relative ELOD is numerically almost the same as the ratio of the corresponding expected information (the relative statistical efficiency).

For the mating type discussed above, Table 7.2 shows the relative ELOD, R, associated with various values of penetrance, f, and recombination fraction, r. It strongly depends on the penetrance but comparatively little on the recombination fraction. For example, with a penetrance of 50%, the ELOD is reduced to approximately ⅓ of its value under full penetrance. Consequently, one needs three times as many observations with $f = 50\%$ than with full penetrance to obtain the same ELOD. Generally, with a relative ELOD of R, the number of observations required must be multiplied by $1/R$. As another example, at $f = 0.20$, Table 7.2 shows $R \approx 0.1$, so that $1/R = 10$ times the number of observations are required for the same ELOD as under full penetrance. Of course, these calculations are based on the assumption of unselected offspring phenotypes. If affected offspring are sampled preferentially as it is customary for most disease loci, results may be somewhat different from the ones presented above. Also, it has been assumed here that penetrance is known but this is rarely the case. When penetrance in the analysis is different from the true penetrance, the recombination fraction estimate tends to be biased (see Section 11.3). In particular, when penetrance is incomplete yet full penetrance is assumed in the analysis, the estimate of the recombination fraction is biased upwards. This will be discussed in Chapter 11.

Table 7.2. Ratio of Expected Lod Scores at True Recombination Fraction, r, Under Incomplete Penetrance, f, versus Full Penetrance

f	Recombination Fraction, r					
	0^a	0.01	0.05	0.10	0.20	0.50^a
1	1	1	1	1	1	1
0.95	0.855	0.867	0.883	0.891	0.899	0.905
0.90	0.758	0.769	0.787	0.798	0.809	0.818
0.80	0.610	0.618	0.634	0.644	0.656	0.667
0.50	0.311	0.314	0.319	0.323	0.328	0.333
0.20	0.108	0.108	0.109	0.110	0.110	0.111

[a] Limiting values.

In principle, there is no lower bound on the penetrance below which linkage analysis could not be carried out. With a very low penetrance, one simply needs a much larger set of data. For example, the gene for dystonia was successfully mapped to the long arm of chromosome 9 although penetrance is only about 30%.

7.3. Estimating Penetrance and Recombination Fraction

With respect to diseases, penetrance is the probability that a susceptible individual is affected. In principle, therefore, the penetrance f is estimated as the proportion of affecteds among susceptible individuals. The problem is that it is not always easy to find a collection of susceptible individuals and to estimate the proportion of affecteds in an unbiased manner. While a detailed coverage of penetrance estimation is beyond the scope of this book (such a topic falls into the realm of segregation analysis; see example in Section 7.5), a few simple approaches are given below. Initially, only the penetrance for genetic cases is considered, with the penetrance for phenocopies taken to be zero.

Penetrance for Genetic Cases. When a rare dominant disease segregates in a sibship, only one of the parents is expected to carry the disease allele, and that parent may or may not be affected. On average, half of the offspring will receive the disease allele and, of those, a proportion f will develop the disease. The proportion of affected offspring is thus $p_A = \frac{1}{2}f$ so that $2p_A$ may be taken as an estimate of f. The relevant procedure for estimating f would then be to find affected individuals and count affected and unaffected individuals among their offspring, including sibships without affecteds. The penetrance estimate is simply double the estimate of p_A (or four times the estimate of p_A for a recessive disease). If the estimate of f exceeds 1, then 1 is taken to be the penetrance estimate.

In practice, it is far easier to collect sibships through an affected sibling, the proband. That way, however, one misses sibships not containing any affected individuals, which would lead to an *ascertainment bias,* if estimation of f is carried out as described in the previous paragraph. Properly correcting for ascertainment biases is difficult (Greenberg, 1986; see also Section 7.5 on age-dependent penetrance; for an overview of ascertainment biases and their statistical treatment, see Ewens, 1991). The easiest ascertainment correction is to leave off the proband from all calculations, which is known as Weinberg's (1927) proband method. If

k_i is the number of affecteds in the ith sibship of size n_i, the corrected estimate for the proportion of affecteds is given by

$$\hat{p}_A = \frac{\sum_i (k_i - 1)}{\sum_i (n_i - 1)}. \tag{7.1}$$

In large pedigrees segregating a dominant disease, when pedigrees are collected on the basis of one or a few probands (and not because they contain a large number of affecteds), effects of ascertainment are probably small (Elston, 1973). Thus, one may estimate the penetrance numerically using one of the programs for linkage analysis. This may be done by repeatedly calculating the likelihood with respect to f until an approximate maximum likelihood estimate of f is found (the ILINK program can estimate penetrances iteratively although obtaining reasonable estimates for more than one penetrance has in practice appeared difficult).

Thus far, our discussion of penetrance estimation has focused on one locus only (the one with possibly incomplete penetrance). However, it is often useful to incorporate in these estimates information from phenotypes at a closely linked marker locus. This may be beneficial, for example, when in a large pedigree some parents are unaffected so that it is unclear with what probability offspring are susceptible. Marker information may then be able to help identify the carrier status of unaffected individuals.

In a collection of large pedigrees, or whenever else ascertainment biases can be ignored, the joint estimation of penetrance f and recombination fraction θ is carried out best by calculating the likelihood, $L(f, \theta)$, for various pairs of values, (f, θ). $L(f, \theta)$ may then be pictured as the height above a plane with coordinates f and θ, and estimates of f and θ are determined by the maximum of $L(f, \theta)$. An example of such an estimation may be found in Rossen at al. (1980). Notice that it is the likelihood (or log likelihood) that is to be maximized, not the lod score (but see Chapter 15 for a discussion of the mod score).

When a test for linkage is carried out, one generally compares the maximum of the likelihood $L(\theta)$ under linkage with the likelihood, $L(\frac{1}{2})$, under absence of linkage, the relevant test statistic being the maximum lod score, $Z_{max} = \log[L(\hat{\theta})/L(\frac{1}{2})]$. If penetrance is incomplete, an analogous test statistic is

$$Z_{max} = \log[L(f, \hat{\theta})/L(f, \frac{1}{2})]. \tag{7.2}$$

In regular cases, under no linkage, $4.6 \times Z_{max}$ then corresponds to a chi-square variable with 1 df. This involves no particular problem when the penetrance is known. In practice, however, penetrance is often estimated and estimates may be correlated. Then, a suitable approach is to treat the penetrance as a nuisance parameter, that is, to obtain separate estimates of f under linkage $(\hat{f})$ and under no linkage $(\tilde{f})$ so that the maximum lod score is given by

$$Z_{max} = \log[L(\hat{f}, \hat{\theta})/L(\tilde{f}, \tfrac{1}{2})], \tag{7.3}$$

where $L(\hat{f},\hat{\theta}) = \max_{f,\theta}L(f, \theta)$ and $L(\tilde{f}, \tfrac{1}{2}) = \max_f L(f, \tfrac{1}{2})$.

To construct a support interval for θ, lod scores at various values of θ from 0 through $\tfrac{1}{2}$ must be available. According to the principle leading to equation (7.3), at any given θ, lod scores should be computed as $Z(\theta, \cdot) = \log[L(\hat{f}_\theta, \theta)/L(\tilde{f}, \tfrac{1}{2})]$. That is, the likelihood in the numerator is maximized over f at each θ value. A 3-lod-unit support interval then consists of all those θ values for which $Z(\theta, \cdot) \geq Z(\hat{\theta}, \cdot) - 3$. If a fixed value of f in numerator and denominator is used for the construction of a support interval, the resulting interval tends to be too small; such a support interval is appropriate only for a known penetrance value.

All Penetrances Nonzero. In many diseases, there is incomplete penetrance (for genetic cases) and occurrence of phenocopies. Estimating these penetrances, particularly in selected pedigrees, is difficult and not considered here any further (but see Chapter 15). In analogy to the discussion above, one might consider treating both penetrances—that for genetic and nongenetic cases—as nuisance parameters, but this is not usually feasible in practice. For example, the ILINK program does not allow restrictions such as $f_{DD} > f_{Dd}$. A particular approach is from Curtis and Sham (1995a). These authors treat penetrances as nuisance parameters but do so under suitable restrictions, for example, that the penetrance for genetic cases should be larger than that for phenocopies, and all parameters are restrained by the condition of a fixed population prevalence of the disease. This method has been implemented in a computer program, MFLINK (Curtis and Sham, 1995a). Another approach is to maximize the lod score (rather than the likelihood) over multiple penetrances. This so-called mod score method is discussed further in Section 15.4.

The remainder of this section is devoted to two rather theoretical aspects of the joint estimation of penetrance and recombination fraction and might only be relevant to readers interested in statistical genetics. The first point of discussion is that generally these estimates are correlated. The section will conclude with a demonstration that these estimates must generally be biased.

Correlation between Estimates. For offspring of a particular simple mating type such as the phase-known double backcross considered in the previous section, it is straightforward to calculate the asymptotic correlation coefficient, $\rho(\hat{f}, \hat{\theta})$ via the inverse of the information matrix [equation (5.9)]. One obtains

$$\rho = \frac{f(1 - 2r)\sqrt{r(1 - r)}}{\sqrt{1 - f + 2f^2r(1 - r)(1 - 2r)[1 - r])}}, \tag{7.5}$$

where f and r refer to true parameter values. The correlation coefficient is positive for $r < \frac{1}{2}$ and equal to 0 for $r = \frac{1}{2}$. For given r, ρ is largest at $f = 1$. At small values of r, the correlation coefficient is equal to 0.70 for $f = 1$ and gradually drops to 0.12 for $f = 0.70$ and to 0.03 for $f = 0.30$.

Analogous calculations may be carried out for larger families. For example, assume a family composed of a phase-known double backcross mating $D1/d2 \times d2/d2$, with a daughter of this mating married to a $d2/d2$ man, and their son. When the correlation coefficient between $\hat{f}$ and $\hat{\theta}$ is calculated from the joint phenotype distribution of the daughter and her son, that correlation turns out to be negative but, in the range $0 < f \leq 1$, $0 < r \leq \frac{1}{2}$, is never larger than 0.32 in absolute value. In practice, correlation coefficients between estimates of f and r may be obtained numerically from the curvature of the log likelihood surface at the joint ML estimates (VARCO6 program; see Section 9.5).

Biased Estimates. A statistically interesting aspect of jointly estimating f and r is that, in simple situations, estimates can be obtained analytically as transformations of multinomial proportions. For example, for the phase-known double backcross mating $D1/d2 \times d1/d1$ considered previously in this section and the previous section, there are four types of offspring, $D1$, $d2$, $D2$, $d1$ (Table 7.1), with respective probabilities of occurrence $p_1 = \frac{1}{2}(1 - r)f$, $p_2 = \frac{1}{2}(1 - rf)$, $p_3 = \frac{1}{2}rf$, and $p_4 = \frac{1}{2}(1 - f + rf)$. Consider the first three proportions, p_1, p_2, and p_3 (p_4 is just their complement to 1). Because of the linear constraint, $p_2 + p_3 = \frac{1}{2}$, the three proportions are defined by two degrees of freedom. Thus, the parameters r and f may be directly expressed in terms of two of the multinomial proportions (class probabilities). Solving p_1 and p_3 for f and r leads to

$$f = 2(p_1 + p_3), \quad r = p_3/(p_1 + p_3). \tag{7.6}$$

Estimates of f and r are obtained when the p's in (7.6) are replaced by their estimates. Equation (7.6) provides a striking example of biased MLEs in human genetics. The existence of the bias may be seen as follows: Estimates of the multinomial probabilities, p_i, are unbiased and assume values ranging from 0 through 1. However, the limited ranges of f and r in (7.6) impose severe restrictions on the ranges of p_1 and p_3, which induces bias. First, the requirement, $0 \le f \le 1$, imposes the restriction, $p_1 \le \frac{1}{2} - p_3$. In Figure 7.1, this limits the range of possible values of p_1 and p_3 to points underneath the line, $p_1 = \frac{1}{2} - p_3$. In addition, the requirement for $0 \le r \le \frac{1}{2}$ imposes the restriction, $p_1 \ge p_3$, which corresponds to points above the line, $p_1 = p_3$. The two conditions together limit the range of possible values for p_1 and p_3 to the hatched triangle in Figure 7.1. These restrictions must bias the resulting estimates of f and r. However, for large sets of observations, the bias is expected to be small as MLEs generally are consistent.

7.4. Factors Influencing Penetrance

As it is outlined in Section 9.2, penetrance (the conditional probability of a phenotype given a genotype) forms an integral part of the pedigree likelihood. In many applications, penetrance depends on a number of covariates such as age or sex. In linkage analysis, the effect of such variables is generally taken into account by forming so-called liability classes (penetrance classes) and, for each class, defining an appropriate set of penetrances. Likelihoods are then generally calculated with parameter values assumed to be known. For example, sex differences in penetrance may be taken into account by distinguishing two sets of age classes,

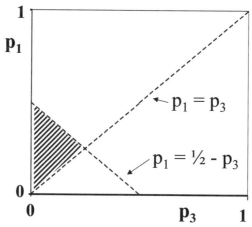

Figure 7.1. Restricted ranges of p_1 and p_3 in the estimation of f and θ.

one for males and one for females. Another example is presence or absence of cytogenetic abnormalities in the fragile X syndrome. The important case of age-dependent penetrance will be covered in the next section.

Incomplete penetrance for a disease implies randomness in the occurrence of the disease. It is usually assumed that unspecified environmental factors determine the probability with which a susceptible genotype expresses the disease. Alternatively, other genes might epistatically interact with the disease gene such that genetic factors at other loci are responsible for incomplete penetrance at the disease locus. Computer simulation experiments have shown (Greenberg and Hodge, 1989) that the source of the reduction in penetrance has little influence on the outcome of linkage analyses.

Occurrence of phenocopies represents a type of heterogeneity (i.e., genetic versus nongenetic cases). Among phenocopies, one may distinguish two forms, genetic and nongenetic forms, where "genetic phenocopies" or "genocopies" represent individuals whose disease is due to a gene other than the one being studied, whereas "nongenetic phenocopies" are affected due to some unspecified environmental agent. In linkage analysis, both forms are generally accounted for in a single-locus disease model although, ideally, a two-locus model would be more appropriate for genetic phenocopies. Durner et al. (1996) investigated effects of both forms of phenocopies on single-locus linkage analysis and concluded that in the presence of nongenetic phenocopies, the actual value of the penetrance for phenocopies matters little as long as it is positive. With genetic phenocopies (when a two-locus trait is analyzed under single-locus assumptions), it depends on the actual genetic model what value of the phenocopy penetrance is appropriate for optimal linkage information but the specific choice of phenocopy penetrance does not lead to an increase in false positive linkage results. Durner et al. (1996) recommended testing a few small values of the phenocopy penetrance for their effect on the maximum lod score, which is reminiscent of the mod score method covered in Chapter 15.

7.5. Age-Dependent Penetrance and Segregation Analysis

Several genetic traits, for example, breast cancer, are not expressed at birth and develop only later in life. That is, penetrance is age dependent. If penetrance for genetic *and* nongenetic cases is positive and age-dependent, estimating these penetrances must be carried out in a careful segregation analysis (for some simple approaches, see below). Segregation analysis refers to a collection of methods and techniques that fall into the realm of (genetic) epidemiology and are not covered in this book. A few aspects of segregation analysis are mentioned here only in passing. An excellent example is that of breast cancer, which is outlined in the following paragraphs on segregation analysis.

Segregation Analysis. Using data from a large population-based, case-control study conducted by the Centers for Disease Control (usually referred as the CASH study) (Wingo et al., 1988), Claus et al. (1991) carried out a segregation analysis on approximately 4700 breast cancer cases and about the same number of matched control individuals. In addition, mothers and sisters of cases and controls were included. Segregation analysis was performed using the POINTER program (Lalouel and Yee, 1980), which is commonly used for this purpose. For nuclear families, it determines the likelihood under various modes of inheritance and allows for the estimation of genetic parameters and statistical comparison among modes of inheritance. Claus et al. (1991) concluded that an autosomal dominant model provided the best fit to the data and that the effect of genotype on risk was greatest at a young age and declined with increasing age. Risk of breast cancer to a mother or sister of a breast cancer case was seen to increase with decreasing age at disease onset of the proband; that is, heritability of the trait is greatest with early onset age, which is a common observation for many diseases. These conclusions were beautifully confirmed by the localization of a breast cancer gene, *BRCA1,* to chromosome 17q (Hall et al., 1990) (the Claus et al. [1991] paper was submitted before the Hall et al. [1990] finding was published). Now, several loci influencing breast cancer and different disease alleles with different penetrances are known. In the analysis of Hall et al. (1990), families with a low mean age of disease onset showed much clearer evidence for linkage than families with an elevated mean of onset ages.

An earlier analysis of the same data showed that there was a genetic correlation between breast and ovarian cancer, and that endometrial cancer was genetically unrelated (Schildkraut et al., 1989), which is another example of how epidemiology can sometimes usefully predict genetic circumstances.

Simple Approach: Onset Age Unknown. As outlined previously, penetrance is the conditional probability of being affected given an individual is genetically susceptible (has a ''disease genotype''). If penetrance varies with age, then penetrance at age x, $F(x)$, is the conditional probability of becoming affected, that is, of developing the disease, by age x, where F is usually referred to as a *penetrance curve*. A conceptually easy approach is then to define age classes, where the kth class comprises individuals between the ages of x_{k-1} and x_k. At the lower bound of the kth age class, penetrance is $F(x_{k-1})$, and at the upper bound it is $F(x_k)$, which generally exceeds $F(x_{k-1})$ owing to those susceptible developing disease in the given age interval. The graph of F is a step function with jumps at each class boundary. In practice, for all ages in the kth age class, penetrance is usually taken to be constant,

$$f(x_k) = \tfrac{1}{2}[F(x_{k-1}) + F(x_k)]. \tag{7.7}$$

For different age classes, values of $f(x_k)$ are generally used as (narrow sense) penetrances in computer programs such as LINKAGE (where penetrance classes are called liability classes). In the LIPED program, which uses penetrances in the general sense, values of $f(x_k)$ are penetrances for affecteds; the corresponding penetrances for unaffecteds are given by $1 - f(x_k)$.

If phenocopies are assumed to be absent, affecteds are known to carry the disease allele, no matter what their age. Hence, only one penetrance class for affecteds is needed, provided that, for a given age, all susceptible genotypes have the same penetrances. Generally, whenever penetrances for one phenotype or penetrance class can be obtained from those for another by multiplication by a constant factor, these two sets of phenotypes require only one penetrance class (multiplication by a constant changes the likelihood but leaves the lod score unchanged). For example, consider genotypes d/d, D/d, and D/D and, for some age class, assume a penetrance array of $(0, 0.17, 0.17)$ for affecteds. At high age, assume full penetrance (i.e., a penetrance array of $[(0, 1, 1)]$). This array of values can be obtained from $(0, 0.17, 0.17)$ by multiplying values in the latter by $1/0.17$. That is, for linkage analysis, only one penetrance array for affected individuals in these two classes is needed. For unaffected individuals, the corresponding two penetrance arrays are $(1, 0.83, 0.83)$ and $(1, 0, 0)$, and the former cannot be translated into the latter by multiplication by a constant. That is, different penetrance classes are required for unaffecteds.

In a given study, how should a suitable penetrance curve be set up? Practice shows that the particular penetrance curve in a linkage study is not crucial as long as age-dependent penetrance is somehow allowed for. Thus, a crude but often adequate approach is to work with straight lines as follows: Define x_1 and x_2 as the respective earliest and latest ages at which anyone ever expressed disease, and assume that penetrance rises linearly from 0 to 1. This leads to the penetrance curve,

$$F(x) = \begin{cases} 0 & \text{if } x \leq x_1 \\ (x - x_1)/(x_2 - x_1) & \text{if } x_1 < x < x_2 \\ 1 & \text{if } x \geq x_2. \end{cases} \tag{7.8}$$

Estimating Age-of-Onset Curves. Ideally, age-dependent penetrances are estimated on the basis of a sample of susceptible individuals. In practice, one usually proceeds in a retrospective rather than prospective way by focusing on a collection of affecteds whose ages at disease onset are recorded. The cumulative distribution of these onset ages is then used as an age-of-onset curve, F. This method suffers from serious drawbacks (Heimbuch et al., 1980; Chen et al., 1993) because effects of population age distribution (age-dependent mortality) and penetrance are confounded, but it nonetheless is often applied in practice. For sophisticated determination of penetrances, methods of genetic epidemiology must be applied (see breast cancer example, above).

To apply approximate methods based on known affected individuals, one may proceed by recording ages, x, at disease onset for these individuals. Age classes are then formed as shown above so that x_k is the upper boundary of the kth age class. $F(x_k)$ is then estimated by the proportion of all affecteds who developed the disease by age x_k, $\hat{F}(x_k)$. The graph of $\hat{F}(x_k)$ will usually take a sigmoid shape. As a simple example, consider the four age categories taken from Table 3 in Bird and Kraft (1978), which presents age at onset of Charcot–Marie–Tooth disease (the example is for illustration purposes only and disregards the known genetic heterogeneity in this disease). Among the 53 affected individuals, 18 had onset by age 10, so that $\hat{F}(10) = 18/53 = 0.34$. By age 15, $18 + 21 = 39$ had onset so that $\hat{F}(15) = 39/53 = 0.74$. By age 20, $18 + 21 + 9 = 48$ had onset so that $\hat{F}(20) = 0.90$. The remaining five individuals developed disease at a later age, say, by age 30, so that $\hat{F}(30) = 1$. Penetrances appropriate for the different age classes would then be computed according to equation (7.7). For the given example, one obtains $f(x_1) = \frac{1}{2}(0 + 0.34) = 0.17$ (for age class 1), $f(x_2) = \frac{1}{2}(0.34 + 0.74) = 0.54$, $f(x_3) = 0.82$, and $f(x_4) = 0.95$.

Instead of estimating penetrances in different age classes, one may determine the functional form of an age-of-onset curve $F(x)$, for example, the cumulative normal or lognormal distribution function. A particularly suitable curve is the logistic distribution,

$$F(x) = \cfrac{1}{1 + \exp\left(-c\cfrac{x - \mu}{\sigma}\right)}, \qquad (7.9)$$

where μ and σ are the respective mean and standard deviation of age at onset, and $c = \pi/\sqrt{3} = 1.8138$ is a constant. For example, in Bird and Kraft (1978), mean and standard deviation for age at onset are estimated as 12.2 and 7.3 years, respectively. With this, equation (7.9) yields for a susceptible individual at age 5 a disease penetrance of $F(5) = 0.143$. A convenient property of the logistic distribution (7.9) is that it has a closed-form inverse,

$$F^{-1}(\cdot) = x = \mu - (\sigma/c) \ln[(1 - F)/F], \qquad (7.10)$$

which yields the onset age corresponding to a given penetrance. For example, with $\mu = 12.2$ and $\sigma = 7.3$, a penetrance of $F = 0.99$ leads to $x = 30.7$; that is, it is expected that, by age 31, 99% of all *susceptible* individuals will have expressed the disease.

Other functional forms for the age-of-onset distribution have been used. These curves are generally characterized by a small number of parameters which may be estimated numerically from pedigree data using one of the linkage programs. Estimating parameters from pedigree data rather than from a sample of unrelated affected individuals tends to be more reliable as information from unaffecteds is used as well. Notice, however, that such estimates do not incorporate any ascertainment corrections.

Allowing for Age at Disease Onset. Thus far, the disease phenotype has been considered as a qualitative trait with two outcomes, affected and unaffected, with penetrances for affected being age-dependent. Age at disease onset has not been used in pedigree likelihood calculations except perhaps to estimate an age-of-onset curve. For many diseases with genetic and nongenetic forms, genetically susceptible individuals tend to have an earlier age of onset than phenocopies. Thus, it is advantageous to incorporate age at disease onset into the pedigree likelihood. This amounts to replacing the qualitative affected status phenotype by a quantitative variable, $x = $ age at disease onset (a general discussion of quantitative traits is given in Chapter 8). Age of onset is then treated as a random variable and the age-of-onset curve, $F(x)$, discussed above is the so-called distribution function of x, while $f(x)$ is its density (generally bell-shaped), that is, the height of the curve $F(x)$ at age x. Statistically, $F(x) = \int_{-\infty}^{x} f(t)dt$. For example, the distribution function defined by (7.8) corresponds to a uniform age-of-onset density, $f(x) = 1/(x_2 - x_1)$ for $x_1 < x < x_2$ and $f(x) = 0$ otherwise, with mean $\mu = \frac{1}{2}(x_2 - x_1)$ and standard deviation $\sigma = (x_2 - x_1)/\sqrt{12}$. In the pedigree likelihood (4.17), penetrance for the qualitative disease phenotype is replaced with the density, $f(x)$. Much of the treatment of age of onset in these sections is based on survival analysis methods (Elston, 1973). The following phenotypes must be distinguished:

- Affected individual with known age, x, at disease onset: The phenotype is x and the corresponding conditional likelihood, given a susceptible genotype, is $f(x)$. In computer programs, one usually groups individuals into age classes and, in each class, uses the average of $f(x)$ as the density representative for each individual in that class. In the LINKAGE programs, such classes would still be called penetrance or liability classes. However, the values of $f(x)$, being densities, may assume values larger than 1 and cannot be interpreted the same way as penetrances.
- Affected individual, age of onset unavailable: The phenotype is qualitative ("affected") with the penetrance being determined by the current age (or age last seen), a. For given age, a, affected status is a binomial variable, that is, the probability of being affected is $F(a)$, which is the penetrance. When current age is unavailable it should be estimated, for example, from the ages of siblings.
- Unaffected individual, current age is a: Disease status is censored at current age (or age last seen). Penetrance for being unaffected is $1 - F(a)$.

Penetrance at high age may never reach 100% but may stay at some lower level, t. Then, the age at onset distribution may be defined as $G(x) = F(x)$ with probability t, and $G(x) = 0$ with probability $1 - t$, where, for example, $F(x)$ is the straight-line age at onset distribution (7.8). This leads to the following straight-line age-of-onset distribution with incomplete penetrance, t, at high age:

$$G(x) = \begin{cases} 0 & \text{if } x \leq x_1 \\ t(x - x_1)/(x_2 - x_1) & \text{if } x_1 < x < x_2 \\ t & \text{if } x \geq x_2. \end{cases} \tag{7.11}$$

When the age x at disease onset is known, the density corresponding to (7.11) is given by $g(x) = t/(x_2 - x_1)$ if $x_1 < x < x_2$ and $g(x) = 0$ otherwise.

These parametrizations have been implemented in the PC-LIPED program. When age-of-onset curves are to be used with other programs, one must make certain that the phenotype of each individual is associated with the corresponding appropriate penetrance. Actual age at disease onset is relevant only when disease can occur with different nonproportional penetrances for different genotypes. If this is not so (in many cases it is not), then one may just use current age and disregard the age at disease onset (this is how age-of-onset curves are usually handled). This is incorrect, however, in the presence of phenocopies unless, at any age, penetrances for nonsusceptible genotypes are constant multiples of those for susceptible genotypes. Of course, if the age-at-onset distribution is to be estimated from family data, then age at disease onset (not current age) should be used whenever it is known.

As an example, in an analysis of familial osteoarthrosis (Palotie et al., 1989), equation (7.8) was used as the age-at-onset distribution for individuals with a genetic predisposition ($x_1 = 0$ and $x_2 = 60$ years of age; full penetrance at age 60 and above). In addition, for nongenetic cases (phenocopies), onset was also assumed to be age dependent [equation (7.11)] with $t = 0.80$, $x_1 = 40$, and $x_2 = 100$ years of age because, at high age, close to 80% of individuals in the Finnish population suffer from osteoarthrosis. Discrimination between genetic and nongenetic cases is modeled primarily through the difference in ages of onset and to a lesser degree through incomplete penetrance in nongenetic cases. Positive values for the densities of age at onset for genetic and nongenetic cases overlap only for ages 40 through 60. Thus, with this parametrization, any onset at age below 40 must be a genetic case, and any onset above age 60 must be a nongenetic case. Within the age range of $x = 40$ through 60 years, the (uniform) density $g(x)$ for genetic cases is 25% higher than that for phenocopies. That is, a priori, an individual with onset age between 40 and 60 years of age is somewhat more likely to be a genetic than a nongenetic case. The positive linkage finding of this study was later confirmed by the detection of a base-pair substitution in the type 2 collagen gene, which was present in all affected members of a large family and absent in unaffected individuals (Ala-Kokko et al., 1990).

Based on the analysis of Claus et al. (1991) (see paragraph on segregation analysis, above), Easton et al. (1993) used slightly modified penetrance functions in a linkage analysis of a large set of breast cancer families. They assumed a dominant mode of inheritance with age-dependent penetrance and disease allele frequency of 0.0033. Figure 7.2 shows the penetrance curves (distribution functions) applied by these authors for unaffected females, where $G(x)$ is the conditional probability of being affected by age x, with penetrances at high age of $t = 0.801$ for genetic cases and $t = 0.082$ for phenocopies. While tables published by Easton et al. (1993) contain constant average values of $G(x)$ within each

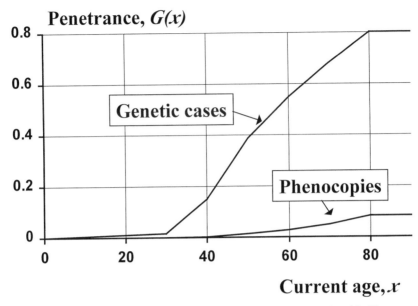

Figure 7.2. Age-of-onset curve $F(x)$ from small sample of affecteds with Charcot–Marie–Tooth disease. x = age of onset.

(typically 10-year) age interval, Figure 7.2 shows linear increases in each interval such that the average per interval, except for the last interval, is as given by Easton et al. (1993). Figure 7.3 shows the corresponding densities for affected females with onset age, x.

7.6. Penetrance for Monozygotic Twins

Fraternal or dizygotic (DZ) twins are generally handled in linkage analysis just like any other siblings, that is, any special environmental effects common to DZ twins are usually disregarded. However, this is different for monozygotic (MZ) twins. They represent two phenotypic expressions of a single genotype. Whereas the MENDEL program has a provision for handling MZ twins, this is not the case for other linkage programs such as LIPED and LINKAGE.

For simplicity, assume that the phenotypes of the two MZ twins are conditionally independent given a disease genotype. This is perhaps unrealistic but allows for a rather simple way of dealing with this situation. Let x_1 and x_2 be the phenotypes observed on two MZ twins. For example, x_1 = "affected" and x_2 = "unaffected." Given a disease genotype, g,

Density for age at onset

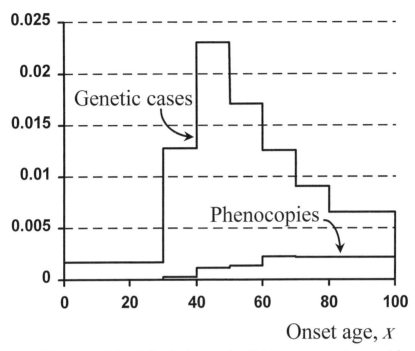

Figure 7.3. Density $f(x)$ and distribution function $F(x)$ for age at onset assumed for familial osteoarthrosis. (Data from Palotie et al., 1989.)

the associated conditional penetrances are $P(x_1|g)$ and $P(x_2|g)$. Under our assumption of independence, the penetrance for the two observations jointly is given by the product, $P(x_1|g)P(x_2|g)$. In a linkage program not explicitly allowing for MZ twins, one may replace a pair of MZ twins by a single contrived individual with phenotype x such that $P(x|g) = P(x_1|g)P(x_2|g)$ for each genotype. A worked example is given in Section 11.2 of Terwilliger and Ott (1994). Note that analogous considerations apply to quantitative phenotypes. Penetrances are then simply replaced by densities.

7.7. Problems

Problem 7.1. For some disease with age-dependent penetrance, assume a straight-line age-of-onset curve, starting with $F(x_1) = 0$ at age

$x_1 = 5$ years and ending with $F(x_2) = 1$ at age $x_2 = 40$ years. At what age are 80% of all susceptible individuals expected to have expressed the disease?

Problem 7.2. Based on Figure 7.2, for a healthy woman at 60 years of age, what is her probability of remaining free of breast cancer (through age 80) if she is (a) genetically susceptible or (b) genetically nonsusceptible?

Problem 7.3. Under the same assumptions as in Problem 7.2, what is the desired probability if susceptibility status is unknown?

Disclaimer: Calculations for Problems 7.2 and 7.3 are made under simplified assumptions (e.g., of only a single breast cancer gene and homogeneity). These problems are for illustration purposes only and are not recommended for genetic counseling situations unless all known factors are taken into account.

8.

Quantitative Phenotypes

A quantitative trait is a phenotype with a continuous (rather than a discrete) distribution. The normal and lognormal distributions are typical of such distributions. For example, the cholesterol level in the blood is often assumed to range between 0 and infinity. Distributions are characterized by their statistical moments, particularly by mean and variance. These moments may depend on factors such as age and sex. If they depend on the genotype of a mendelian gene locus, then such a locus is called a quantitative trait locus (QTL). For example, the QTL may have two alleles, a normal allele, t, and a disease allele, T, where the latter has a low population frequency, such as 0.01. The phenotype may follow a normal distribution with a fixed variance but with means being genotype dependent. For instance, means may be 100, 100, and 150 for the respective genotypes t/t, T/t, and T/T, so that the T allele is recessive; homozygotes T/T have phenotype values that are shifted upwards by 50 units.

Although it is usually the mean of the QTL that is taken to depend on mendelian genotypes, traits have been described in which the means are unvarying and the genetic message lies in other aspects of the distribution such as the variance (Murphy and Trojak, 1986). In a series of papers, E.A. Murphy has developed theory for the analysis of such traits.

More than one observation may be made on an individual, in which case the phenotype is called multivariate. For example, in the LINKAGE programs, the genotype-specific component of a QTL may follow a multivariate normal distribution with a mean vector and a variance–covariance matrix.

A multivariate phenotype may consist of quantitative and qualitative variables (e.g., cholesterol level and affection status) but analysis of such QTLs is not directly possible with the current implementation of the LINKAGE programs. An ad hoc way of handling this situation has been described (Ott, 1995a) but is not considered here.

Section 8.1 will discuss the notion of a mixture of distributions. In Sections 8.2 and 8.3, a simple treatment of QTLs for linkage analysis is given (more sophisticated approaches are by way of variance components). Several other methods for using quantitative phenotypes in linkage analyses have been proposed, for example, by Haseman and Elston (1972), Hill (1975), Smith (1975), and Cockerham and Weir (1983). In Section 8.5, variance components for quantitative traits will be introduced.

8.1. Mixed Distributions

Consider a quantitative measurement, x, such as stature (body height). If measured on a large number of men, for all practical purposes, stature follows a normal distribution, $f_1(x)$, with a certain mean, μ_1. Stature of women also is normally distributed, $f_2(x)$, but with a somewhat smaller mean, μ_2. In the population, for men and women together, the distribution of body height is a mixture of two components,

$$f(x) = p_1 f_1(x; \mu_1) + p_2 f_2(x; \mu_2), \tag{8.1}$$

where the weights, $p_1 + p_2 = 1$, represent the relative proportions of individuals in the two components. Analogously, a QTL under the control of a mendelian locus may have a mixed distribution, where the "normal" or "unaffected" component has mean μ_1 and the "abnormal" component has mean μ_2. For example, in familial hypercholesterolemia, $\mu_2 > \mu_1$. As another example, in osteoporosis, the quantitative measurement is bone mineral density, where $\mu_2 < \mu_1$. For rare diseases, $p_2 \ll p_1$. For practical reasons, the standard deviation, σ, is often assumed to be the same for the two components. Depending on the distance, $d = (\mu_2-\mu_1)/\sigma$, between the two components, the mixed distribution may be bimodal or unimodal. With $p_1 = p_2 = \frac{1}{2}$, the distribution is bimodal when $d > 2$ (see Problem 8.1).

The next two sections introduce a simple approach at estimating parameters of mixture distributions for unrelated individuals and for family members. In practice, quantitative phenotypes are often analyzed by defining a cutoff point separating abnormal (high) from normal (low) values, which creates a qualitative phenotype with two classes, affecteds and unaffecteds. In principle, removing the overlap by creating two distinct classes leads to an increase in misclassifications and to a bias in parameter estimates. Mixed observations should be analyzed under a model of a mixture of distributions whenever possible. On the other hand, forming distinct classes obviates the need for estimating means and standard deviations.

8.2. Parameter Estimation for Unrelated Individuals

The first step in a QTL analysis is to establish whether there is good evidence for a mixture of components versus a single component of the phenotype. This involves obtaining parameter estimates under the assumption of one, two, or more components. In this section, presence of a set of unrelated individuals is assumed. If the analysis procedures covered in this section are applied to family members, results are only approximate because familial relationships are disregarded; refinement of the results must then be obtained, for example, by procedures discussed in the next section.

Once evidence for the presence of two components is obtained (perhaps in the form of a bimodality), the question is how to interpret this finding. One possibility might be that the data are heterogeneous; for example, we may have measured stature and have had males and females in our pool of data. When the interest is on genetic effects, differences due to such concomitant variables as age and sex are uninteresting. Although there are sophisticated approaches to take such covariates into account in the analysis (see Section 8.5), a common simple procedure is to adjust all data to a common age and sex prior to analysis. This is often done by linear regression on the basis of a sample from the general population sample.

In many situations, the most interesting case of admixture is that of two components, where the "abnormal" component may have an elevated or a low mean and may be associated with an "abnormal" genotype (an example may be found in Ott, 1979b). The abnormal component may correspond to one genotype, T/T (recessive case), or to two genotypes, T/t or T/T (dominant case). For unrelated individuals, these two cases cannot be distinguished.

To test for the presence of two components versus a single component, consider the null hypothesis, $H_0 : \mu_1 = \mu_2$, and the alternative hypothesis, $H_1 : \mu_1 \neq \mu_2$, where μ_i is the mean of the ith component. To test whether H_1 fits a sample of observations significantly better than H_0, one looks at the log likelihood obtained under each hypothesis. Under two components, the log likelihood is given by $L_1 = \Sigma \log[f(x_i)]$, where $f(x_i)$ is the density (8.1) for the ith observation. Under one component, one has $p_1 = 1$, which is equivalent to $\mu_1 = \mu_2$. Then, one forms the statistic, $G^2 = 2(L_1 - L_0)$, where L_i is the maximum log likelihood obtained under the ith hypothesis.

Because $\mu_1 = \mu_2$ forces $p_1 = 1$, G^2 does not have an asymptotic chi-square distribution. Often, it is nonetheless taken to approximately be chi-squared with 2 df. Computer simulations show that the p-value so obtained is somewhat too small, that is, the test based on the chi-square distribution with 2 df is liberal (nonconservative) (Thode et al., 1988). For a chi-square test with 2 df at the 5% significance level, the threshold of the test statistic is equal to 5.99. Instead of this limit, according to Thode et al. (1988), the somewhat higher limit, $6.08 + 4.51/\sqrt{n}$, should be used, where n is the number of observations (see also Section 10.4).

Parameter estimation under two components may be carried out numerically by iterative maximization of the log likelihood. A form of the EM algorithm has been implemented in the NOCOM program (available at http://linkage.rockefeller.edu), which carries out the analyses described in this section (references may be found in Ott, 1979b). For iterative likelihood maximization, suitable starting values for parameters are required. They are easiest to obtain from a histogram of observed x values.

A large normal component with a small abnormal component with slightly elevated mean will appear in the population as a trait phenotype with a skewed distribution. It is not easy to distinguish true skewness from a mixture of distributions. Also, the components in a mixture may themselves be skewed. Skewness may be allowed for by a suitable transformation, for example,

$$y = (x^\lambda - 1)/\lambda + \lambda. \tag{8.2}$$

In this power transformation, the limiting value of $\lambda = 0$ corresponds to $y = \log_e(x)$, and $\lambda = 1$ is equivalent to $y = x$. Although equation (8.2) requires $x \geq 0$, a constant c may be added to x to ensure that $x + c \geq 0$ (MacLean et al., 1976).

With unrelated individuals, a measure for the discrimination power between the two components of a distribution mixture is the standardized difference between the two means. A decreased standardized difference is indicative of a reduced discrimination power. Another measure is the difference in log likelihood achieved under each of the two hypotheses (one versus two components). When means and variance of a mixture are estimated based on pedigree members (related individuals), some individuals may be known to be in one or the other of the two components. For example, under dominant inheritance with low values corresponding to "disease," when a child has an extremely low value, one of the parents is expected to also have a low value. In that case, even a moderately low value of a parent will almost certainly identify that value as coming from the low component. Thus, knowledge of the mendelian rules adds information not available to analysis of unrelated individuals. The above example also demonstrates that the standardized difference between the two means no longer is a good indicator of discrimination power—a moderately low value (perhaps decreasing standardized difference) may be known to be in the low component and thus adds as much information as an extremely low value of an unrelated individual. Therefore, with related individuals, the only reliable measure of discrimination power is the difference in log likelihoods. This is discussed in the next section.

8.3. Parameter Estimation in Family Data

Estimates of mixture parameters based on unrelated individuals tend to be somewhat imprecise. Much information may be gained by the availability of observations on relatives. For example, under a mixture of two components for a rare dominant QTL with high values being abnormal, both parents may have low trait values. If an offspring has intermediate trait values, based largely on parental phenotypes, his phenotype most likely belongs to the low rather than the high component. Thus, misclassification tends to be much lower with observations on relatives than with independent observations.

Parameter estimation for family data cannot be carried out with the procedures described in the previous section, or only as a preliminary step. Computer programs such as ILINK of the LINKAGE package are available that allow the estimation of means and variances in the presence of observations on family members. Component weights are then given in terms of allele frequencies, which determine genotype probabilities of founder individuals in a family pedigree. Details may be found in Terwilliger and Ott (1994). Typically, initial parameter estimates are obtained with the NOCOM program in which observations on family members are treated as if they were independent. Then, refined estimates are furnished by the ILINK program that takes relationships among family members into account. For example, in a sample of 7 families comprising 37 individuals, the ILINK program estimated mean bone mineral density scores of $\mu_1 = -0.004$ and $\mu_2 = -1.656$ with a common standard deviation of $\sigma = 0.917$. This resulted in a standardized difference between the means of $d = (\mu_2 - \mu_1)/\sigma = -1.80$ (Spotila et al., 1996).

8.4. Informativeness of Overlapping Distributions

To elucidate the properties of the lod score method for quantitative traits, Lange, Spence, and Frank (1976) carried out a simulation study, in which susceptible and nonsusceptible genotypes were associated with two normal distributions separated by a certain difference in their mean values. They found that the peak lod score dropped from 4.5 for practically complete separation of the phenotype distributions to a value of about 1.7 when the difference between the means was 2 units of standard deviation. Although a drop of 2.8 units of lod score seems like a dramatic loss in information, one must remember that the sum of two normal distributions with a standardized mean difference of 2 or less is no longer multimodal. It is thus encouraging that, even with strongly overlapping distributions, one can still expect positive lod scores.

An overlap of quantitative phenotypes gives rise to misclassification, even when they are analyzed taking the overlap into account. Therefore, overlap of quantitative phenotypes leads to a reduction in the amount of information that data are capable of furnishing on the recombination fraction r. To quantify this loss of information, assume a normally distributed phenotype with standard deviation 1, divided into a large number, c, of classes. The density $f(x_i; \mu_g)$ is then replaced by a histogram, with one bell-shaped histogram for each of the two means, which are separated by $\Delta\mu = \mu_2 - \mu_1$. The conditional probability of occurrence of the phenotype x_i is its penetrance.

In addition to the main locus, assume a dominant marker locus with two alleles and two phenotypes, B and b. Consider a phase known double backcross mating $AB/ab \times ab/ab$. For the ith phenotype at the main locus let the penetrance be q_i when a given genotype contains the A allele, and p_i otherwise. With $\Delta\mu = 0$, one has $p_i = q_i$. The phenotypes, considered jointly at the two loci, occur with probabilities

$$P(x_i, B) = \tfrac{1}{2}[rp_i + (1 - r)q_i]$$
$$P(x_i, b) = \tfrac{1}{2}[(1 - r)p_i + rq_i], \tag{8.3}$$

where $i = 1 \ldots c$, and r is the true recombination fraction. From this, with a given difference $\Delta\mu$ of the means, Fisher's expected information per offspring is obtained as

$$i(r) = \tfrac{1}{4}\sum_{i=1}^{c} (p_i - q_i)^2[1/P(x_i, B) + 1/P(x_i, b)]. \tag{8.4}$$

For complete separation of the two distributions ($\Delta\mu = \infty$), $i(r)$ (8.4) becomes $1/[r(1 - r)]$ as it should be. Sample values of the relative efficiency, $i(r; \Delta\mu)/i(r; \Delta\mu = \infty)$, are given in Table 8.1. As one can see, as long as $\Delta\mu \geq 3$, the relative efficiency is no less than 47%; that is, the loss of information due to such an overlap may be compensated for by approximately doubling the number of observations. The values in Table 8.1 were obtained under the assumption of known means and variances. When these have to be estimated, efficiency is presumably lower.

Table 8.1. Relative Efficiency of the Recombination Fraction Estimate with Two Overlapping Distributions of the Phenotype at the Main Trait

$\Delta\mu$	Recombination Fraction, r				
	0.01	0.05	0.10	0.20	0.50
∞	1	1	1	1	1
5	0.92	0.96	0.97	0.97	0.97
4	0.77	0.85	0.88	0.90	0.92
3	0.47	0.62	0.69	0.74	0.78
2	0.15	0.30	0.39	0.46	0.52
1	0.02	0.06	0.10	0.14	0.19

8.5. Variance Components

The methods outlined above for quantitative traits are based on a very simple model. There are only two sources of variability, genetic variance due to differences in means between genotypes at a single locus, and variability around these means due to random environmental deviations. In this section, a few methods are briefly mentioned that go beyond the simple model considered thus far.

An early approach to allowing for additional sources of variability consisted of a model that allowed for a single major gene acting on a background of polygenes and random environmental variation (complex segregation analysis; Morton and MacLean, 1974). An alternative approach to working with a major gene and polygenic background was introduced by Hasstedt (1982).

Under an additive model for the effects of single genes, polygenes, common family environment, and other factors, the relative influences of these factors were more generally treated in terms of variance components (Ott, 1979a). As mentioned in Section 4.8, that formulation formed the basis for Bonney's (1984) regressive models and may be seen as an early version of today's sophisticated variance components methods. That early variance components approach was implemented in a computer program and applied to *IgE* levels in members of nuclear families, but computer time was prohibitively long for an efficient application of this method (Ott, 1979a).

Amos (1994) developed a variance-components approach, in which variability among trait observations from individuals within pedigrees is expressed in terms of fixed effects from covariates and effects due to an unobservable trait-affecting major locus, random polygenic effects, and residual nongenetic variance. The method allows for recombination between the major trait locus and a genetic marker.

Almasy and Blangero (1998) extended variance components methods to include multipoint linkage analysis in pedigrees of arbitrary size and complexity. They developed a general framework for multipoint identity-by-descent (IBD) probability calculations. The general IBB pedigree variance component and IBD estimation methods have been implemented in the SOLAR (Sequential Oligogenic Linkage Analysis Routines) computer package (Almasy and Blangero, 1998).

8.6. Problem

Problem 8.1. Show analytically that, in a mixture of two normal distributions with equal weights, there are two modes only when the standardized difference between the two component means exceeds 2. *Hint:* In $f(x)$ [equation (8.1)], assume $p_1 = p_2 = \frac{1}{2}$, $\mu_1 = 0$, $\mu_2 = m$. Then take the second derivative of $f(x)$ *w.r.* to x and evaluate it at the midpoint between the two component means, i.e. at $x = \frac{1}{2}m$, to find those values of m for which the second derivative is positive (i.e., where $f(x)$ is a minimum rather than a maximum).

9.

Numerical and Computerized Methods

Human linkage analysis applies statistical procedures to observations of family members. As in many applications of classical statistical methods such as analysis of variance, linkage analysis may involve extensive calculations. This aspect of linkage analysis will be covered in this chapter. It would be a mistake, however, to assume that carrying out a linkage analysis is basically a matter of using a computer program.

In some simple situations, it is possible to obtain the solution to a linkage problem by analytical means (see Section 9.1). In more complicated cases, analytical solutions may still be possible but are simply too tedious to carry out. One may then write a computer program or use one of the commercially available spreadsheet programs to find the desired solution. An example is provided in the second half of Section 9.1. Often, however, analytical solutions are not feasible, in which case so-called numerical methods may be applied, which generally result in any desired accuracy. Examples may be found in Section 9.4. Finally, some problems are so complex or time consuming to carry out that even numerical solutions are inappropriate, in which case one may resort to computer simulation (see Section 9.7).

9.1. Calculating Lod Scores Analytically

In Chapter 4, some simple lod scores were calculated. Below, for a few specific families (Ott and Frater-Schröder, 1981), it is demonstrated in detail how to derive two-point lod scores analytically. Instructive examples may also be found in Morton (1956). Four two-generation families have been selected for these exercises (Table 9.1). One of the loci used is that coding for transcobalamin II (TCN2, now known to be on chromosome 22), a vitamin B_{12} binding protein, whose alleles are numbered 1, 2, and 3. The marker locus is either HLA, whose haplotypes are designated by

Table 9.1. Four Families from a Linkage Investigation of TCN2

Family	Individual[a]	Phenotype	Possible Genotypes
Bu	F	⅓; a/b	(I) *1a/3b* or (II) *1b/3a*
	M	⅔; c/d	*3c/3d*
	S	⅔; a/c	*3a/3c*
	D	⅔; b/c	*3b/3c*
De	F	—	(I) *1a/3b* or (II) *1b/3a*
	M	⅔; c/d	*3c/3d*
	S	⅓; a/c	*1a/3c*
	D	⅓; b/c	*1b/3c*
	D	⅔; a/d	*3a/3d*
A47	F	⅓; O	*1o/3o*
	M	⅓; A	(I) *1a/3o* or (II) *1o/3a*
	S	⅓; O	*1o/3o*
	S	⅓; O	*1o/1o*
	S	⅔; A	*3a/3o*
B5	F	—	$(p)^2$ *3a/3o* or $(2p(1-p))$[*3a/xo* or *3o/xa*]
	M	⅓; O	*1o/1o*
	D	⅓; O	*3o/1o*
	S	⅓; A	*3a/1o*
	S	⅓; O	*3o/1o*

Source: Data from Ott and Frater-Schröder (1981).
[a] M = mother, F = father, D = daughter, S = son.

a, b, c, and *d,* or the ABO locus with alleles *a, b,* and *o* with phenotypes (blood types) *A, B, AB,* and *O.* Phases are distinguished by roman numerals, I, II, and so on.

Family Bu. Of the four individuals in family Bu, three unequivocally exhibit their genotypes through the phenotypes. In the father, however, a double heterozygote, two phases can be distinguished. Under phase I, the son is a recombinant and the daughter is a nonrecombinant, while the reverse is true under phase II. The phases are assumed to occur with equal frequencies in the population so that the likelihood is proportional to

$$L(\theta) = \tfrac{1}{2}\theta(1 - \theta) + \tfrac{1}{2}(1 - \theta)\theta = \theta(1 - \theta).$$

With θ set equal to ½, this leads to $L(\tfrac{1}{2}) = \tfrac{1}{4}$, so that the lod score is obtained as

$$Z(\theta) = \log[4\theta(1 - \theta)].$$

This is the same lod score as the one for a phase-known double backcross family with one recombinant and one nonrecombinant offspring. In family Bu there is one known recombinant, but because the phase of the father is unknown, one cannot tell which of the children is the recombinant.

The maximum of Z occurs at $\theta = \frac{1}{2}$, that is, all other lods in this family are negative.

Family De. Although the phenotype of the father is unknown, his single-locus genotypes may be inferred from those of the other family members. The mating type in this family turns out to be the same as that in the previous family. In phase I, there are one nonrecombinant and two recombinants, and the reverse is true in phase II. The likelihood is thus proportional to

$$L(\theta) = \frac{1}{2}(1 - \theta)\theta^2 + \frac{1}{2}\theta(1 - \theta)^2 = \frac{1}{2}\theta(1 - \theta).$$

It differs from the likelihood for family Bu by a constant that cancels in the likelihood ratio, so that the lod score for family *De* is identical to that for family *Bu*. The three children in family *De* are as informative for linkage as the two children in family *Bu*.

Family A47. Both parents are heterozygous at the TCN2 locus. As one can infer from the occurrence of children with blood type O, the mother is also heterozygous at the ABO locus. Under phase I, the first son is a recombinant if the *1o* haplotype was received from the mother and a nonrecombinant if that haplotype was received from the father; the reverse is true under phase II. Given either of the two phases, the first son's phenotype occurs with probability $\frac{1}{2}[\frac{1}{2}\theta + \frac{1}{2}(1 - \theta)] = \frac{1}{4}$; that is, all he contributes to the likelihood is a constant factor, which will cancel in the likelihood ratio. In this family, therefore, such a phenotype is not informative for linkage (there were two such children in this family, but only one is listed in Table 9.1). Under phase I, sons 2 and 3 are both recombinants; under phase II, however, they are both nonrecombinants. The likelihood is thus proportional to

$$L(\theta) = \theta^2 + (1 - \theta)^2. \tag{9.1}$$

Family B5. As in family *De*, the father's phenotype is unknown. From the other family members it can be concluded that his ABO genotype must be *a/o*. The first son is a double heterozygote; the phase of his genotype is known because the mother is doubly homozygous. At the TCN2 locus, the father may have one of several genotypes whose probabilities depend on the population allele frequencies. As will be seen, one may simply consider the *3* allele and lump the other alleles together into an unspecified allele, *x*. The gene frequencies at the *ABO* locus are not relevant because the *ABO* genotypes are known in both parents.

Let p denote the frequency of the *3* allele at the TCN2 locus. For the father, the following three genotypes at the TCN2 locus must then be distinguished: (1) If he has genotype *3/3*, each of the children's genotypes occurs with probability ½, that is, the conditional likelihood is equal to 1/8. In this case, the family is uninformative for linkage, but this possibility must still be taken into account. It occurs with probability p^2. (2) If the father has one *3* allele (the other TCN2 allele is denoted by x), then in phase I the daughter, son 1, and son 2 are a recombinant, a nonrecombinant, and a recombinant, respectively, and the reverse holds in phase II. Hence, under phase I, the likelihood is equal to $(1/8)\theta^2(1 - \theta)$, and under phase II it is equal to $(1/8)\theta(1 - \theta)^2$. Because each phase occurs with probability ½, the conditional likelihood for case 2 turns out to be equal to $\theta(1 - \theta)/16$, and this case occurs with probability $2p(1 - p)$. (3) The father must have at least one *3* allele so that the genotype x/x need not be considered. The total likelihood is then proportional to the weighted average of the two conditional likelihoods,

$$L(\theta, p) = (1/8)p^2 + (1/8)p(1 - p)\theta(1 - \theta), \tag{9.2}$$

so that the lod score is given by

$$Z(\theta; p) = \log\{4[\theta(1 - \theta)(1 - p) + p]/(1 + 3p)\}. \tag{9.3}$$

The maximum of Z occurs at $\theta = $ ½ so that all other lod scores are negative. For instance, with $p = 0.52$ and $\theta = 0.10$, $Z(0.10) = -0.055$. Equation (9.3) is an example of a lod score whose value depends on parameters other than θ alone. In a large pedigree the gene frequencies influence genotype probabilities of the founder members only and will not usually have much effect on the lod score; in this small family, however, varying p greatly affects the lod score. For example, at $\theta = 0$ the lod score (8.3) is given by $Z(\theta = 0; p) = \log[4p/(1 + 3p)]$, which is equal to -0.09 for $p = 0.52$ and equal to $- 3.08$ for $p = 0.10$. The reason for this dependency on p may be seen as follows: Because only the ratio between $2p(1 - p)$ and p^2 matters, the relative probability of the father's being a double heterozygote—and thus being informative for linkage—is given by $2p(1—p)/[2p(1–p) + p^2] = 2(1–p)/(2–p)$, and this is largest as $p \rightarrow 0$.

9.2. The Elston–Stewart Algorithm

As mentioned in Section 4.1, calculating lod scores in large families by hand is extremely tedious and becomes prohibitive in the multilocus case. Early on, therefore, attempts were made to have computers carry out this task (see Section 9.3), but family sizes were restricted to at most three generations. A particular representation of the likelihood, published by Elston and Stewart (1971), made it possible to calculate likelihoods for large families in a recursive (or telescopic) manner. The resulting method for rapidly calculating pedigree likelihoods is called Elston–Stewart (ES) algorithm and is the subject of this section, which is necessarily somewhat technical. A special issue of *Human Heredity* in 1991 was devoted to the celebration of the twentieth anniversary of the publication of this algorithm (Stewart, 1992; Elston et al., 1992). As outlined at the end of this section and in Section 4.8, other methods of calculating pedigree likelihoods have since been developed. As an aside, it is interesting to note that the term ''algorithm'' goes back to an astronomer, al-Khorezmi, who lived in Uzbekistan in the ninth century (Stewart, 1996).

Consider a human pedigree of size m. Let x_i denote the phenotype and g_i a particular genotype of the ith pedigree member, where phenotype and genotype may refer to several loci simultaneously. The pedigree likelihood is then expressed as given by equation (4.17), with $P(x|g) = \Pi\ P(x_i|g_i)$, where $P(x_i|g_i)$ refers to the penetrance (perhaps penetrances at multiple loci) for the ith family member. Assuming absence of phenotypic interactions at different loci, each $P(x_i|g_i)$ factors into the corresponding single-locus terms. For qualitative traits, $P(x_i|g_i)$ is given by the penetrance discussed in Chapter 7; for a quantitative trait (QTL), $P(x_i|g_i)$ is the density (height of bell-shaped curve) at the point x_i of the distribution with mean g_i.

The pedigree likelihood is usually calculated conditional on various known variables such as age and sex (see Section 7.4). In particular, birth order is assumed given.

To evaluate the likelihood (4.17), one would have to take a multiple sum over all possible combinations of genotypes, which can be very complex (Bailey, 1961) and too time-consuming for even a modern computer. The Elston–Stewart (1971) algorithm provides a means of evaluating the multiple sum (4.17) in a streamlined fashion. This is particularly suitable for implementation in computers if pedigrees are of the so-called simple type, as follows: Consider the commonly used graphical representation of pedigrees as shown, for example, in Figure 6.1, with lines connecting related and/or married individuals. A path is said to exist between two individuals (e.g., two unrelated mates) when they are connected by an uninterrupted sequence of lines. A *loop* is said to exist in a pedigree when a path consists of a complete circle, leaving an individual by one line and returning to that individual by a different line. One loosely distinguishes two types of loops: a *consanguinity loop* contains at least two mates who are blood related; in a *marriage loop,* however, no mating of related individuals exists. A commonly encountered marriage loop exists when, in two pairs of siblings, each sib of one pair is married to one sib in the other pair (an example is shown in Figure 1 of Sandkuyl and Ott, 1989). Genetically, two individuals (whether married or not) form a mating only when they have offspring. With these terms, a *simple pedigree* is defined as any family in which no loops occur and in which, for any mating, at most one of the mates has his or her parents in the pedigree. A pedigree not falling into this category is termed a *complex pedigree*.

In a simple pedigree, consider the individuals ordered such that parents precede their children. The pedigree likelihood (4.17) may then be represented as the telescopic sum

$$L(\theta) = \Sigma P(x_1|g_1)P(g_1|\cdot) \ldots \tag{9.4}$$
$$\Sigma P(x_{m-1}|g_{m-1})P(g_{m-1}|\cdot)\Sigma P(x_m|g_m)P(g_m|\cdot)$$

(Elston and Stewart, 1971), where $P(g_i|\cdot)$ represents either the ith child's genotype given the parental genotypes, in which case it may involve the recombination fraction, or the probability that a founder individual (no parents in pedigree) has genotype g_i. Calculating a pedigree likelihood (9.4) by the Elston–Stewart algorithm starts with the innermost (rightmost) sum, which is evaluated for each genotype in the next outer sum, and each summation result is "tagged on" to the appropriate term corresponding to that genotype in the outer sum. Once the summations have been carried out for all genotypes in the outer loop, the rightmost sum is no longer required (for a detailed description, see Ott, 1974a). This recursive procedure is seen to "clip off" or "peel" branches (sibships) from the pedigree and is thus called a *peeling algorithm*. It evaluates one sibship after another, starting at the bottom and finishing at the top of the pedigree. One such round of calculations yields the pedigree likelihood for given values of the recombination fraction and other parameters. To evaluate $L(\theta)$ at other θ values, the procedure must be repeated.

The ES algorithm proved to be very effective in practical applications (see next section). It was extended to nonlooped complex pedigrees (Ott, 1974a) and to general complex pedigrees (Lange and Elston, 1975). The latter extension is based on the following principle. For example, consider an individual who is both an offspring and a mate. If his or her genotype (including phase) is known or can be inferred, one may for calculation purposes represent that individual as two separate individuals, one being an offspring and one being a mate, and treat these as if they were two separate individuals, each with the same single known genotype(s). This "doubling" of individuals results in at most a multiplication of the likelihood by a constant factor, which may involve gene frequencies but no recombination fractions, and this factor is easily accounted for in a computer program. Consider now a special representation of the likelihood,

$$L(\theta) = P(x) = \sum_{gi} P(x, g_i), \tag{9.5}$$

where each term in the sum is calculated jointly with one (multilocus) genotype of the ith individual and the sum is evaluated over all genotypes of that individual. In each evaluation, the exact genotype of the ith individual is known; therefore, that individual can be "doubled" or "tripled" as described above. The original form of this technique has been implemented in the LIPED program (see below) to allow the processing of complex pedigrees by the ES algorithm. Clearly, this extension is purchased at a price: the likelihood must be evaluated a number of times, this number being equal to the number of possible genotypes of the ith individual. It is thus beneficial, for example, to perform this calculation for an individual (the so-called loop breaker) whose phenotype or pedigree relationships exhibit as much as possible of the underlying genotype, so the sum in (9.5) must be calculated over as small a number of terms as possible.

Recursive algorithms other than ES, allowing pedigree traversal in any direction, have been developed, for example, by Cannings, Thompson, and Skolnick (1978). In the MENDEL program (see below), a particular peeling algorithm has been implemented, which corresponds to moving the summation signs in equation (9.4) inward (to the right) as much as possible. This way, loops are handled in the framework given by equation (9.4) and not by conditioning on the genotypes of a specific individual. A modified Elston–Stewart algorithm has been implemented in the LINKAGE programs: Free-ending branches of a pedigree (not involved in a loop) are peeled upward or downward as needed, and loops are handled by conditioning on an individual's genotypes [equation (9.5)].

9.3. Computer Programs for Parametric Linkage Analysis

After a slow start some 25 years ago, quite a few linkage programs are available now and are still being developed. I am familiar with some but not all of them, so the programs discussed in this section necessarily represent a subset of the existing programs. A list of programs is available at URL http://linkage.rockefeller.edu/soft/list.html. For nonparametric linkage analysis (Chapter 13), Davis and Weeks (1997) provided comparisons among a large number of available programs. Several of the programs mentioned below are discussed in greater detail in the book by Terwilliger and Ott (1994).

Early Programs. Most linkage programs in current use compute lod scores by calculating pedigree likelihoods numerically for a set of parameter values, whereas early approaches consisted of calculating some lod scores by hand for certain well-defined family types and simply storing them on a computer. The first lod scores for nuclear families were tabulated on a vacuum-tube predecessor of the IBM 650 computer (Morton, 1955).

A remarkable program was developed by Renwick (Renwick and Schulze, 1961). Based on a fully efficient likelihood formulation by C.A.B. Smith, it was implemented on an IBM 7094 in Baltimore and calculated lod scores for large pedigrees. Being written in machine language, it was unfortunately not transportable. Its flow chart may be found at URL http://linkage.rockefeller.edu/ott/renwick.html.

In later approaches, lod scores were calculated numerically for linkage analysis in three-generation families (Falk and Edwards, 1970; Edwards, 1972). In the PEDIG program (Heuch and Li, 1972), genetic risks were calculated via pedigree likelihoods. The MOSM program (Gedde-Dahl et al., 1972), used in Oslo and Copenhagen until the early 1990s, computed lod scores for two-generation families (family types 1–18; Morton, 1956) and posterior linkage probabilities based on Smith (1959). It was first applied in the discovery of the Gm-PI linkage (Gedde-Dahl et al., 1972).

LIPED. The first generally available program to compute likelihoods numerically in large pedigrees was LIPED (for LIkelihood in PEDigrees) (Ott, 1974a, 1976). It is based on the Elston–Stewart algorithm (Elston and Stewart, 1971) and extensions of it (Lange and Elston, 1975) and allows calculation of two-point lod scores. As the source code is freely available—it is written in FORTRAN—several groups have made modifications to the original version. The only version currently supported by me is PC-LIPED for IBM type microcomputers, available at URL ftp://linkage.rockefeller.edu/software/liped/. I have generalized it to allow for allelic association and age-dependent penetrance (onset age known or unknown). It was first applied to a large kindred of over 90 individuals, where linkage relationships between familial hypercholesterolemia (LDLR) and 16 genetic markers were estimated (Ott et al., 1974a). The results showed a weak suggestion of linkage between LDLR and complement C3, which was later confirmed by other groups (Berg and Heiberg, 1976; Elston et al., 1976; Berg and Heiberg, 1978).

The LIPED program is still used by many researchers because it has been error free for more than 20 years and because it is able to detect a large percentage of errors in the input data by carrying out many checks for data consistency. LIPED works with penetrances in the wide sense. At each locus the user must furnish a table of penetrances such as the one given in Table 1.1. The program produces lod scores at predetermined values of θ or (θ_m, θ_f) (male and female recombination fractions jointly), but it does not iteratively find maximum likelihood estimates.

The LIPED program (as well as most other linkage programs) makes very restrictive assumptions on the genetic models for the phenotypes. Although these are allowed to be qualitative or quantitative, they are assumed to consist of two components only—a genetic component due to a mendelian gene and a random environmental deviation.

PAP. Many traits may be influenced by polygenic effects and nonrandom environmental factors contributing to the similarity among relatives. A computer program approximately taking such effects into account was developed by Hasstedt (1982): The PAP program extends linkage analysis to several (currently four) loci jointly. It is being used by many researchers. For details, the reader is referred to its original description (Hasstedt and Cartwright, 1981).

LINKAGE. The original purpose of developing the LINKAGE programs (Lathrop et al., 1984) was for gene mapping. Presently, they exist in two versions: a set of programs for general pedigrees and a specialized version for the analysis of codominant markers in the CEPH panel of reference families (Dausset et al., 1990). As pointed out in the previous section, the LINKAGE programs basically use the Elston–Stewart algorithm but can peel upward or downward in a pedigree. The specialized LINKAGE version for CEPH families employs a technique of factorizing the multilocus likelihood (Lathrop, Lalouel, and White, 1986), which, in comparison with the version for general pedigrees, allows more rapid analysis and joint processing of a greatly increased number of loci. The description below focuses on the version for general pedigrees.

The LINKAGE package consists of three analysis programs, each of which calculates two-point or multipoint likelihoods in human pedigrees. MLINK calculates likelihoods by stepwise variation of the recombination fraction in one of the interlocus intervals. It also computes genetic risks. The LINKMAP program assumes a fixed map of markers and calculates likelihoods for a new locus at various points in each interval along the known map. The third program, ILINK, iteratively estimates recombination fractions and other model parameters. Except for three-locus analysis, these programs (like most other linkage programs) assume absence of interference in the calculation of gamete probabilities given parental genotypes (see Chapter 6). The three analysis programs have been extended to allow for a two-locus mode of inheritance of a qualitative phenotype, which is of particular interest for linkage analysis of complex disease loci (Lathrop and Ott, 1990). The LINKAGE programs are written in PASCAL and are available, for example, at URL ftp://linkage.rockefeller.edu/software/linkage/.

A major difference between LIPED and the LINKAGE programs is in the definition of penetrance (see Section 7.1). Whereas LIPED uses penetrance in the general (wide) sense, penetrance in the LINKAGE programs is the probability of being affected given a genotype. A table of penetrances such as Table 1.1 is suitable for direct input to LIPED. To use such penetrances in the LINKAGE programs, it is easiest to treat such a locus as an ''affection status locus,'' to call each individual affected at this locus and to consider each phenotype (column in Table 1.1) as representing a so-called liability or penetrance class (examples and more detailed explanations are provided in the manual accompanying the LINKAGE programs).

Another difference between the two program sets is in the way they handle male (θ_m) and female (θ_f) recombination fractions. Whereas LIPED directly uses these two parameters and the LINKAGE programs output both θ_m and θ_f, for input the LINKAGE programs work with the two parameters θ_m and the ratio, $R = x_f/x_m$, of female-to-male map distances. Using the Haldane mapping function (absence of interference), conversions between θ_f and R (with given θ_m) may be accomplished by the following two formulas:

$$R = \ln(1 - 2\theta_f)/\ln(1 - 2\theta_m), \tag{9.6}$$

$$\theta_f = \tfrac{1}{2}[1 - (1 - 2\theta_m)^R], \tag{9.7}$$

where ln denotes the natural logarithm (base e). These conversions may also be carried out by the SEXDIF utility program.

FAP. The Family Analysis Package (FAP; Neugebauer and Baur, 1991) is a set of programs originally developed for the estimation of allele and haplotype frequencies at the HLA locus. It has been extended to carry out many other tasks including linkage analysis.

MAPMAKER. MAPMAKER (Lander et al., 1987) is a user-friendly linkage program specializing in analyzing codominant loci in CEPH-type families. Using the EM algorithm (for a review on EM, see Weir, 1996), it maximizes the likelihood recursively over loci rather than over individuals in a pedigree, which allows analysis of a large number of loci jointly but limits the size of the pedigrees it can handle. For families with unambiguous genotypes, MAPMAKER evaluates likelihood at an impressive speed, but it can be slow for phase unknown matings. Also, it does not seem to make full use of all of the data (White et al., 1990).

CRI-MAP. Developed by Dr. Phil Green to analyze codominant marker systems in small families, CRI-MAP has been extended to more general pedigrees and to simple dominant systems (Goldgar et al., 1989). Single-locus genotypes must be known (through phenotypes or inference) or else some information will be lost in the analysis. When family structures are incomplete, CRI-MAP tries to infer the genotypes of missing individuals. If it cannot infer the genotype at a particular locus in a particular individual, the meiotic information at that locus in that individual is lost. Focusing on known recombination events can lead to a bias in the estimated recombination fraction (see Section 11.1).

MENDEL. The MENDEL program (Lange, Weeks, and Boehnke, 1988) is comparable in its capabilities to the general version of the LINKAGE programs. It is written in FORTRAN and provides routines for special tasks such as risk calculation and estimating parameters for homogeneity tests. Loops in pedigrees are handled by basically condensing pedigree information onto individuals in the loops and analyzing data with the loops unbroken. This method of handling loops appears to be more efficient and leads to shorter analysis times than, for example, the method implemented in LIPED and LINKAGE. On the other hand, for analyzing the same problem, MENDEL tends to require more memory than the LINKAGE program, which is particularly problematic on microcomputers. Like LINKAGE, the MENDEL program can analyze phenotypes under the joint control of two loci (Spence et al., 1993).

In linkage analysis, the likelihood is maximized over θ values and perhaps other parameters. Some programs such as LIPED do this by simply evaluating the likelihood at a predefined set of parameter values, while other programs use various iterative numerical maximization techniques. For example, in ILINK, the GEMINI routine (Lalouel, 1979) for numerical maximization of the likelihood is implemented. The MAPMAKER program makes use of the EM algorithm (Dempster, Laird, and Rubin, 1977), which is known to be very stable and to converge quickly when parameter values are far away from their estimates, but it tends to be slow close to the maximum of the likelihood. In MENDEL, a hybrid technique is implemented in that the EM algorithm is used first, which is later switched to a quasi-Newton algorithm (Lange and Weeks, 1989).

MAP+. MAP+ (Collins et al., 1996b) is an updated version of an older program based on the method of Rao et al. (1979) for combining two-point lod scores into a multipoint framework. The MAP+ program uses the Rao mapping function (see Section 1.5). It has been written to construct high resolution linkage maps. Its description may be found at URL ftp://cedar.genetics.soton.ac.uk/public_html/guide.html.

HOMOZ. HOMOZ is a program for rapid multipoint mapping of recessively inherited disease genes in nuclear families (this includes so-called homozygosity mapping). Multipoint analysis with dozens of markers can be carried out in minutes on a personal workstation (Kruglyak et al., 1995).

VITESSE. The VITESSE program (O'Connell and Weeks, 1995; see also Ott, 1995b) is based on novel methods to recode each person's genotype (''set-recoding'') and infer transmission probabilities (''fuzzy inheritance''). VITESSE allows extremely rapid computation of exact multipoint likelihoods for large numbers of highly polymorphic markers.

GENEHUNTER. GENEHUNTER (Kruglyak et al., 1996) carries out parametric and nonparametric linkage analysis in a unified manner, where the latter represents an extension of the method implemented in MAPMAKER/SIBS (see Section 13.1) to affected pedigree members. It allows for rapid multipoint analysis with large numbers of marker loci but is limited to relatively small families. Currently, GENEHUNTER assumes equal recombination fractions in males and females; that is, it does not allow for sex-specific map distances. It also does not permit analysis of quantitative phenotypes. With missing data, GENEHUNTER performs suboptimally. An improved algorithm has been developed and implemented by Kong and Cox (1997). The optimized program is available at ftp://galton.uchicago.edu/pub/kong/.

ASPEX. ASPEX is Dr. Neil Risch's multipoint program for nonparametric linkage analysis (Schwab et al., 1995) and is available from ftp://lahmed.stanford.edu/pub/aspex.

Loki. Loki (Heath, 1997, 1998) permits linkage and segregation analysis of oligogenic traits in large pedigrees with multiple marker loci. This is achieved by approximating the pedigree likelihood through Markov chain Monte Carlo (MCMC) methods. The program is available at ftp:// ftp.u.washington.edu/pub/user-supported/pangaea/PANGAEA/LOKI_V2.1/.

9.4. Special Applications of Linkage Programs

Linkage programs are generally designed to estimate recombination fractions. Because they calculate pedigree likelihoods for various genetic parameters other than recombination fractions, they also lend themselves to the maximum likelihood estimation of these parameters. For example, the ILINK program can numerically estimate gene frequencies, haplotype frequencies, penetrances, ratios of female-to-male map distances, and so on. Notice, however, that such estimates are obtained without ascertainment corrections, which may represent serious problems. For example, for linkage analyses involving a disease locus, families are often collected to contain as many affected individuals as possible. In those cases, uncorrected estimates of penetrance based on the collected families tend to yield inflated values.

The purpose of this section is not to discuss parameter estimation but to point out some less well known applications of linkage programs, which can be of considerable value to linkage analysts. The first examples outlined below involve tricking a program into carrying out analyses for which it was not directly designed. Later examples will show how to numerically obtain some probability distributions, whose calculation would be very tedious if not impossible to carry out in any other way (an example is also given in Section 5.10).

Pseudoautosomal Loci. Linkage programs perform analyses between autosomal loci or between X-linked loci, but there is generally no provision for an analysis between an X-linked and a pseudoautosomal locus, between an X-linked and a Y-linked locus, or between two Y-linked loci. No new programs are required, however. Linkage investigations involving pseudoautosomal loci can be handled with an appropriate use of penetrances (Ott, 1986a). The principle applied here is to emulate X- and Y-linked inheritance as special forms of autosomal inheritance. For the pseudoautosomal regions, recombination in females occurs when two X chromosomes pair up, whereas recombination in males takes place when the X and Y chromosomes unite. As described below, several cases must be distinguished.

Loci located in the pseudoautosomal regions (see Section 1.4) behave in their inheritance pattern exactly like autosomal loci. Hence, linkage analyses among pseudoautosomal loci may be carried out as if the loci followed an autosomal mode of inheritance except that a low female-to-male map distance ratio of approximately 0.066 should be applied (see Section 1.6). With genetic marker loci, it may often be possible to count recombinations and nonrecombinations so that a linkage analysis need not be carried out with a computer program. For example, Gough et al. (1990) analyzed families for linkage between the granulocyte-macrophage colony-stimulating factor (GM-CSF) receptor gene in the pseudoautosomal region and the gender phenotype (male/female), which is thought to be the expression of a sex-determining locus. One of their families is depicted in Figure 9.1, where X and Y refer to the pseudoautosomal portions of the X and Y chromosomes, respectively. This family provides a good object for studying the inheritance of pseudoautosomal loci.

To assess linkage relationships involving pseudoautosomal as well as X- and Y-linked loci, it is easiest to model X linkage and Y linkage

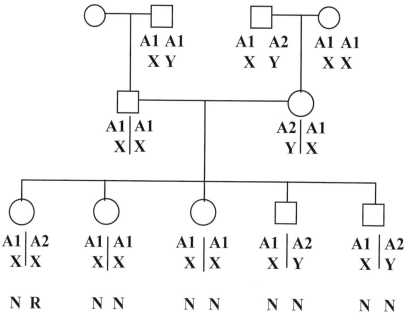

Figure 9.1. A family showing linkage between the GM-CSF receptor gene and gender. (Data from Gough et al., 1990.)

Table 9.2. Penetrances at an X-Linked Locus with an Emulated Autosomal Inheritance Pattern

Genotype	Female Phenotypes				Male Phenotypes		
	A	*Aa*	*a*	Unknown	*A*	*a*	Unknown
A/A	1	0	0	1	0	0	0
A/a	0	1	0	1	0	0	0
A/y	0	0	0	0	1	0	1
a/a	0	0	1	1	0	0	0
a/y	0	0	0	0	0	1	1
y/y	0	0	0	0	0	0	0

in the framework of autosomal inheritance. This is achieved by adding a dummy allele to each locus (*x* in Y-linked loci and *y* in X-linked loci) and setting penetrances in such a way that, for instance, no male can ever have a genotype *x/x* or *y/y*. As an example, assume a codominant X-linked locus with alleles *A, a,* and *y,* with the corresponding gene frequencies being taken as p_A, p_a, and ½ (the gene frequencies then sum to 1.5). Similarly, assume a Y-linked locus with alleles *D, d,* and *x.* Tables 9.2 and 9.3 show the penetrances required in this situation. Pairwise analyses between an X-linked and a pseudoautosomal locus or between a Y-linked and a pseudoautosomal locus will yield correct lod scores under this scheme (the likelihoods will be incorrect by a constant factor). For multipoint analyses, haplotypes instead of alleles must be defined (Ott, 1986a), but this can be tricky. The methods outlined above are easiest to use in two-point linkage.

As an example for a linkage investigation between an X-linked and a pseudoautosomal locus, consider the artificial pedigree shown in Figure

Table 9.3. Penetrances at a Y-Linked Locus with an Emulated Autosomal Inheritance Pattern

Genotype	Any Female Phenotype	Male Phenotypes		
		D	*d*	Unknown
D/D	0	0	0	0
D/d	0	0	0	0
d/d	0	0	0	0
D/x	0	1	0	1
d/x	0	0	1	1
x/x	1	0	0	0

9.2. Phenotypes are made up to allow counting recombinants and nonrecombinants. Shown in Figure 9.2 are the genotypes including phase where known. The estimated male recombination fraction is $\hat{\theta}_m = 1/6$, and the female recombination fraction is $\hat{\theta}_f = 2/6$ (as pointed out above, θ_m is expected to be much larger than θ_f because at least one crossover occurs in the pseudoautosomal region). One may verify the correct operation of this coding scheme by running the example pedigree with one of the usual linkage programs. Needless to say, one must be extremely careful when applying such a scheme. Linkage programs have no way of detecting an error in coding (e.g., when a male phenotype is used in a woman or vice versa), and such errors easily lead to completely wrong results.

Family-Specific Expected Statistics. To calculate the expected lod score (see Section 5.2) or the risk distribution (see Section 12.5) in a given family, one must evaluate all possible values of the lod score or the genetic risk and calculate the probability of occurrence of each value. Even when the number of values is not too large, evaluating their probabilities is often impossible by analytic means. As these probabilities are

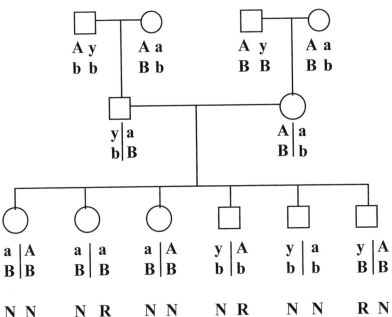

Figure 9.2. Theoretical example for the linkage analysis between a pseudoautosomal locus (alleles *A*, *a*) and an X-linked locus (alleles *B*, *b*). *R* and *N* indicate recombinant and nonrecombinant haplotypes.

proportional to the pedigree likelihood, linkage programs may conveniently be used to obtain the required outcome probabilities. The example below was pointed out to me by Drs. Leena Peltonen and Irma Järvelä.

Infantile neuronal ceroid lipofuscinosis (CNL1; Santavuori disease, MIM no. 25673) is a recessive disorder that leads to blindness by the age of 2 years and to brain death by 3 years and that is fatal by 10 years of age. CNL1 has been mapped to the short arm of chromosome 1 (Järvelä et al., 1991). Two parents with an affected child wanted to know with what precision geneticists could predict the risk to a future child. Blood was drawn from the parents (who are obligate carriers of the disease gene) and from their affected child, and genotypes were determined for the two genetic markers nearest the disease, the locus order being *CNL1-D1S62-D1S57* with interval recombination rates of 0.02 and 0.082. Father, mother, and affected child turned out to have the following respective marker phenotypes: 2/2, 1/2, and 2/2 at *D1S62* and 1/2 each at *D1S57*.

To evaluate the range of risks to a future child, one compiles a list of all possible marker phenotypes for that child. At *D1S62,* an offspring can be either 1/2 or 2/2, and at *D1S57,* it can be 1/1, 1/2, or 2/2. Hence, there are a total of six possible phenotypic outcomes at the two marker loci. At each of these outcomes, a risk can be calculated, and each occurs with a certain conditional probability given the known phenotypes of parents and affected child. Using the MLINK program, assuming linkage equilibrium and equal male and female recombination fractions, the pedigree likelihood (the antilog of the log likelihood) and a risk of being affected are then computed. Also, a likelihood must be obtained under the assumption that the future child has unknown phenotype at each of the two markers—that likelihood should be the sum of the likelihoods over all six outcomes, which serves as a check that the outcomes are mutually exclusive and exhaustive. The likelihoods are then divided by their sum, which yields the probabilities of the various outcomes.

Table 9.4 displays the various risks that may be given to a future child, as determined by the marker phenotypes it can have. The probabilities of the different outcomes appear simple, but it is in general difficult to compute these by hand. The weighted average of the risks is ¼, which is the risk without marker information. The following answers may now be given to the parents: The risk to a future child is generally low (i.e., ¼). When marker information is available on a new fetus, there is a 50% chance that the test will result in a much lower risk of 1% to 3%. Otherwise, there is an equal chance that the test is uninformative (no change to the expectation of a risk of ¼) or that it increases the risk to 70%. The test will never result in a risk higher than 70%, but that does not, of course,

Table 9.4. Example of Determining the Distribution of Risks, *R,* to a Future Child in a Specific Family (see text)

DIS57	DIS62	R	L	Probability L/ΣL
1/1	1/2	0.028	1.4324	0.125
1/1	2/2	0.264	1.4324	0.125
1/2	1/2	0.011	2.8648	0.250
1/2	2/2	0.697	2.8648	0.250
2/2	1/2	0.028	1.4324	0.125
2/2	2/2	0.264	1.4324	0.125
Total			11.4592	1

Note: L = likelihood, multiplied by 10^9.

mean that a future child could not be affected. Obviously, such probabilistic details are not generally useful for counselees, but they can be very valuable for counselors.

In larger families, generally many different risks to a proband can occur. In these cases, risk distributions may be approximated using computer simulation (see Section 9.7). Techniques analogous to the one described above may be used to find the distribution of lod scores, their average, and the probability that they exceed a certain threshold. But, as mentioned before, this is feasible only when the number of possible outcomes is not too large. For these problems, too, one would in general use computer simulation. On the other hand, Section 5.10 quotes an example in which all possible outcomes for a small family type are evaluated with the aid of a computer program.

9.5. Linkage Utility Programs

In linkage analysis, calculations are sometimes required that would be somewhat tedious to carry out on a calculator. A set of small computer programs called linkage utility programs is available at URL ftp://linkage. rockefeller.edu/software/utilities/. They have proven useful in a linkage analyst's daily routine. Some of them are discussed elsewhere; for example, the ASSOCIATE program is mentioned in Section 13.4. This section briefly describes some of these programs. Details are given in the manual available at URL http://linkage.rockefeller.edu/ott/linkutil.htm. Programs for analyzing genetic heterogeneity are discussed in Chapter 10.

The BINOM program computes binomial class frequencies and exact confidence intervals (not support intervals) for binomial proportions for values of *n* up to 8000. A typical application is as follows: In $n = 20$

recombination events, assume that $k = 3$ recombinations have occurred. The corresponding recombination fraction estimate is $3/20 = 0.15$ with a maximum lod score of $Z_{max} = 2.35$. The empirical significance level associated with this Z_{max} is the probability of obtaining under $\theta = \frac{1}{2}$ three or fewer recombinants. It is obtained from the BINOM program as $p = 0.0013$.

In the 2BY2 program, Fisher's exact test (Armitage and Berry, 1987, p. 129) is carried out for a comparison between two binomial proportions. For example, two recombination rates obtained from different meiosis counts may be compared and tested for equality. One-sided and two-sided *p*-values are calculated as described in Weir (1996).

The CHIPROB program computes *p*-values for given values of chi-square and number of degrees of freedom. A useful application is as follows: When *p*-values from n independent investigations should be combined into one *p*-value, Fisher's (1970) method specifies that one should transform each value of p into $c = -2 \times \ln(p)$. The resulting n *c*-values are added together. Their sum, Σc, represents a chi-squared variable with $2n$ df. So, if Σc is entered in the CHIPROB program with $2n$ df, the *p*-value returned is the overall observed level of significance. For example, assume that three independent tests (not necessarily chi-square tests) have furnished the respective *p*-values 0.011, 0.047, and 0.35. The corresponding *c*-values are 9.02, 6.12, and 2.10. Their sum, 17.24, with 6 df, yields a combined *p*-value of 0.008. Researchers do not have to carry out these various steps manually—the PVALUES program can do this for them.

EQUIV computes equivalent observations (see Section 4.5), either from Z_{max} and $\hat{\theta}$ or from a pair of lod scores, Z_1 and Z_2 at θ_1 and θ_2. It also computes lod scores for given numbers of recombinants and fully informative meioses.

For given allele frequencies at a locus, the HET program calculates maximum likelihood and unbiased estimates for heterozygosity, and maximum likelihood estimates for PIC (polymorphism information content). Both are computed from allele frequencies, that is, as expected under Hardy–Weinberg equilibrium. For the heterozygosity estimate, the standard error is computed as the square root of the estimated variance (based on Nei and Roychoudhury, 1974). From this, a 95% confidence interval for heterozygosity is obtained.

The MAPFUN program converts recombination fractions into map distances and vice versa using seven different map functions, while SEX-DIF converts (θ_m, θ_f) into (θ_m, R) and vice versa (using Haldane or Kosambi map functions), where $R = x_f/x_m$ is the female-to-male map distance ratio.

NOCOM analyzes a mixture of distributions by estimating means, variances, and proportions of the single components (Ott, 1979b). The distributions are taken to be normal with optional power transformation of the observations, which accommodates the lognormal and a range of other distributions (see Chapter 8).

For the normal distribution, NORPROB computes the p-values associated with a given normal deviate, while NORINV finds the normal deviate associated with a given p-value and furnishes the density at the normal deviate.

Approximate Variances. Lod scores are usually computed at each of a set of θ values. One may then want to carry out interpolation and approximately find the maximum lod score and its curvature, the latter being used to compute a standard error for $\hat{\theta}$. The VARCO programs (for *var*iance *co*mponents) perform these tasks for univariate (VARCO3, three θ points) or bivariate (VARCO6, six points) lod scores.

In the univariate case, the observed likelihood is taken to approximately represent a normal density with mean at $\hat{\theta}$, provided that $0 < \hat{\theta} < \frac{1}{2}$. The lod score is then quadratic in θ,

$$Z(\theta) \approx c - m(\theta - \hat{\theta})^2/(2\sigma^2), \tag{9.8}$$

where c is a constant additive term and $m = 1/\ln(10) = 0.4343$ [for $\log_e(\theta)$ rather than $Z(\theta)$, replace m by 1 in equations (9.8)–(9.13)]. On the θ axis, as shown below, any three points θ_i with their corresponding lod scores Z_i determine (9.8). The first and second derivatives of (9.8) with respect to θ are given by

$$Z' \approx -m(\theta - \hat{\theta})/\sigma^2 \text{ and} \tag{9.9}$$

$$Z'' \approx -m/\sigma^2. \tag{9.10}$$

Now, pick $\theta_1 < \theta_2 < \theta_3$ with respective lod scores, Z_1, Z_2, and Z_3, such that Z_2 is the largest of the three (this is to ensure numerical stability). From the three pairs of (Z_i, θ_i), derivatives may be numerically approximated as

$$Z' \approx (Z_3 - Z_1)/(\theta_3 - \theta_1) \text{ and} \tag{9.11}$$

$$Z'' \approx 2[(Z_3 - Z_2)/(\theta_3 - \theta_2) - (Z_2 - Z_1)/(\theta_2 - \theta_1)]/(\theta_3 - \theta_1). \tag{9.12}$$

The standard error may now be approximated by rearranging (9.10),

$$\sigma \approx \sqrt{(-m/Z'')}, \tag{9.13}$$

and inserting (9.12) for Z'' in (9.13). Furthermore, it can be shown that, by virtue of (9.11), Z' is the exact first derivative of the quadratic (9.8) at the point $\frac{1}{2}(\theta_1 + \theta_3)$. Inserting this for θ in (9.9) and equating (9.9) with (9.11) leads to

$$\hat{\theta} \approx \frac{1}{2}(\theta_1 + \theta_3) - Z'/Z''. \tag{9.14}$$

At small θ values, the lod score curve is often not well approximated by a quadratic, particularly when the points of θ_i are not closely spaced. Then, it is advisable to transform the θ values such that the lod score curve on the transformed scale, x, is quadratic. Consider the power transformation, $x = \theta^\lambda$ (Box and Cox, 1964), for example, $x = \sqrt{\theta}$ for $\lambda = \frac{1}{2}$, where λ is a real-valued exponent of θ. For the binomial case of scoring k recombinants and $n - k$ nonrecombinants, the appropriate value of λ can be determined as follows: One requires that, on the transformed scale, $Z(x) = n \log(2) + k \log(\theta) + (n - k)\log(1 - \theta)$ is quadratic at $\theta = \hat{\theta}$, where $\theta = x^{1/\lambda}$. This is equivalent to postulating that the third and higher derivatives be equal to zero. Lengthy algebraic manipulations lead to the simple result,

$$\lambda = \frac{1}{3}(1 + \hat{\theta})/(1 - \hat{\theta}), \tag{9.15}$$

where $\hat{\theta} = k/n$. Thus, the appropriate transformation is given by the observed recombination fraction estimate. For example, $\lambda = \frac{1}{3}$ for $\hat{\theta} = 0$, and $\lambda = \frac{1}{2}$ for $\hat{\theta} = 0.20$. Equations (9.11) through (9.14) are then used with $x_i = \theta_i^\lambda$ instead of θ_i, and the resulting value, $\hat{x}$, is transformed back into $\hat{\theta} = \hat{x}^{1/\lambda}$. All of these manipulations have been incorporated into the VARCO programs.

Applying analogous considerations to the bivariate case, the likelihood $L(s, t)$ is taken to represent a bivariate normal density, where, for example, s and t stand for the male and female recombination fractions. The log likelihood is then quadratic in s and t,

$$\ln L(s, t) = c - \frac{1}{2}[S^2 - 2\rho ST + T^2]/(1 - \rho^2), \tag{9.16}$$

where $S = (s - \hat{s})/\sigma_s$, $T = (t - \hat{t})/\sigma_t$, and c is a constant additive term. The six parameters c, $\hat{s}$, t, σ_s, σ_t, and ρ in (9.16) can be determined by six suitably chosen points (L_i, s_i, t_i). A particular layout of six such points in the (s, t) plane has been incorporated in the VARCO6 program.

Only one additional utility program shall be mentioned here: The VaryPhen program (Xie and Ott, 1990), available at URL ftp://linkage. rockefeller.edu/software/varyphen/, carries out a sensitivity analysis by varying the disease phenotype of each individual in a family, for example, by temporarily setting it to unknown. For each such change, a linkage analysis is run and the resulting change in lod score and $\hat{\theta}$ (due to making the ith individual unknown) are recorded. The resulting list tells an investigator, which of the family members' diagnostic accuracy is most crucial for the analysis.

9.6. Paternity Calculations

In cases of disputed paternity, when an alleged father of a child claims not to be the father, the traditional approach has been to compare blood groups and other genetic markers among mother, alleged father, and child. When this comparison does not clearly exclude the man as the child's father, statistical methods are used to assess the probability with which the man might be the father. Several types of statistical analyses have been used for paternity calculations (Weir, 1996). Here, only the so-called paternity index will be considered (Baur et al., 1986; Rao, 1989). Also, discussion of genetic systems will be restricted to those with a clearly mendelian mode of inheritance. The so-called DNA fingerprinting technique (Jeffreys, Wilson, and Thein, 1985) detects several hundred mini- or microsatellite loci and is often used for individual identification, but its treatment is beyond the scope of this book (see Brookfield, 1989; Hampe et al., 1997).

Consider two rival hypotheses, (1) that a given man is the father, and (2) that he is not the father, and assume that marker typing has been carried out on the man, the mother, the child, and perhaps other relatives of the child and/or the man. Under each of the two hypotheses, a pedigree likelihood can be computed. If the markers are unlinked, the likelihood for all markers is just the product of the likelihoods for the individual markers; when they are linked, the likelihood must be calculated in a multipoint fashion, for example, with the aid of a linkage program. When the man is not the father, he still must appear in the calculations (as an individual unrelated to the child). Denote the likelihoods under the two hypotheses by $P(F|\text{father})$ and $P(F|\text{not father})$, where F stands for the observed phenotypes. The likelihood ratio, $R = P(F|\text{father})/P(F|\text{not father})$, is called the *paternity index*.

When it is known or can be assumed with what probability an alleged father is the biological father, then the posterior probability of his being the father may be expressed as

$$P(\text{father}|F) = \frac{R \times P(\text{father})}{1 - P(\text{father}) + [R \times P(\text{father})]},$$

where $P(\text{father})$ is the prior probability (frequency) that an alleged father is the biological father. In practice, prior probabilities are not usually specified. Instead, the value ½ is chosen, which leads to the posterior "probability," $P(\text{father}|F) = R/(1 + R)$.

On the basis of a large set of family data, it may be of interest to estimate the proportion of children whose biological father is not the legal father (nonpaternity rate). For a man who is not the biological father of a child, genetic markers have a limited probability of excluding this man as being the father. Thus, estimates of nonpaternity rates cannot simply be equated with exclusion rates, the latter typically being lower than the former. Many papers have dealt with this problem. Several methods for the estimation of paternity rate based on exclusion rate have been discussed by Sasse et al. (1994). Nonpaternity rates tend to range from one to several percentages (Sasse et al., 1994; see also the papers quoted by these authors).

9.7. Computer Simulation Methods

Computer simulation (Monte Carlo method) is a numerical technique that is often used as a substitute for analytical calculations that are too complex to be carried out. Computer simulation then yields approximate solutions. For example, to model traffic flow in cities, computer simulation is the method of choice to predict the effect of a temporary street closure. This section provides examples of computer simulation methods applied in human linkage analysis. Technical aspects will be discussed first, followed by a review of the rationale and purposes of computer simulation in human genetics.

Random Numbers. Monte Carlo or computer simulation methods are based on random numbers, which are uniformly distributed in the interval (0, 1). As they are generated by computer programs, they are not truly random but pseudorandom. With the same starting value ("seed"), the sequence of pseudorandom numbers produced by a random number generator is always the same. Good random number generators produce numbers with low serial correlations and a long period before the same sequence is repeated. In my experience, the approach by Wichman and Hill (1982) is highly reliable.

With Monte Carlo methods, real-life events are simulated on the computer so that the simulated and real events share their most important properties. In human pedigree analysis, the process most often simulated is the flow of alleles and gametes from one generation to the next. Such a simulation usually starts with a founder, that is, an individual assumed to be randomly drawn from the population. Consider a single locus with three alleles, *1*, *2*, and *3*, with the respective frequencies 0.04, 0.32, and 0.64. These numbers are also the probabilities with which an allele randomly drawn from the population will occur in an individual. To pick one of the two alleles in an individual randomly, one draws a pseudorandom number on the computer. Then, allele *1* is selected if that number is less than 0.04, allele *2* is selected if the number is between 0.04 and 0.36, and allele *3* is taken when the number exceeds 0.36. For the second allele in a founder, this process is repeated. Analogously, one may simulate passing a single locus or multilocus gamete from parents to offspring. Computer simulation methods were proposed for certain problems in pedigree analysis many years ago (Ott, 1974b, 1979a), but it is only relatively recently that practical applications have been developed.

Unconditional Simulation of Genotypes and Phenotypes. In Chapter 5, expected lod scores $E[Z(\theta)]$ are calculated for some family types. These calculations can be carried out analytically because the phenotypes in those families occur in a limited number of classes with known probabilities of occurrence. For general pedigrees, analogous calculations may be approximated by Monte Carlo methods as follows: One starts by randomly assigning genotypes at, say, two loci to all founders in the pedigree, as described above. With given genotypes of two founding mates and an assumed (''true'') recombination fraction *r* between the two loci, a haplotype (gamete) is randomly produced for each founder. The two haplotypes then represent the genotype of a child. This process is repeated for each child and each parental mating. Given the genotype of each individual, a phenotype is assigned which may be the same as the genotype in the case of codominant loci, or it may have to be produced randomly in the case of incomplete penetrance. This completes one round (one *replicate*) of unconditionally simulating genotypes and phenotypes. Computer programs such as SIMULATE (Terwilliger et al., 1993) can rapidly generate thousands of such replicates. For multiple loci, in addition to generating alleles and genotypes, what must also be simulated are crossovers. This is usually accomplished by assuming independence and uniform distribution of crossovers over a chromosome.

Each replicate is now analyzed as if it had been observed in reality. Assume that phenotypes at a disease and a marker locus have been generated (the ''unknown'' phenotype is obtained by simply deleting generated phenotypes for unavailable individuals). For each replicate generated, one now computes lod scores $Z(\theta)$ at various assumed values of θ (notice the difference between true and assumed recombination fractions!). To obtain a representative random sample of phenotype arrays in the family members, a reasonably large number of replicates is required, for example, $n = 500$. Being randomly sampled, each such generated array has probability of occurrence $P_i = 1/n$ in the sample. In analogy to equation (5.11), at each θ, an expected lod score is now calculated as the average of the lod scores generated. Once this is done at each θ value, one obtains the expected (average) lod score curve. With a very large number of replicates, it should have its maximum at the true recombination fraction, $\theta = r$, under which the replicates were generated.

In most applications, not the whole expected lod score curve is of interest but only the ELOD (see Chapter 5), that is, the expected lod score at $\theta = r$. It has the nice property of being additive over families and provides a measure for the linkage informativeness of pedigree structures.

Unconditional Simulation of Marker Genotypes with Given Disease Phenotypes. The above application of computer simulation is of rather theoretical interest. In practice, one might want to know, for example, the false positive rate (type 1 error) associated with an observed maximum lod score at a single locus (see Section 4.6) or in a genome screen of hundreds of marker loci. Assume that linkage analysis has resulted in an observed maximum lod score, Z_{obs}. How likely is it to obtain such a result by chance? The probability of finding a maximum lod score, Z_{max}, as high or higher than Z_{obs}, given no linkage, is termed the empirical significance level associated with Z_{obs}. It may conveniently be approximated by computer simulation in a manner analogous to the procedure outlined above. The only difference here is that disease phenotypes are already known and do not have to be generated. Because the disease locus is assumed to be unlinked with the marker loci, unconditional simulation of marker genotypes is possible, for example, with the SIMULATE program available at ftp://linkage.rockefeller.edu/software/simulate/. In each replicate, a complete analysis is carried out as if marker genotypes has been observed in reality. Thus, each replicate furnishes a maximum lod score. The proportion, p, of replicates with a maximum lod score equal to or greater than Z_{obs} approximates the empirical significance level (the p-value).

Computer simulation methods allow approximating the empirical significance level p associated with an observed Z_{obs} even when that has been obtained under unusual circumstances and cannot be interpreted in the usual manner, for example, because of the application of multiple diagnostic schemes. A well-known example is a linkage analysis carried out for schizophrenia and chromosome 5 markers (Sherrington et al., 1988). Three diagnostic schemes and a range of different penetrance values under each diagnostic scheme were tried. As one usually reports the overall maximum lod score obtained under any model tried, this practice amounts to maximizing the lod score over model parameters. The resulting maximum lod score must be inflated as compared to the distribution of Z_{max} values evaluated under fixed parameter values (maximized only over θ values). This was indeed shown by Weeks et al. (1990) and Clerget-Darpoux et al. (1990), who computed p-values associated with the maximum lod score observed in the study. A locus-specific p-value of 0.0001 asymptotically corresponds to a "real" maximum lod score criterion of 3. In genome-wide analysis, a p-value of 0.05 is generally considered evidence for significant linkage, which corresponds to locus-specific lod score thresholds somewhat higher than 3 (see Section 4.7).

A value of p obtained in a simulation is an estimate for the true but unknown significance level. What number n of replicates is required for an accurate estimate of p? Often, p is a small number, and if n is chosen too small, p will tend to be estimated as zero (no Z_{max} exceeds Z_{obs}). It is therefore important to determine the confidence interval for p based on the number n of replicates carried out. Detailed instructions on how to compute confidence intervals are provided in Section 3.6. In principle, a linkage should be declared significant when not only p but also the upper bound of its associated confidence interval is smaller than 0.0001 (locus-specific) or 0.05 (genome-wide). As mentioned in Section 3.6, confidence intervals are conveniently determined using the BINOM program. For example, let k denote the number of maximum lod scores generated which exceed Z_{obs}, and assume that in $n = 500$ replicates, no replicate showed a maximum lod score exceeding Z_{obs}. Thus, with $k = 0$, the estimated p-value is equal to zero and its 95% confidence interval extends from 0 through 0.0060, which is much larger than 0.0001. Hence, one will even in the best situation ($k = 0$) never be able to declare a linkage significant when only 500 replicates are used. With $k = 0$ out of n replicates, the upper endpoint of the $100(1 - \alpha)\%$ confidence interval is equal to $p_U = 1 - \alpha^{1/n}$. Solving this for n yields $n = \log(\alpha)/\log(1 - p_U)$, which is the number of replicates required such that, with $k = 0$, the confidence interval for the p-value extends from 0 through p_U. For example, with $\alpha = 0.10$ (90% confidence interval) and $k = 0$, $n \approx 23{,}000$ replicates are required for the upper confidence limit of p to be smaller than 0.0001, and $n \approx 45$ for $p_U \leq 0.05$ (genome-wide significance level).

Simulation of Marker Genotypes Given Observed Disease Phenotypes. Whereas randomly generating genotypes for family members is relatively straightforward, it is more difficult to generate marker genotypes conditionally, that is, at a marker locus given observed phenotypes at a disease locus, when the two loci are genetically linked. In that case, as pointed out by Boehnke (1986), sampling must be carried out from the conditional distribution of the genotypes given phenotypes. Conditional sampling is relevant, for example, if one requires an answer to the question: Given a set of families with known disease phenotypes already collected, what maximum lod score can one expect from these families if marker typing is to be carried out on family members? Answers to such questions are obviously of importance in the planning of a linkage study. A computer program, SIMLINK, has been developed to carry out the required simulations. Its original version (Boehnke, 1986) required knowing the disease genotypes for each individual, but an extension of it is applicable to more general situations (Ploughman and Boehnke, 1989).

Another program, SLINK, was developed based on a method exploiting the ability of linkage programs to carry out risk calculations (Ott, 1989b). The SLINK (Weeks, Ott, and Lathrop, 1990) and FastSLINK (ftp://watson.hgen.pitt.edu/pub/slink/) programs implement a particular form of such "risk" calculations on marker genotypes. These programs are applicable to a wide range of situations, for example, that some individuals may already have known marker genotypes. Given that some but not all individuals in a particular family are typed and only a portion of the remaining untyped individuals can still be investigated, one may ask who should be typed next. One way of answering this question would be to determine the increase in expected lod score due to typing each one of the remaining untyped individuals, which can be evaluated with SLINK. One would then choose that individual leading to the highest increase in ELOD. Owing to its generality, this method of generating marker genotypes is relatively slow compared with the more specialized genotype simulation procedures discussed above.

Conditional simulation of marker genotypes is usually used for the estimation of power. For known disease phenotypes in family members, marker genotypes are generated under some postulated recombination fraction such as $r = 0.01$. Also, characteristics of the marker must be specified, for example, that it has four equally frequent alleles (corresponding to a heterozygosity of 0.75). There are usually two numbers obtained from such a simulation. The first is the proportion of replicates in which the maximum lod score exceeds some threshold. This estimates power (corresponding to the significance level under no linkage); that is, the probability that the given data will find a significant linkage. The second number is just the average of the maximum lod scores obtained in each replicate, the so-called EMLOD. It tends to be somewhat higher than the

ELOD and is not quite additive over families. Approximately, a maximum lod score equal to or exceeding the EMLOD will be found with probability of 50%.

Maximum or Average Lod Scores. If evidence for linkage has been found, one may want to carry out a simulation under the assumption of linkage, generating marker genotypes under an assumed true recombination rate equal to that estimated in the real data. One would then expect that generated maximum lod scores will be in the neighborhood of Z_{obs}, that is, finding a lod score as high or higher than Z_{obs} should no longer be a rare event. In other words, if linkage is what caused the high value, Z_{obs}, then the probability of finding a maximum lod score at least as high as Z_{obs} should be around 50%. Otherwise, one has to suspect that there are reasons other than linkage which have led to the high value of Z_{obs} in the data. For example, the model for the disease might be incorrect although this would not generally be expected to lead to false evidence for linkage. Other possible explanations might include: (1) The observations were subject to some sort of bias, for example, preferential scrutiny of recombinants but not nonrecombinants, which tends to eliminate true recombinants; (2) The disease model was chosen to fit the data; or (3) The lod score was maximized over model parameters and this was only partially (or not at all) taken into account in the simulation. A simulation under $r < \frac{1}{2}$ (linkage) may thus serve as a check for the plausibility of the observations but, to my knowledge, such analyses are not often carried out.

Rather than considering the average lod score as recommended above, researchers sometimes focus on the largest possible lod score under linkage (the largest Z_{max} value in all replicates). This overall maximum represents the highest lod score one is able to obtain from the given data. It may, however, be very unlikely to ever find this high of a lod score, so that relying on that overall maximum might be misleading. This question is extensively discussed in Section 5.10. Here, computer simulation is used to demonstrate the difference between the overall maximum lod score and the expected (average) lod score. For two pedigrees such as the one shown in Figure 9.3, genotypes were generated for a marker with five equally frequent alleles, completely linked with a dominant disease. Penetrances at the disease locus were 0.01 and 0.90 for phenocopies and genetic cases, respectively, and the disease allele frequency was set to 0.0001. Two thousand replicates were generated in such a way that the marker was effectively fully informative (the unaffected top parent was always given the genotype *1/1*, the affected top parent *2/3*, and the remain-

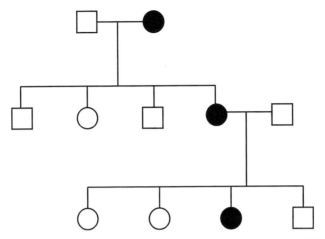

Figure 9.3. Artificial family for simulation of maximum and average lod scores.

ing founder individual *4/5*). Each replicate was analyzed by evaluating assumed recombination fractions in steps of 0.02. The average lod score turned out to be 1.03 with an overall maximum lod score of 3.12. Clearly, there is a huge discrepancy between average and maximum lod scores despite full marker informativeness and complete linkage. For these two pedigrees, the probability of finding a maximum lod score exceeding the threshold of 3 was estimated as 0.069. There is nothing an investigator could do to achieve the maximum lod score of 3.12—the variability of maximum lod scores in those families is random. It depends on marker inheritance and is beyond the control of the investigator.

Tips and Tricks. Based on the uniformly distributed random variables, *U,* variables with other distributions may be generated through suitable *transformations.* If *X* is a random variable with distribution function $F(\cdot)$ that has an explicit inverse, $F^{-1}(\cdot)$, then the probability integral transformation (Parzen, 1960) furnishes a convenient way to obtain values of *X* from values of *U*. For example, based on equation (7.10), the transformation

$$X = \mu - \frac{\sigma}{c}\ln\frac{1-U}{U} \tag{9.17}$$

furnishes values of a variable, *X,* with a logistic distribution whose respective mean and standard deviation are μ and σ, with $c = 1.8138$ being a constant.

The discrete analog of the probability integral transformation provides a way to generate random variables with discrete distributions such as the binomial. Assume that this distribution is defined for a finite number of integers (classes) with associated probability p_i for the ith class. The standard approach is to draw a random number, U, and assign an individual to class 1 if $U < p_1$, assign the individual to class 2 if $U < (p_1 + p_2)$, to class 3 if $U < (p_1 + p_2 + p_3)$, and so on, stopping as soon as the inequality is satisfied. Obviously, it is most efficient to arrange the p_i's in such a way that large class probabilities are tested first. A quick method (also known as the table look-up method) requires truncating the p_i to, say, two or three decimal places. For example, let $p_1 = 0.03$, $p_2 = 0.15$, $p_3 = 0.09$, and so forth. Then one fills an integer array, V_i, $i = 1 \ldots$ 100, as follows: The first three elements of V are assigned the value 1, that is, $V_1 = V_2 = V_3 = 1$. The next 15 elements of V, V_4 through V_{18}, are assigned the value 2, the next nine elements of V are assigned the value 3, and so on. Now, if a random number is drawn, it is multiplied by 100 and rounded to the nearest integer so that one obtains $W = [100U + 0.5]$, where $[r]$ is the nearest integer for the real number r. Then, $V(W)$ is the number of the class into which this observation should fall. Clearly, for small numbers of classes, the standard approach is faster because it requires only a small number of ''if'' evaluations, while the table look-up method requires multiplication and truncation.

To obtain a normally $N(0, 1)$ distributed variable, X, one makes use of the fact that the sum of independent uniform variables, U, quickly approaches normality as the number of terms in the sum increases. The transformation

$$X = \tfrac{1}{2}\left(\sum_{i=1}^{48} U_i \right) - 12 \tag{9.18}$$

generates normal variables with zero mean and unit variance (Newman and Odell, 1971).

To generate multivariate normal variables, $X \sim N(0, \Sigma)$, with zero means and $n \times n$ variance covariance matrix, Σ, the easiest approach is through a certain factorization, $\Sigma = AA^T$, where A is a lower triangular matrix and A^T its transpose (all material in this paragraph is based on Newman and Odell, 1971, with some errors corrected). The elements, a_{ij}, of A can be computed recursively from Σ, where i refers to rows and j to columns, and the recursion proceeds by columns as follows:

$$a_{11} = \sigma_{11}^{1/2},$$

$$a_{i1} = \sigma_{i1}/a_{11}.$$

When a given column is done, the next (jth) column is started with the diagonal element,

$$a_{jj} = \left(\sigma_{jj} - \sum_{k-1}^{j-1} a_{jk}^2 \right)^{1/2},$$

and the column completed with

$$a_{ij} = \left(\frac{\sigma_{ij} - \sum_{k-1}^{j-1} a_{ik}a_{jk}}{a_{jj}} \right)$$

for $i = j + 1, \ldots , n$. The example given by Newman and Odell (1971) is

$$\Sigma = \begin{bmatrix} 4 & 2 & 2 \\ 2 & 5 & 1 \\ 1 & 1 & 5 \end{bmatrix}, \quad A = \begin{bmatrix} 2 & 0 & 0 \\ 1 & 2 & 0 \\ 1 & 0 & 2 \end{bmatrix}.$$

To reliably approximate small p-values, such a large number of replicates may be required that it might not be feasible to carry out. Under linkage, the probability of exceeding some threshold lod score is expected to be much higher than under no linkage. Thus, a possible solution is to generate data under the alternative hypothesis, that is, under linkage and appropriately correct the probability of the resulting random observations. Such a procedure was once suggested to me by Dr. Kenneth Lange (Ott, 1979a). It later became known as *importance sampling* (Hammersley and Handscomb, 1983; Ott and Terwilliger, 1992; Kong et al., 1992). However, its drawback is that parameters under the alternative hypothesis of linkage may not be well specified for complex traits.

For some applications, random permutations must be formed. That is, n observations should be put into a random order. A simple approach is to take the first observation and put it at random into one of the n new places. Then take the second observation and put it at random into one of the remaining $n - 1$ places, and so forth. To randomly assign an observation to one of k equally likely places, one draws a random number, U, and finds $[kU + 0.5]$ is the associated random place number. For methods to list all possible permutations of a set of n numbers, see Lehmer (1964) or Nijenhuis and Wilf (1978). The method described in Lehmer (1964) is implemented in the PERMUTE program of the Linkage Utilities.

The Monte Carlo methods presented here are all based on so-called simple random sampling. When the calculation of a replicate is time consuming, one may want to generate only a small number of replicates and apply to them one of the numerical resampling techniques such as the jackknife or the bootstrap (Efron, 1982; Weir, 1996; Terwilliger and Ott, 1992a).

9.8. Problems

Problem 9.1. Write down the lod score corresponding to the likelihood given in equation (9.1).

Problem 9.2. For family *B5* covered in Section 9.1, write down the lod scores for the two limiting cases, $p = 0$ and $p = 1$.

Problem 9.3. An animal breeder wants to localize a recessive disease gene. She has various possibilities of setting up suitable matings to score offspring for linkage. In particular, she is considering the following two mating types in which all individuals have known phase at the disease locus (alleles $+$ and *d*, *d* = disease allele) and an assumed marker locus (alleles *1, 2, . . .*).

I. Both parents are doubly heterozygous, that is, have genotypes *d1/+2* and *d3/+4* (both unaffected). The advantage of this mating type is that both parents are informative for linkage but unaffected offspring are of ambiguous genotype.

II. One parent is doubly heterozygous, *d1/+2* (unaffected), whereas the other is doubly homozygous, *d3/d3* (affected). Only the doubly heterozygous parent is informative for linkage but all offspring, affected and unaffected, can unambiguously be scored for linkage.

Given the same number of offspring per mating, which provides more linkage information? *Hint*: Compute expected lod scores for different values of the recombination fraction, *r*.

10.

Variability of the Recombination Fraction

Thus far, variation in the estimates, $\hat{\theta}$, of the recombination fraction have been attributed to random fluctuation about the true unknown recombination rate, r. In this section, situations will be discussed in which r is not constant but depends on other variables. Two principally different situations will be distinguished: (1) r varies between recognizable classes of families and is constant within each class, and (2) families with different values of r form a mixture and cannot be differentiated as to which ones share the same r value. In statistics, the two cases are referred to as fixed effects and random effects situations, respectively. Sections 10.1 through 10.3 address case 1, Section 10.4 covers the mixture case, and Section 10.5 discusses the mixed situation, in which random effects occur within fixed categories of families. Section 10.6 addresses efficiency of analyses due to incorporation of biological variables.

10.1. Male and Female Recombination Fractions

According to a rule by Haldane (1922), crossing over is more frequent in the homogametic sex (e.g., XX) than in the heterogametic sex (e.g., XY). This rule applies in many animal species. An extreme case is that of the fruit fly *Drosophila*, where the male does not show any recombination at all. In humans, a clear sex difference in the recombination fraction was first shown for the linkage between ABO and the locus for the nail-patella syndrome (NPS1), with a lower estimate of the recombination rate in males, $\hat{\theta}_m = 0.084$, than in females, $\hat{\theta}_f = 0.146$ (Renwick and Schulze, 1965). Since then, the ratio θ_f/θ_m of female to male recombination rate has been found to vary in the human genome from region to region (Donis-Keller et al., 1987). On some chromosomes, there is a male excess at one or both telomeres and a female excess elsewhere, for example, on chromosomes 12 (O'Connell et al., 1987) and 16 (Keith et al., 1990). On other chromosomes, recombination in females is uniformly more frequent (e.g., on chromosome 21; Warren et al., 1989). Differences in recombination rates between the two sexes are a form of *heterogeneity,* which should be taken into account in the analysis. In a linkage analysis, it is thus important to estimate θ_m and θ_f separately. The two-point case will be considered first.

It is easiest to obtain separate two-point estimates of θ_m and θ_f when one can distinguish families in which only fathers are informative for linkage (doubly heterozygous) from those with only mothers as the informative parents. The former families will yield lod scores $Z_m(\theta_m)$ for the recombination fraction in males, and the latter will result in "female" lod scores, $Z_f(\theta_f)$. Bivariate lod scores with respect to male and female recombination rates are then simply the sum,

$$Z(\theta_m, \theta_f) = Z_m(\theta_m) + Z_f(\theta_f). \tag{10.1}$$

The graph of the joint lod score (10.1) may be pictured as a mountainous surface above a plane with coordinates, θ_m and θ_f, with $Z(\theta_m, \theta_f)$ being the height above the plane at the point (θ_m, θ_f).

Generally, matings cannot be separated by the sex of the informative parent. Instead one must estimate sex-specific recombination rates by calculating joint lod scores, $Z(\theta_m, \theta_f)$, for example, using the LIPED program. Consider the results shown in Table 10.1, which were obtained in a linkage analysis of a large multigenerational family (Vogel and Motulsky, 1986). The values along the diagonal (italicized) are lod scores calculated under the assumption of equal male and female recombination fractions, $Z(\theta, \theta)$, $\theta = \theta_m = \theta_f$, with a maximum lod of $Z(\theta, \theta) = 6.84$ at $\theta = 0.10$. The overall maximum lod score is 7.88 with sex-specific recombination fraction estimates of $\hat{\theta}_m = 0.05$ and $\hat{\theta}_f = 0.20$.

The significance of an observed heterogeneity in recombination frac-

Table 10.1. Sex-Specific Lod Scores in a Pedigree with Dentinogenesis Imperfecta and GC Blood Types

θ_m	Female Recombination Fraction, θ_f				
	0.05	0.10	0.20	0.30	0.50
0.50	0.28	0.70	1.19	1.01	*0*
0.30	2.74	3.98	4.73	*4.68*	3.42
0.20	4.30	5.62	*6.42*	6.37	5.08
0.10	5.50	*6.84*	7.64	7.59	6.26
0.05	*5.74*	7.08	**7.88**	7.83	6.48

Source: Adapted from table A9.3 in Vogel and Motulsky, 1986.

tion estimates is determined by the difference between the maximum lod scores achieved under the two hypotheses, H_0 : homogeneity ($\theta_m = \theta_f$), and H_1 : heterogeneity ($\theta_m \neq \theta_f$). Asymptotically,

$$X^2 = 2 \times \ln(10) \, [Z(\hat{\theta}_m, \hat{\theta}_f) - Z(\hat{\theta}, \hat{\theta})] \qquad (10.2)$$

follows a chi-square distribution on 1 df. For the example in Table 10.1, one finds $X^2 = 4.6 \times (7.88 - 6.84) = 4.784$, with an associated empirical significance level of $p = 0.029$ (obtained from the CHIPROB program). The difference between male and female recombination fraction estimates is thus significant at the 5% level but not at the 1% level.

Table 10.1 demonstrates that it is generally easier to find a high lod score when θ_m and θ_f are distinguished than when they are kept equal. Hence one should in such cases set a higher critical lod score. This situation is analogous to multiple comparisons (two comparisons in this case) discussed in Section 4.7. The appropriate critical lod score should thus be raised from $Z_0 = 3$ to approximately $Z_0 + \log(2) = 3.3$. In practice, this is not often done. When a strong difference between male and female recombination rates exists, lod scores at $\theta = \theta_m = \theta_f$ may all be much lower than the overall maximum. One may then miss detecting a linkage by not allowing for a difference between θ_m and θ_f.

Male and female recombination fraction estimates are independent when the bivariate lods can be represented as the sum of two terms,

$$Z(\theta_m, \theta_f) = Z(\theta_m, \tfrac{1}{2}) + Z(\tfrac{1}{2}, \theta_f), \qquad (10.3)$$

which is analogous to equation (10.1). The first term on the right side of (10.3) corresponds to the lod scores in the rightmost column (at $\theta_f = \tfrac{1}{2}$) of Table 10.1, and the second term corresponds to the top row (at $\theta_m = \tfrac{1}{2}$). If θ_m and θ_f are independent, the two terms on the right side of (10.3) represent male and female lod scores, respectively, and lod scores at any point in the plane are equal to the sum of the corresponding two marginal lods. This condition can serve as a useful verification for the independence of male and female recombination rates. For example, with independence in Table 10.1, one would expect that $Z(0.05, 0.20)$ should be equal to $Z(0.05, \tfrac{1}{2}) + Z(\tfrac{1}{2}, 0.20) = 6.48 + 1.19 = 7.67$. In fact, it is equal to 7.88, so that the estimates are not independent, but nearly so. Nonindependence of the estimates may occur, for example, when an offspring demonstrates a recombination, but it is unknown in which parent it occurred. In such cases, one cannot estimate θ_m without specifying θ_f, and vice versa. Hodge et al. (1998) reported an interesting example of an extreme case, in which the design of a linkage study in rats made θ_m indistinguishable from θ_f.

In practice, bivariate lods such as those shown in Table 10.1 are not usually published. Instead, one records the univariate lods, $Z(\theta, \theta)$, at the usual θ values. In addition, one indicates the overall maximum lod score and the values of θ_m and θ_f at which it occurred. Sometimes, male and female lods are read off a table such as Table 10.1 along the margins, that is, as $Z(\theta_m, \frac{1}{2})$ and $Z(\frac{1}{2}, \theta_f)$. As pointed out by Morton (1978), when the estimates are in any way correlated, this manner of defining sex-specific lod scores is inappropriate.

As pointed out in Section 9.3, the LINKAGE programs use a different parametrization from that described above. They work with the two parameters θ_m and R, where $R = x_f/x_m$ is the ratio of female-to-male map distance. Equations (9.6) and (9.7) provide conversion formulas between θ_f and R (the SEXDIF utility program allows for conversion between many different parameters). The use of R instead of separate male and female recombination fractions is most useful in multipoint linkage analysis. In maps of whole chromosomes, three hypotheses are often distinguished. Consider $n + 1$ marker loci and n map intervals, with R_i referring to the female-to-male map distance ratio in the ith interval. Then the three hypotheses are:

1. $R_i = 1$, that is, female and male map distances are the same in each interval (n parameters)
2. $R_i = R_j \neq 1$, that is, the value of R is the same in each interval but is different from 1 ($n + 1$ parameters)
3. $R_i \neq R_j$, that is, male and female recombination fractions are different in each interval ($2n$ parameters)

On many chromosomes, a plot of R_i reveals a trend along the chromosome. Low order (linear, quadratic cubic) trends of R or $Q = (x_f - x_m)/(x_f + x_m)$ have been investigated statistically (Fann and Ott, 1995). Such trends correspond to hypotheses intermediate between hypotheses 2 and 3 considered above. For example, chromosome 4 shows a quadratic trend of R with $R < 1$ at chromosome ends and $R > 1$ in the middle of the chromosome (Li et al., 1998).

10.2. Recombination Fraction and Age

Several methods have been used to investigate whether the recombination fraction changes with age but, overall, the question of age dependency of the recombination fraction has not received much attention.

Haldane and Crew (1925) investigated offspring of phase-known matings in poultry. They had obtained five cocks that were doubly heterozygous *BS/bs* for two sex-linked mendelian loci, and mated them with *bs* hens. The four possible offspring types could all be distinguished phenotypically. Based on a total of 648 chicks, the estimated recombination fraction turned out to be 0.229, 0.369, and 0.476 in the first, second, and third breeding years, respectively. Thus, linkage became progressively weaker with advancing age of the cocks.

A thorough analysis for the ABO-NPS1 linkage was carried out by Elston, Lange, and Namboodiri (1976). These authors estimated by maximum likelihood the parameters of regression lines, regressing the recombination fraction on age a, $\theta = \alpha + \beta a$, separately for males and females. In fifteen large families comprising a total of 289 individuals, achieving a maximum lod score of 15.5, they found that age was more significant than sex in its effect on the recombination fraction, but neither factor was formally significant; the empirical significance level was much larger than 0.05. The age effect observed by Elston, Lange, and Namboodiri (1976) seemed to be limited to males. Under the restriction $0 \leq \theta \leq \frac{1}{2}$, they estimated a decrease in θ_m of $\beta = 0.003$ per year. This means that, for example, in 20 years, θ_m for ABO versus NPS1 is expected to drop by 6 cM.

For 27 markers spanning 102 cM on the long arm of chromosome 21, Tanzi et al. (1992) compared patterns of recombination in specific regions with regard to both parental sex and age. They found a statistically significant downward trend in the frequency of recombinations in the most telomeric portion of chromosome 21 with increasing maternal age. A less significant decrease in recombination with increasing maternal age was observed in the pericentromeric region of the chromosome. These results have not been confirmed and the question of a general age-dependency of the recombination fraction in humans is still somewhat unclear.

10.3. Heterogeneity between Classes of Families

A phenotype, in particular a disease, is genetically heterogeneous when it has a genetically different etiology in different individuals, for example, when in some individuals or families a disease is due to a single gene, whereas in other individuals the same disease phenotype is caused by an environmental agent. In the context of linkage analysis, two types of heterogeneities are distinguished, allelic and nonallelic heterogeneity; the latter is also referred to as locus heterogeneity. With allelic heterogeneity, individuals differ from each other by having different alleles at the same locus responsible for the disease; in nonallelic heterogeneity, however, the disease is caused by different loci. The two types of heterogeneity may be characterized as outlined below. Assume that some pathway of biochemical steps leads to the production of an enzyme which, when missing, results in disease. If several of the steps in the pathway are susceptible to being interrupted, the disease may show locus heterogeneity. On the other hand, if all but one of the steps are stable, but the single step accumulates different mutations, each leading to an interruption of the pathway, the disease may exhibit allelic heterogeneity. An example of the latter is cystic fibrosis: A fairly large number of different mutant alleles have been found in affected individuals, all at the same locus on chromosome 7 (Davies, 1990). An example of a disease with locus heterogeneity is Charcot–Marie–Tooth disease, which may be caused by at least a locus on chromosome 1 or a locus on chromosome 17 (Ouvrier, 1996) and is discussed further in Section 10.4. Also, retinitis pigmentosa may be caused by various loci; linkage studies of large families and candidate-gene screening of known retinal genes have identified 59 independent genetic loci that can cause retinal degeneration such as retinitis pigmentosa and macular degeneration (Sullivan and Daiger, 1996). A classical case of locus heterogeneity is that between elliptocytosis and the Rh blood group (Morton, 1956).

A striking example for locus heterogeneity was reported by Trevor-Roper (1952) (quoted by McKusick, 1990; MIM no. 203200, autosomal recessive albinism). Two albino parents had four normally pigmented children, which suggests the presence of two different genes for albinism in the parents.

When a disease is relatively rare and mutation rates are low, individuals within a family are generally homogeneous. Locus heterogeneity then leads to the situation that the recombination fraction between disease phenotype and marker will be different in different families, whereas allelic heterogeneity does not lead to such differences. Hence, only locus heterogeneity, not allelic heterogeneity, can be detected through linkage analysis. In the absence of any biochemical clues for heterogeneity, linkage analysis has more than once proved to be a powerful tool for unraveling such situations.

In this section, the rather simple case of heterogeneity between recognizable classes of families is discussed. The next section covers the more complex situation in which heterogeneity in θ is the only means of differentiating between families. The principles will be outlined below for two-point linkage analysis.

By various criteria, families may be grouped into a number c of classes, among which the recombination fraction may vary. For example, families may have been contributed to an analysis by different investigators, or they may come from different countries. One may also want to distinguish simplex from multiplex families (families with one or several affecteds); or $c = 2$ classes may be formed based on whether a disease is associated with HLA haplotypes or not (as in Hodge et al., 1983). Analogously, recombination events may be distinguished as to whether they occurred in males or females (see Section 10.1). Of course, each family may be considered to form its own class so that c is equal to the number of families, which is the situation originally considered by Morton (1956). To test whether the recombination fraction varies between classes, one compares the likelihood under homogeneity with that under heterogeneity. The hypothesis H_1 of linkage and homogeneity specifies $r_1 = r_2 = \ldots = r_c < \frac{1}{2}$, where r_i denotes the true value of the recombination fraction in the ith class. Under heterogeneity, $H_2 : r_1 \neq r_2 \neq \ldots$, the recombination fraction is potentially different in each class. Notice that H_1 is obtained from H_2 by imposing $c - 1$ linear restrictions, for example, $r_2 = r_1, r_3 = r_1, \ldots, r_c = r_1$. To test H_1 against H_2, Morton (1956) introduced the likelihood ratio test described below into linkage analysis. To distinguish it from other homogeneity tests discussed later, in this book Morton's test is called the *M-test*.

Let $Z_i(\theta)$ denote the total lod score of the families in the ith class, and let $\hat{\theta}_i$ be the MLE of the recombination fraction in the ith class, that is, that value of θ at which $Z_i(\theta)$ is largest. Adding up the lod scores at given θ values over classes leads to the grand total $Z(\theta) = \Sigma_i Z_i(\theta)$, with an associated maximum at the estimate $\hat{\theta}$ of the overall recombination fraction. With this, one computes

$$X^2 = 2 \times \ln(10)[\Sigma Z_i(\hat{\theta}_i) - Z(\hat{\theta})]. \tag{10.5}$$

Asymptotically, under the assumption of homogeneity (H_1), X^2 follows a chi-square distribution with $(c - 1)$ df, that is, the test is considered significant, and homogeneity is rejected, when X^2 is larger than the appropriate critical chi-square value. The test is easy to carry out by hand, or one may use the MTEST computer program.

For medium values of the recombination fraction $(r \approx 0.20)$ and large family sizes, the M-test tends to be nonconservative (actual significance level exceeds the formal significance level predicted on the basis of the chi-square distribution) (Risch, 1988). For example, with $c = 10$ families of eight recombination events each, the formal critical value of χ^2_{c-1} is 16.9 for a significance level of 5%. However, when the true recombination fraction is equal to 0.20 in each family, the test will be significant with a probability of roughly 10%.

As a practical example, consider the lod scores in 29 families between polycystic kidney disease and the 3'HVR locus on chromosome 16, which are displayed in Table 10.2. Inspection of the table shows that the θ estimates in each family range from 0 to 0.20 with one family having all negative lod scores ($\hat{\theta} = 0.50$). Application of the M-test yields a sum of the 29 maximum lod scores of 64.28, and the maximum of the sum of lod scores at the same θ values over families is equal to 56.96. With this, application of equation (10.5) results in $X^2 = 33.71$ with 28 df, which approximately corresponds to a p-value of 0.21. This result suggests that no difference in the true recombination fractions in the 29 families exists. Further analysis of these families is presented in the next section.

Table 10.2. Two-Point Lod Scores of Polycystic Kidney Disease (PKD1) versus the Marker 3'HVR and Conditional Probability w of Being of the Linked Type

| Family i | \multicolumn{7}{c}{Recombination Fraction} | | | | | | | w_i |
	0	0.001	0.05	0.10	0.20	0.30	0.40	
1	−2.15	−1.46	0.04	0.23	*0.28*	0.19	0.07	0.963
2	*5.19*	5.19	4.76	4.30	3.31	2.19	0.93	1.000
3	−∞	0.25	1.69	*1.71*	1.41	0.90	0.30	0.999
4	2.92	2.91	2.66	2.39	1.81	1.18	0.49	0.999
5	*1.09*	1.09	0.99	0.88	0.64	0.38	0.12	0.995
6	2.24	2.24	2.03	1.81	1.32	0.78	0.24	0.999
7	−∞	−1.13	0.37	*0.46*	0.37	0.20	0.05	0.982
8	*0.90*	0.90	0.81	0.72	0.52	0.30	0.09	0.993
9	*0.26*	0.26	0.24	0.22	0.15	0.08	0.02	0.976
10	*1.28*	1.28	1.17	1.04	0.73	0.40	0.10	0.997
11	*2.61*	2.61	2.33	2.06	1.50	0.90	0.30	0.999
12	−∞	0.02	2.51	*2.78*	2.27	1.54	0.72	0.999
13	*0.60*	0.60	0.53	0.46	0.32	0.17	0.05	0.987
14	*1.77*	1.77	1.59	1.41	1.01	0.59	0.21	0.998
15	−∞	7.26	*8.04*	7.37	5.62	3.63	1.51	1.000
16	−∞	0.53	2.04	*2.11*	1.84	1.31	0.62	0.999
17	2.93	2.92	2.66	2.38	1.77	1.09	0.38	0.999
18	−∞	0.50	1.94	*1.97*	1.67	1.17	0.53	0.999
19	*0.60*	0.60	0.53	0.46	0.32	0.17	0.05	0.987
20	2.71	2.70	2.44	2.17	1.61	1.02	0.42	0.999
21	−∞	−0.71	0.82	*0.95*	0.88	0.66	0.36	0.993
22	−∞	0.06	2.99	*3.08*	2.60	1.76	0.76	1.000
23	−∞	−0.41	1.10	*1.20*	1.05	0.74	0.45[a]	0.996
24	*3.50*	3.49	3.21	2.92	2.27	1.55	0.77	1.000
25	−∞	1.76	4.59	*4.59*	3.87	2.72	1.25	1.000
26	−∞	−2.14	1.09	1.47	*1.52*	1.38	0.56	0.996
27	−∞	0.23	3.23	*3.38*	2.96	2.11	0.99	1.000
28	*3.61*	3.16	3.32	3.02	2.38	1.67	0.89	1.000
29	−∞	−9.29	−2.76	−1.68	−0.72	−0.28	−0.06	0.040
Sum	−∞	27.19	*56.96*	55.86	45.28	30.50	13.17	

Sources: Families 1–28 from Reeders et al. (1987); family 29 from Romeo et al. (1988).
[a] Value interpolated.

In practice, one often investigates several linked marker loci simultaneously and calculates multipoint lod scores or location scores (see Chapter 6) for various positions of a disease locus along a map of marker loci. The M-test may then be carried out as before, using equation (10.5), where the constant, $\ln(10)$, must be dropped if natural logarithms instead of logarithms to the base 10 are used. Notice, however, that multipoint lod scores are generally multimodal, and it is unclear whether the same asymptotic approximations hold as in the two-point case. With multipoint lod scores, therefore, asymptotic empirical p-values must be taken to be very approximate, or they should not be used at all. Instead one may simply report the observed likelihood ratio R between the two hypotheses H_1 and H_2, which may be obtained from equation (10.5) as

$$R = \exp(\tfrac{1}{2}X^2). \tag{10.6}$$

Of course, R may have to be interpreted differently depending on the number of classes (degrees of freedom) investigated, for it is easier to obtain a large likelihood ratio with an increased number c of classes. For example, $X^2 = 33.71$ obtained from the 29 families in Table 10.2 translates into a likelihood ratio of approximately $R = 2.09 \times 10^7$, which appears impressive. Per degree of freedom, however, one obtains $X^2/\mathrm{df} = 33.71/28 = 1.204$, corresponding to a likelihood ratio of only $\exp(1.204/2) = 1.8$. This result may also be obtained as the geometric mean per degree of freedom of $R = 2.09 \times 10^7$; it is $(2.09 \times 10^7)^{1/28} = 1.8$.

With a single degree of freedom, various critical levels R_0 have been used as thresholds for determining "significance" or "meaningful difference." Table 10.3 lists the R_0 values commonly used along with the corresponding differences $\Delta\ln(L)$ and $\Delta\log_{10}(L)$, where L stands for likelihood. Parameter values with an associated $\ln(L)$ larger than $\ln(L_{max}) - \Delta\ln(L)$ then belong to the "$\Delta\ln(L)$"-unit support interval. Edwards (1992) recommends constructing 2-unit support intervals ($\Delta\ln(L) = 2$; see Section 3.6). In human genetics, the narrowest support interval generally used is

Table 10.3. Likelihood Ratios R_0 and Corresponding Differences $\Delta\ln$ (Likelihood) and $\Delta\log_{10}$ (Likelihood)

R_0	$\Delta\ln L$	$\Delta\log L$
10	2.3	1.0
20	3.0	1.3
50	3.9	1.7
100	4.6	2.0
1000	6.9	3.0

that corresponding to a critical level of $R_0 = 10$, but often more stringent criteria are applied.

Tests for heterogeneity are usually carried out at the 5% or 1% level of significance. In tests for linkage, however, one requires more stringent criteria, that is, a maximum lod score of at least 3, corresponding to a *p*-value of 0.0001. Assume now that for a particular set of families, the maximum of the total lod score (under homogeneity) stays below 3 yet a test of homogeneity results in a *p*-value of 0.02. Declaring the heterogeneity significant would amount to saying that in some of the families the recombination fraction is significantly smaller than 0.5. This is the same as accepting a significant linkage for some families, which contradicts the conclusion of no significant linkage based on a maximum lod score of less than 3. The solution to this dilemma is that, in the absence of a proven linkage, the test for heterogeneity should only be declared significant when the empirical *p*-value is no larger than 0.0001 or when the likelihood ratio (perhaps on a per df basis) is at least 1000 : 1.

The M-test requires the estimation of a separate parameter, θ_i, in each of the *c* families (or classes). A more powerful (bayesian) approach was proposed by Risch (1988) in the form of the so-called *B-test*. For this test, the θ values in the different families are assumed to follow a beta distribution with two parameters. These two parameters are then estimated from the posterior distribution of θ. The test statistic is constructed on the basis of the difference of the maximum log likelihoods under H_1 and H_2 and is associated with 1 df (a computer program to carry out the B-test is available from Dr. Risch). The B-test is generally conservative and often more powerful than the M-test (Risch, 1988).

An example of two distinct disease forms are Usher's syndrome types I and II, where type I is characterized by a profound hearing loss and absence of vestibular functions, and type II has a milder hearing loss and normal vestibular function. The two forms are genetically heterogeneous, because Usher's syndrome type II is linked with markers on chromosome 1 but type I is not (Kimberling et al., 1990). In this case, clinical heterogeneity runs parallel to genetic heterogeneity. As will be seen below, however, in other diseases this is not necessarily the case.

10.4. Heterogeneity due to a Mixture of Families

In the homogeneity tests considered thus far, the alternative to the hypothesis of homogeneity is that the recombination fraction is potentially different in each family (or family class). In many situations, however, a more plausible alternative is the presence of two types of families, those with linkage ($\theta_1 < \frac{1}{2}$) and those without linkage ($\theta_2 = \frac{1}{2}$) (Smith, 1961). The two family types are mixed such that an unequivocal assignment of a given family to one or the other type is impossible. A common situation leading to this kind of heterogeneity is as follows. In some families a disease is caused by a gene located in the vicinity of a marker locus, whereas in other families the same disease phenotype is due to a disease gene located elsewhere, or the disease is not due to a single gene. In this situation, linkage to the given marker will exist only in the first type of family and not in the others. A good example of a heterogeneous disease that is due to a large number of disease loci is retinitis pigmentosa. For the non-syndromal form alone (only the retina is affected), 18 loci have been found thus far (Wright et al., 1997).

Smith (1963) considered still other cases, for example, three family types, one with recombination fraction $\theta_1 < \frac{1}{2}$, another with θ_2 ($\theta_1 < \theta_2 < \frac{1}{2}$), and a third with $\theta_3 = \frac{1}{2}$, and treated the hypotheses of homogeneity and heterogeneity in a bayesian framework. In this book, the various hypotheses are evaluated by maximum likelihood rather than by bayesian methods (Ott, 1983). A simple introduction to the test procedures will be given first, followed by some theoretical explanations towards the end of this section. In the remainder of this section, the different heterogeneity models are discussed under headings that refer to the names of the corresponding appropriate computer programs.

HOMOG. Consider a mixture of two types of families, one with linkage and one without linkage. It may be tempting to somehow separate the families into two groups, corresponding as much as possible to the two family types, and to analyze the two groups under a known classification scheme as in Section 10.3. This would be fallacious, however, because an investigator would use his judgment to form groups from the mixture of families, thereby adding extra information not contained in the data. This additional information may well inflate the evidence for the presence of two family types. Instead of separating families, it is better to analyze the families as a whole under a model allowing for a mixture. In the simplest such model, two family types exist, with α denoting the proportion of type 1 families and $1 - \alpha$ the proportion of type 2 families. The recombination fraction in the type 1 families is equal to θ_1 and that in the type 2 families is $\theta_2 = \frac{1}{2}$. The bivariate likelihood of the ith family is then given by (Smith, 1961)

$$L_i(\alpha, \theta_1) = \alpha L_i(\theta_1) + (1 - \alpha)L_i(\frac{1}{2}), \qquad (10.7)$$

where $L_i(\theta_1)$ is the likelihood, evaluated at $\theta = \theta_1$. To formulate equation

(10.7) in terms of likelihood ratios, one divides each likelihood by $L_i(\frac{1}{2})$ and thereby adjusts the bivariate likelihood to be equal to 1 at $\theta = \frac{1}{2}$. Thus, one obtains

$$L_i^*(\alpha, \theta_1) = \alpha L_i^*(\theta_1) + (1 - \alpha), \tag{10.8}$$

where $L_i^*(\theta_1)$ is the antilog of the usual lod score in the ith family. The overall (adjusted) log likelihood is then given by

$$\log L(\alpha, \theta_1) = \Sigma_i \log[L_i^*(\alpha, \theta_1)], \tag{10.9}$$

which is a function of the two parameters, α and θ_1. Graphically, the log likelihood (10.9) may be represented as the height above a plane with coordinates α and θ_1. The hypothesis of heterogeneity is then formulated as $H_2 : \alpha < 1, \theta_1 < \frac{1}{2}$, and homogeneity is obtained from H_2 by a single restriction, $H_1 : \alpha = 1$; that is, the families share a common recombination fraction.

The evaluation of (10.9) for given lod scores is straightforward but somewhat time consuming. The HOMOG computer program may conveniently be used to evaluate (10.9) for various values of α and θ_1. Under H_2, estimates of α and θ_1 are obtained as that pair of points for which (10.9) is a maximum. Under H_1 (homogeneity), the restricted estimate, $\hat{\theta}_r$, is obtained. For example, for the 29 families in Table 10.2 with polycystic kidney disease (PKD1) versus the 3′HVR locus on chromosome 16 (Reeders et al., 1987; Romeo et al., 1988), the HOMOG program evaluates the log likelihoods (10.9) as given in Table 10.4. The unrestricted

Table 10.4. Log_e Likelihoods for the 29 Families in Table 10.2

α	Recombination Fraction, θ							
	0	0.001	0.05	0.10	0.20	0.30	0.40	0.50
1.00	$-\infty$	62.61	*131.16*	128.62	104.26	70.23	30.33	0
0.99	10.09	80.49	132.82	128.76	104.06	70.02	30.17	0
0.98	19.42	81.82	133.18	128.78	103.86	69.81	30.02	0
0.97	24.86	82.66	133.30	128.74	103.65	69.60	29.87	0
0.96	28.70	83.28	*133.32*	128.66	103.44	69.38	29.71	0
0.95	31.65	83.76	133.28	128.55	103.22	69.17	29.56	0
0.94	34.04	84.15	133.19	128.42	103.00	68.95	29.40	0
0.92	37.75	84.72	132.95	128.10	102.55	68.51	29.08	0
0.90	40.56	85.13	132.62	127.73	102.09	68.05	28.76	0
0.80	48.64	85.77	130.42	125.42	99.56	65.65	27.06	0
0.70	52.51	85.21	127.59	122.53	96.64	62.96	25.21	0
0.50	55.24	81.91	120.08	114.94	89.29	56.39	20.92	0
0.30	53.48	75.39	108.71	103.50	78.47	47.12	15.38	0
0.10	44.25	60.93	85.89	80.66	57.53	30.41	7.18	0
0.01	24.20	35.84	48.15	43.48	26.47	9.96	0.99	0

estimates are $\hat{\alpha} = 0.96$ and $\hat{\theta}_1 = 0.05$. Under homogeneity ($\alpha = 1$), one obtains $\hat{\theta}_r = 0.05$ which happens to be equal to $\hat{\theta}_1$; generally, $\hat{\alpha}$ and $\hat{\theta}_1$ are positively correlated so that $\hat{\theta}_r > \hat{\theta}_1$. For more accurate estimates, one may apply quadratic interpolation using the VARCO3 and VARCO6 programs. The test of the hypothesis of homogeneity is carried out by calculating

$$X^2 = 2[\log_e L(\hat{\alpha}, \hat{\theta}_1) - \log_e L(1, \hat{\theta}_r)], \tag{10.10}$$

which asymptotically has a chi-square distribution with 1 df with probability ½, and is equal to 0 with probability ½ (one-sided test). From Table 10.4, one evaluates $X^2 = 2 \times (133.32 - 131.16) = 4.32$. The corresponding p-value is approximately equal to $p = 0.019$ (half of the $2p$ value obtained from the CHIPROB program). Heterogeneity of θ among the PKD1 families is thus significant at the 5% level but not at the 1% level. Declaring the test result significant on the basis of the usual significance levels is warranted because the test for linkage is highly significant (lod score exceeds 3; see Section 10.3). Notice that the M-test carried out in the previous section is not significant.

The homogeneity test based on (10.10) has been termed the *A-test* (Hodge et al., 1983; Ott, 1983), *A* standing for *Admixture*. It is conservative (rate of false-positive results smaller than expected from the p-value) and, under the hypothesis of a mixture of linked and unlinked families, more powerful than the M-test (Risch, 1988). For two-point data, the p-value obtained from the asymptotic chi-square distribution seems to be quite accurate (Ott, 1989b). In multipoint situations, however, when in some families a disease is linked to a map of markers and in other families it is unlinked to the markers, it is unknown whether these asymptotic properties still hold (see discussion of this point in the previous section). In such multipoint cases, the parameter θ_1 is usually replaced by x_1, denoting the map position of the disease locus. Lod scores with respect to θ_1 are then replaced by multipoint lod scores relative to x_1 values.

Given good estimates of α and θ_1, one may compute the estimated conditional probability, given the observations, that the ith family belongs to the linked type,

$$w_i(\hat{\alpha}, \hat{\theta}_1) = \frac{\hat{\alpha} L_i^*(\hat{\theta}_1)}{[\hat{\alpha} L_i^*(\hat{\theta}_1) + 1 - \hat{\alpha}]} \tag{10.11}$$

which for $\hat{\alpha} = 0.96$ and $\hat{\theta}_1 = 0.05$ is given in the last column of Table 10.2. For known parameter values, $w_i > ½$ can be shown to represent an optimal classification rule to identify families of the linked type (Goldstein and Dillon, 1978). However, with estimates for α and θ_1, in small samples, the classification rule

$$w_i(\hat{\alpha}, \hat{\theta}_1) > \hat{\alpha} \qquad (10.12)$$

is generally more reliable (Ott, 1983). Inequality (10.12) is equivalent to $Z_i(\hat{\theta}_1) > 0$, where Z_i is the lod score of the ith family evaluated at the estimate for θ_1 obtained from all families together. Inequality (10.12) is intuitively appealing: when a family provides no information on linkage, then $w_i = \alpha$; evidence for linkage (i.e., for belonging to the linked family type) raises w_i above α. All but one family in Table 10.2 exhibit very high conditional probabilities of linkage. The evidence for heterogeneity apparently stems from family 29, whose lod scores are equivalent to approximately 4 recombinants in eight phase-known meioses (as obtained from the EQUIV program). To be confident of heterogeneity, it is thus important to scrutinize the recombinations in that family.

The number of families required to detect heterogeneity has been investigated for various situations (Cavalli-Sforza and King, 1986; Ott, 1986b). In particular, consider the problem that several families with linkage have been observed, and one is interested in knowing how many families are required to detect a small proportion of unlinked families. For the case of no recombination ($\theta = 0$) in linked families and n phase-known families with m meioses each, a simple solution is obtained, as shown below. Owing to tight linkage in linked families, any recombination is, by assumption, evidence for the presence of unlinked families. Thus, the question is reduced to asking how many families are required to find, with probability (power) P, at least one family with one or more recombinations. The probability that in a family with m offspring none of them is a recombinant is given by $\alpha + (1 - \alpha)(\frac{1}{2})^m$. Therefore, the probability that in n families at least one will have one or more recombinants is given by $P = 1 - [\alpha + (1 - \alpha)(\frac{1}{2})^m]^n$, which is the probability to detect heterogeneity and is easily solved for n (Ott, 1986b). For example, with a power of 90% and families of size $m = 4$, 48 families are required to detect the presence of a proportion of 5% of families with $\theta = \frac{1}{2}$. In the analysis of common diseases, incomplete penetrance increases the required numbers of families substantially (Clerget-Darpoux, Babron, and Bonaïti-Pellié, 1987).

To establish linkage on the basis of a single family, the maximum lod score Z_{max} must exceed the critical limit of 3. If, in a number n of families, all have shown good evidence for linkage between a disease and a marker (no apparent heterogeneity), a smaller critical value for Z_{max} should be sufficient to decide whether a new family is also of the linked type. An heuristic argument may be given as follows (Ott, 1986c): Let a new family be classified as linked when the predicted conditional probability of linkage w_i (10.11) is at least 0.95. Based on the current estimate of the proportion of linked families, $\hat{\alpha} = 1$, the predicted probability of linkage is also equal to 1. Therefore, judgment is based on the lower endpoint of the confidence interval for α, which will also represent the lower endpoint of the confidence interval for w_i. If at least $n = 7$ clearly linked families have been investigated, the 95% confidence interval for α extends from 1 down to $(0.05)^{1/n} = 0.65$ (see Section 3.6). What is the minimum lod score, at the overall $\hat{\theta}$, for a new family so that $w_i \geq 0.95$? Solving equation (10.11) yields $L_i^* = w(1 - \alpha)/[(1 - w)\alpha]$ for the likelihood ratio, which, with $w_i = 0.95$ and $\alpha = 0.65$, translates into a minimum lod score of $Z = 1$. Thus, a lod score of 1 at the θ estimate for all linked families together is sufficient for a new family to be classified as linked, provided that a sufficient number of families (at least seven) have already given unequivocal evidence for linkage homogeneity.

When families are of unequal size and penetrances vary, for example, with family size, estimates of α and θ tend to be biased, which has a negative impact on risk calculations under heterogeneity (Janssen et al., 1997).

Testing for Linkage Given Heterogeneity. Thus far, testing for heterogeneity given linkage has been considered, that is, the (null) hypothesis of homogeneity, $H_1 : \alpha = 1$, is tested against the alternative hypothesis of heterogeneity, $H_2 : \alpha < 1$. The corresponding test statistic is given by equation (10.10). Another approach is to test for linkage given heterogeneity, that is, to test the hypothesis of no linkage, $\theta = \frac{1}{2}$, against the alternative of linkage, $\theta < \frac{1}{2}$, while allowing for heterogeneity under each hypothesis. The relevant likelihood ratio is given by $L(\hat{\theta}, \hat{\alpha})/L(\frac{1}{2}, \tilde{\alpha})$, where $\hat{\theta}$ and $\hat{\alpha}$ are the maximum likelihood estimates under the alternative hypothesis and $\tilde{\alpha}$ is the estimate under the null hypothesis (α is treated as a nuisance parameter). With $\theta = \frac{1}{2}$, the value of α is irrelevant. Thus, the lod score corresponding to the likelihood ratio for linkage given heterogeneity may be written as

$$Z(\theta) = \log 10[L(\theta, \hat{\alpha})/L(\frac{1}{2}, \alpha = 0)]. \tag{10.13}$$

This is often referred to as the *hlod* (for example, in Elmslie et al., 1997). The value of $\hat{\alpha}$ generally changes as θ changes. The *hlod* may be interpreted as measuring the evidence for linkage and/or heterogeneity.

In a test for linkage under heterogeneity, a suitable test statistic is $X^2 = 4.6 \times Z(\hat{\theta})$. Under regular conditions, X^2 would follow a chi-square distribution under the null hypothesis. However, imposing one restriction ($\theta = \frac{1}{2}$) automatically imposes another ($\alpha = 0$). In such irregular situations, asymptotic theory does not hold. Investigations have shown that in this case, the asymptotic distribution of X^2 is given by $\max(X_1, X_2)$, where X_1 and X_2 are independent chi-square variables with 1 df (Faraway, 1993). The null distribution of X^2 may be viewed as a chi-square distribution with a non-integral number of df, which is between 1 and 2 (Chiano and Yates, 1995). Thus, chi-square with 2 df will yield conservative significance levels.

In multipoint analysis, to estimate the position of a disease locus on a map of markers, one may construct a lod score curve for various assumed positions, x, across the marker map. In analogy to the two-point situation considered above, an hlod may be constructed as $Z(x) = \log_{10}[L(x, \hat{\alpha})/L(x = \infty, \alpha = 0)]$, where, again, $\hat{\alpha}$ varies with varying x. It is generally recommended to search for disease genes and test for linkage under this heterogeneity model, that is, by using the hlod.

HOMOG2. In some applications, the model for heterogeneity considered above is not realistic. Instead, a disease may be caused by either of *two* disease loci, where the two loci may be within measurable distance of each other on the same chromosome. One must then estimate not one, but two recombination fractions, θ_1 and θ_2, where θ_1 refers to the disease locus segregating in type 1 families (occurring in the sample with proportion α), and θ_2 refers to the disease locus in type 2 families (proportion $1 - \alpha$). In analogy to equation (10.7), the likelihood for the ith family is then given by

$$L_i(\alpha, \theta_1, \theta_2) = \alpha L_i(\theta_1) + (1 - \alpha)L_i(\theta_2). \tag{10.14}$$

Under heterogeneity, the three parameters α, θ_1, and θ_2 are estimated by maximum likelihood in a manner analogous to that described above. Under homogeneity, the restriction $\alpha = 1$ implies $\theta_1 = \theta_2$ so that the dimensionality of the parameter space drops from 3 to 1. This is a situation commonly encountered in the analysis of mixtures of distributions and is known to lead to unusual distributions of the test statistics. In analogy to testing for linkage given heterogeneity considered above, taking the null distribution of the test statistic,

$$X^2 = 2[\log_e L(\hat{\alpha}, \hat{\theta}_1, \hat{\theta}_2) - \log_e L(1, \hat{\theta}_r)], \tag{10.15}$$

to be chi-squared with 2 df may lead to conservative tests. Maximizing the likelihood over the different parameters is tedious but may conveniently be carried out using the HOMOG2 program. An example of an analysis along these lines was the investigation of multiple loci for retinitis pigmentosa on the X chromosome (Ott et al., 1990a).

HOMOG3R. The basic model of heterogeneity may be extended in still other ways, but only one model of particular importance in practice will be pursued here further. It refers to the situation where a disease (or any other phenotype) is caused in some families by one locus and in other families by another locus, with the disease loci themselves being unlinked with each other but each linked with a marker locus (or map of markers). An example is osteogenesis imperfecta, which may be due to a disease gene on chromosome 7 (OI4) or 17 (Sykes et al., 1990). The general case of any number of disease loci may be handled by the HOMOGM program (see below) whereas HOMOG3R is specialized for two disease loci. The mixture of families is taken to consist of three components as follows. In any given family, its disease gene is linked with one or the other of two markers or maps of markers. In a third proportion of families, the disease is due to a hypothetical third gene located elsewhere. Hence, three family types are distinguished with the respective proportions of α_1, α_2, and $\alpha_3 = 1 - \alpha_1 - \alpha_2$. The recombination fraction between disease locus 1 and the marker linked with it is θ_1, and that between disease locus 2 and its linked marker is θ_2. If instead of a single marker, a map of markers is considered, these recombination fractions are replaced by map positions.

With these assumptions, in analogy to (10.7) the likelihood for the *i*th family is derived as outlined below. For clarity, this derivation is given here in detail; the less mathematically inclined reader may want to skip the next one or two paragraphs. Let y, y_1, and y_2 denote the respective phenotypes for the disease, marker 1 and marker 2. For any family, the joint likelihood for the three phenotypes is obtained by conditioning on each of the three family types:

$$P(y, y_1, y_2; \alpha_1, \alpha_2, \theta_1, \theta_2) = \alpha_1 P(y, y_1; \theta_1)P(y_2) \quad (10.16)$$
$$+ \alpha_2 P(y, y_2; \theta_2)P(y_1) + \alpha_3 P(y)P(y_1)P(y_2).$$

Now, define the likelihood with respect to θ_1, adjusted to be equal to 1 at $\theta_1 = \frac{1}{2}$, as $L(\theta_1) = P(y, y_1; \theta_1)/P(y, y_1; \frac{1}{2}) = P(y, y_1; \theta_1)/[P(y)P(y_1)]$. Hence, we can write $P(y, y_1; \theta_1) = L(\theta_1)P(y)P(y_1)$ and, analogously, $P(y, y_2; \theta_2) = L(\theta_2)P(y)P(y_2)$. With this, the right side of equation (10.16) is rewritten as $\alpha_1 L(\theta_1)P(y)P(y_1)P(y_2) + \alpha_2 L(\theta_2)P(y)P(y_2)P(y_1) + \alpha_3 P(y)P(y_1)P(y_2)$. Dividing through by the common terms shows that the likelihood is proportional to

$$L(\alpha_1, \alpha_2, \theta_1, \theta_2) = \alpha_1 L(\theta_1) + \alpha_2 L(\theta_2) + 1 - \alpha_1 - \alpha_2. \quad (10.17)$$

This expression refers to a single family and is analogous to (10.7). The overall log likelihood is then proportional to the sum of the logarithm of (10.17) over all families. Maximum likelihood estimates of the four parameters may be obtained by an exhaustive search of the parameter space, by varying each parameter in a number of steps (this is how the HOMOG3R program works).

For the example of osteogenesis imperfecta referred to above, 35 of the 38 families reported by Sykes et al. (1990) allow the calculating of lod scores with respect to θ_1 and θ_2, where θ_1 refers to linkage between osteogenesis imperfecta and COL1A1 on chromosome 17, and θ_2 refers to OI4 versus COL1A2 on chromosome 7. With α and θ values incremented between 0 and 1 (or ½) in steps of 0.05 each, maximum likelihood estimates are obtained under various hypotheses. Under heterogeneity, parameter estimates are $\hat{\alpha}_1 = 0.55$, $\hat{\alpha}_2 = 0.45$ (hence, $\hat{\alpha}_3 = 0$), $\hat{\theta}_1 = 0$, and $\hat{\theta}_2 = 0$.

If one is interested only in the α values, for each pair (α_1, α_2), one may simply look at the likelihood maximized over θ_1 and θ_2 with α_1 and α_2 kept fixed. The resulting log likelihoods for α_1 and α_2 are displayed in Table 10.5. A 3.9-unit support interval (likelihood ratio of 50:1) includes all parameter values with $\log_e(L)$ equal to or larger than 26.9 − 3.9 = 23.0; the corresponding log likelihoods in Table 10.5 are set in bold. As one can see, $\hat{\alpha}_1$ and $\hat{\alpha}_2$ are strongly negatively correlated (the support interval is deliberately chosen stringently so that it becomes rather wide and is better visible in the table). Corresponding to the support interval chosen, the support limits for α_1 as well as α_2 extend from 0.30 through 0.70 (for support intervals of α_3, see Problem 10.1).

Table 10.5. $\log_e$ Likelihoods, ln$L$-90, for 35 Families from Sykes et al. (1990) with Respect to a Mixture of Three Family Types

					α_2						
α_1	.20	.30	.35	.40	.45	.50	.55	.60	.65	.70	.80
.80	21.1										
.70	19.2	**25.0**									
.65	18.1	**23.8**	**26.0**								
.60	16.9	22.6	**24.8**	**26.6**							
.55	15.7	21.3	**23.4**	**25.3**	**26.9**						
.50	14.3	19.8	22.0	**23.8**	**25.4**	**26.9**					
.45	12.7	18.2	20.3	22.2	**23.8**	**25.2**	**26.5**				
.40	11.0	16.4	18.5	20.4	22.0	**23.4**	**24.7**	**25.8**			
.35	9.1	14.4	16.5	18.3	19.9	21.3	22.6	**23.7**	**24.8**		
.30	6.9	12.2	14.2	16.0	17.6	19.0	20.2	21.3	22.3	**23.2**	
.20	1.2	6.4	8.4	10.1	11.6	12.9	14.1	15.2	16.1	17.0	18.4

If one is convinced that the genetic markers are candidate loci, one may compute likelihoods only at $\theta_1 = \theta_2 = 0$. In this case, because the recombination fraction estimates turned out to be equal to zero, restricting the parameter space to $\theta_1 = \theta_2 = 0$ furnishes the same estimates for α_1 and α_2 as above, where estimation was carried out over the full parameter space including $0 \le (\theta_1, \theta_2) \le \frac{1}{2}$. There is, however, one difference between the two approaches. If the parameter space is restricted to $\theta_1 = \theta_2 = 0$, the evidence for heterogeneity is inflated, which may be seen in Table 10.6, which presents results obtained by the HOMOG3R program. Allowing for θ_1 and θ_2 to vary between 0 and $\frac{1}{2}$, one will find at least some evidence for homogeneity, although it is comparatively small. The difference in log likelihood between heterogeneity and that hypothesis of homogeneity with the highest likelihood turns out to be equal to $\Delta \ln L = 76.5$. With θ_1 and θ_2 fixed at 0, the corresponding evidence for heterogeneity is $\Delta \ln L = 116.9$, which is much higher than 76.5. Of course, in both cases the conclusion of strong evidence for heterogeneity is the same, but Table 10.6 does show that it is generally prudent to allow for θ_1 and θ_2 to vary.

The approach implemented in the HOMOG3R program turns out to be a good substitute for two-locus linkage analysis (see Section 14.2). If it is used for simultaneous gene mapping of two disease loci jointly causing a disease, special consideration must be given to the rate of false-positive results (see Section 14.2).

HOMOGM. The method implemented in the HOMOG3R program has been extended to any number, *m,* of loci. Again, the assumption is that in any one family, at most one of the disease loci is segregating.

Table 10.6. Parameter Estimates and Evidence for Heterogeneity in a Mixture of Osteogenesis Imperfecta Families

| Hypothesis | Estimates for Parameters | | | | | $\ln L$ | $\Delta \ln L$ |
	α_1	α_2	α_3	θ_1	θ_2		
Estimating θ							
Heter.	0.55	0.45	0	0	0	116.9	76.5
Homog.	1	0	0	0.15	$\frac{1}{2}$	27.9	
Homog.	0	1	0	$\frac{1}{2}$	0.15	40.4	
Homog.	0	0	1	$\frac{1}{2}$	$\frac{1}{2}$	0	
Setting $\theta = 0$							
Heter.	0.55	0.45	0	0	0	116.9	116.9
Homog.	1	0	0	0	$\frac{1}{2}$	$-\infty$	
Homog.	0	1	0	$\frac{1}{2}$	0	$-\infty$	
Homog.	0	0	1	$\frac{1}{2}$	$\frac{1}{2}$	0	

Such an approach has been implemented in the HOMOGM program (Bhat et al., 1999) in which the log likelihood is maximized over parameter values (α_i, θ_i, $i = 1 \ldots m$) by the simplex algorithm.

Whenever more than one disease locus is allowed for, multiple hypotheses of homogeneity may be considered, that is, each of $H_i : \alpha_i = 1$, $i = 1 \ldots m$, represents homogeneity (all families with linkage to the ith marker or ith map of markers). A global hypothesis of heterogeneity (all α values are estimated) may then be tested against the union of all hypotheses of homogeneity, with the log likelihood maximized under heterogeneity and under homogeneity.

Thus far, heterogeneity as a mixture of two or more disease loci was considered between families but it was taken to be excluded within families. For more common diseases, however, so-called bilineal pedigrees are observed in which a disease enters a family through more than one individual. Such cases cannot be handled by the methods outlined above. They require that the likelihood be calculated under a model of heterogeneity for individuals in the same family. Such approaches will be discussed in Chapter 14.

Analytical Treatment. For mathematically inclined readers, a few theoretical aspects of mixtures of families will now be discussed in the remainder of this section. As was mentioned above, in a mixture of linked and unlinked families the estimates of α and θ are often correlated. For a known distribution of the estimates, this correlation can be calculated. For example, consider n families with m phase-known meioses each. A family is of the linked type with probability α and of the unlinked type with probability $1 - \alpha$. Hence, in any family, the probability of occurrence of k recombinants is given by

$$P(k; \alpha, r) = \alpha P(k; r) + (1 - \alpha)P(k; \text{½}), \qquad (10.18)$$

where $P(k; r)$ is the binomial probability, $\binom{m}{k}r^k(1 - r)^{m-k}$, and r is the true recombination rate. As an example, $P(k = 2; \alpha, r) = 3[\alpha r^2(1 - r) + (1 - \alpha)/8]$. Using the methods of Section 5.3, it is then easy to compute the asymptotic variance-covariance matrix (5.8). For $n = 10$ phase-known families of size $m = 3$ each and given parameter values α and r, Table 10.7 shows some resulting values of the correlation $\rho(\hat{\alpha}, \hat{\theta})$ and the standard error $\sigma(\hat{\theta})$. The correlation is small for $\alpha = 1$ and small recombination rates, but it increases rapidly with decreasing α and increasing r. With a decreasing α, the standard error of $\hat{\theta}$ increases, partly owing to the smaller number of families present with linkage.

In most applications, $\hat{\alpha}$ and $\hat{\theta}$ must be found numerically. The subse-

Table 10.7. Asymptotic Correlation ρ between $\hat{\alpha}$ and $\hat{\theta}$ and Standard Error $\sigma(\theta)$ for $n = 10$ Families of Size $m = 3$ Each (r = True Recombination Rate)

	$r = 0.01$		$r = 0.05$		$r = 0.10$		$r = 0.30$	
α	ρ	σ	ρ	σ	ρ	σ	ρ	σ
1.0	.07	.018	.03	.042	.51	.064	.91	.204
.9	.58	.037	.53	.060	.63	.087	.91	.235
.8	.65	.053	.60	.075	.66	.104	.92	.271
.5	.75	.126	.73	.151	.76	.187	.93	.449
.1	.88	.829	.88	.916	.89	1.052	.94	2.244

quent example of an analytic solution nicely shows the structure of such estimates and makes it plausible that the test for heterogeneity should indeed be one-sided, even though values of $\alpha > 1$ are inadmissible. Consider n phase-known families with $m = 2$ offspring each. In each family, 0, 1, or 2 recombinants may occur with the respective trinomial probabilities p_0, p_1, and $p_2 = 1 - p_0 - p_1$. The maximum likelihood estimates of these probabilities are given by $\hat{p}_i = k_i/n$, where k_i denotes the number of families with i recombinant offspring, $k_0 + k_1 + k_2 = n$. Because $p_0 + p_1 + p_2 = 1$, there are two unknown probabilities that may be specified as

$$p_1 = 2\alpha r(1 - r) + \tfrac{1}{2}(1 - \alpha), \quad p_2 = \alpha r^2 + \tfrac{1}{4}(1 - \alpha). \tag{10.19}$$

For example, $\alpha = 0.7$ and $r = 0.1$ lead to $p_1 = 0.276$, $p_2 = 0.082$, and $p_0 = 0.642$. Because the number of parameters to be estimated is equal to the number of degrees of freedom (independent multinomial probabilities), the MLEs of α and r may be obtained from $\hat{p}_1$ and $\hat{p}_2$ simply by solving equations (10.19) (Weir, 1996). Hence, one obtains

$$\begin{aligned} \hat{\theta} &= \tfrac{1}{2}(\hat{p}_1 - 2\hat{p}_2)/(\hat{p}_0 - \hat{p}_2), \\ \hat{\alpha} &= \hat{p}_0 - \hat{p}_2)^2/(\hat{p}_0 - \hat{p}_1 + \hat{p}_2). \end{aligned} \tag{10.20}$$

For $\hat{\theta} = \tfrac{1}{2}$, define $\hat{\alpha} = 0$ and vice versa.

Equations (10.20) demonstrate that many estimates of p_i result in values of $\hat{\alpha}$ and $\hat{\theta}$ outside their range of definition. For example, $\hat{p}_0 = 0.55$, $\hat{p}_1 = 0.40$, and $\hat{p}_2 = 0.05$ lead to $\hat{\alpha} = 1.25$ and $\hat{\theta} = 0.30$. Restricting $\hat{\alpha}$ to the range between 0 and 1 clearly introduces a bias, which, however, tends to vanish with increasing numbers of observations; that is, the estimates will be asymptotically unbiased (and consistent).

10.5. Hierarchical and Mixed Models of Heterogeneity

Often, families are grouped in hierarchical classifications. For example, several investigators may each have contributed some families. With fixed classifications, the overall X^2 (10.5) may then easily be partitioned into components corresponding to the different levels of hierarchy (see, e.g., Morton, 1956). In a similar manner, Rao et al. (1978) analyzed heterogeneity between studies within each sex and heterogeneity between sexes.

In many cases, male and female recombination fractions are different. Taking them to be equal when in fact they are not may introduce an apparent heterogeneity when in some families many more male than female parents are informative for linkage. The appropriate remedy is either to work with the known female-to-male map distance ratio or to allow for heterogeneity both between families and between sexes. The latter possibility has been implemented in the HOMOG1a and HOMOG1b programs, which extend the model of a mixture of linked and unlinked families to allow for a sex difference in each of the family types.

A situation with important practical applications shall be demonstrated with an example of several years ago. Childhood-onset spinal muscular atrophy (SMA) is recessively inherited and may be divided into two classes, an acute form (Werdnig–Hoffmann disease, SMA type I) with onset in infancy and death within the first years of life and chronic forms (e.g., Kugelberg–Welander disease) with onset between 6 months and 17 years of age. Chronic SMA shows clear linkage to chromosome 5 markers (Brzustowicz et al., 1990; Melki et al., 1990). Acute SMA is linked to about the same region on chromosome 5 (Gilliam et al., 1990). Each of the two forms may be heterogeneous in the sense that each may contain unlinked families (perhaps due to diagnostic problems). For a test of homogeneity *between* the two forms, one would like to allow for heterogeneity *within* each form. Assuming homogeneity within each form and carrying out the M-test between them may lead to strongly biased results, for example, when the proportion of unlinked families in the two forms is very different. A solution to this problem is included in Gilliam et al. (1990) and proceeds as outlined below.

To evaluate the log likelihood (adjusted by a constant) under heterogeneity, one computes the log likelihood in each form of SMA independently, allowing for a mixture of linked and unlinked families in each form. This may be done by applying the HOMOG program to each form. Thus, the likelihood is maximized over the parameters x_1, x_2, α_1, and α_2, where x_i is the map position and α_i is the proportion of linked families in each form, with $i = 1$ for the chronic and $i = 2$ for the acute form. The resulting $\log_{10}$ likelihoods turn out to be 8.94 and 2.47 for chronic and acute families, respectively, leading to a total $\log_{10}$ likelihood under heterogeneity of 11.41 (Gilliam et al., 1990). For homogeneity of map position (but possible heterogeneity within each form), one introduces the single constraint that the map locations of the two forms should be at the same position, $x = x_1 = x_2$. At each value of x, for each form, the likelihood is maximized over the other parameter (α_1 or α_2, depending on the family form analyzed) (the current version of the HOMOG program provides such maximized likelihoods as intermediate results). Thus, the likelihood is maximized over parameters x, α_1, and α_2. The sum of the two log likelihoods, maximized separately for each form, represents the log likelihood at map position x. The maximum of these sums over all x values is the maximum log likelihood under homogeneity of map position and turns out to be equal to 11.21 (Gilliam et al., 1990). The antilog of the difference, $11.41 - 11.21$, is 1.6 and is the likelihood ratio for heterogeneity. This represents very little evidence for heterogeneity in map position between the two forms of SMA.

10.6. Covariates in the Test for Admixture

A mixture of linked and unlinked families represents a difficult problem. Statistically, as was shown in the previous section, estimates of α and θ may be strongly correlated so that good quasi-independent estimates of α and θ can be obtained only with a high proportion of linked families and tight linkage in these families. Another problem is that germinal mosaicism or similar effects, when not recognized as such, may mimic heterogeneity. A case in point is an apparent heterogeneity in families with agammaglobulinemia (Ott et al., 1986), which was recognized as an instance of aberrant segregation upon examination with molecular genetics techniques (Hendriks et al., 1989). Another example was reported by Arveiler et al. (1990). In the face of these problems, it would be beneficial to know biological variables (covariates), which could help in assigning families to one or the other type. A particular such variable is age at disease onset; the discussion below is restricted to this important case.

As outlined in Chapter 7, age at disease onset may be regarded as the disease phenotype (or as part of it). If the observed age at onset is a, the conditional likelihood given some genotype is then equal to $f(a)$, the density of the age-of-onset curve. Consider now the investigation of familial osteoarthrosis (Palotie et al., 1989) discussed in Section 7.4. In that analysis, a mixture of two types of individuals in the same large pedigree was assumed: (1) individuals in whom the disease was due to a single gene (genetic or susceptible cases) and (2) individuals whose disease was the consequence of environmental factors (nongenetic or nonsusceptible cases, phenocopies). Genetic cases had an associated age-of-onset curve with low mean and 100% lifetime penetrance, whereas the corresponding curve for nongenetic cases had an increased mean and less than 100% lifetime penetrance. Hence, the age at onset helps discriminate between genetic and nongenetic cases. In this example, the mixture is between individuals in the same pedigree. The discussion below focuses on a mixture of linked and unlinked families, with homogeneity within families.

In conditions with onset after birth, mean onset age can be quite different for different diseases. For example, Alzheimer and Parkinson diseases generally are characterized by high age at onset, whereas Huntington disease tends to manifest in mid-life (average age at onset at 36 to 45 years of age; Folstein, 1989), and still other diseases are expressed shortly after birth. In the presence of heterogeneity such as in familial osteoarthrosis, it appears plausible that for nonmendelian conditions, age at onset is later in life. In two well-known examples, Alzheimer disease (St George-Hyslop et al., 1990) and familial breast cancer (Hall et al., 1990), families with low mean age of onset exhibited linkage to a genetic marker, whereas families with high onset age did not. As this difference is indicative of genetic heterogeneity, onset age may be used as a powerful discriminator between family types. A maximum likelihood analysis might proceed by defining two age-of-onset distributions, one with a low mean μ_1 and one with a high mean μ_2, both perhaps having a common variance σ^2 (Mérette et al., 1992). Families of the linked type (proportion α) are assumed to have mean μ_1 and families of the unlinked type have mean μ_2. Under heterogeneity, the likelihood must be maximized over the five parameters α, θ, μ_1, μ_2, and σ^2. Under homogeneity, the restriction $\alpha = 1$ is equivalent with $\mu_1 = \mu_2 = \mu$, so that only three parameters must be estimated.

If families are divided into, say, three age groups, a test for linkage and perhaps heterogeneity may be carried in each group of families. Other covariates may also be considered so that eventually a rather large number of tests will become necessary. As this technique leads to increased rates of false-positive results (multiple testing problem), the number of subdivisions of families should be kept low.

10.7. Problems

Problem 10.1. In Table 10.5 (Section 10.4), with the support region as indicated by the italicized log likelihood values, what is the support interval for a_3? If a less stringent support region is defined, for example, by $\Delta \ln L = 3.0$ (likelihood ratio $= 20 : 1$), what are then the support limits for α_1, α_2, and α_3?

Problem 10.2. With $n = 10$ phase-known families of $m = 3$ meioses each, given that $\alpha = 0.9$ and $\theta = 0.05$ (Table 10.6), the estimate of θ has a certain precision. How many families does one have to investigate to obtain a θ estimate of equal precision when linked and unlinked families are mixed with a proportion $\alpha = 0.5$ of linked families?

11.

Inconsistencies

The example at the end of Section 10.4 demonstrated a common property of maximum likelihood estimates (MLEs)—they are generally biased. However, in most cases of practical importance, bias and variance of the estimate tend to disappear as sample size increases. This property of an estimate is called *consistency* (see Section 3.3). As long as MLEs are consistent, the presence of a bias is not too serious a problem because it can be remedied by increasing the number of observations.

MLEs may be *in*consistent; for example, because of biased sampling or assumptions of wrong parameter values in the analysis. The extent of the inconsistency may be measured by the *asymptotic bias,* that is, the limit of the bias when sample size tends to infinity. In this chapter, examples of inconsistent estimates are outlined. The first half of each section will introduce a particular problem, with the remainder of the section covering the more theoretical aspects of it.

One way to prove consistency is to show that the expected log likelihood attains its maximum at the true parameter value, which is simple to do for categorical data. The tilde sign will be used to indicate at what parameter value (e.g., $\theta = \tilde{\theta}$) the expected log likelihood is highest. When, in a formula, both true and assumed parameter values of the recombination fraction occur, the true value will be denoted by r, whereas θ will be the symbol for assumed (trial) values.

11.1. Ascertainment Bias

Owing to their easily recognizable mode of inheritance, X-chromosomal loci were among the first to be analyzed for linkage. Because most X-linked diseases are rare recessives, implying that sons can be affected whereas daughters may or may not be carriers (Vogel and Motulsky, 1986), a common way of analyzing families has been to score sons

236

only. Also, to be able to count recombination events, sometimes only those families are used in which it is known or can be inferred that the mother is doubly heterozygous. Many of these ascertainment schemes have been shown to lead to biased estimates of the recombination fraction, and appropriate ascertainment corrections have been devised (Edwards, 1971). Nowadays, because families are routinely analyzed in an unselected manner, there is less of a need for these ascertainment corrections.

Observing the following two rules ensures unbiased estimation of the recombination fraction:

1. *Sequential sampling*. On the basis of the data already collected, one may freely decide which individuals to ascertain next. However, once ascertained, each individual so selected must be included in the analysis, and no individual can be deleted from the analysis (Cannings and Thompson, 1977).

2. *Selection at a single locus*. One may select and possibly remove from the analysis any individual as long as such a decision is based on the phenotype at only one of the loci between which recombination is to be estimated (Fisher, 1935b). For example, with respect to a monogenic disease, one may ascertain family pedigrees containing a minimum of two or three affecteds. This will not bias the results as long as this selection is carried out irrespective of the phenotypes at the marker loci. There are some caveats, however. For analyses involving diseases, one often ascertains so-called high-density pedigrees containing as many affecteds as possible. If in such pedigrees penetrance is estimated in a direct manner, the estimates are bound to be much higher than in pedigrees ascertained from a single proband only. Using an inflated penetrance estimate may very well lead to a bias in the recombination estimate. This is not to say that rule 2 is violated; rather, rule 2 cannot be invoked in this case as it does not apply to segregation analysis (it applies only to linkage analysis).

Even when rule 2 is applied properly, one should recognize that different sampling strategies may yield different degrees of informativeness for linkage. For example, in a dominant disease with incomplete penetrance, when a sibship contains a high proportion of affecteds, one of the parents may well be homozygous for the disease allele and thus uninformative for linkage. In recessive diseases, too, when a high number of affected individuals occurs in a pedigree, some of them may be parents but will be uninformative for linkage (when only one parent is affected, the other is still informative, of course). Owing to assortative mating, situations in which one or both parents are uninformative for a recessive disease are not too infrequent; examples may be found in families with

Usher's syndrome (e.g., Smith et al., 1989). The question of sampling strategies in linkage analysis has received considerable attention (e.g., Durner et al., 1992; Moldin, 1997a).

In a linkage analysis between two loci, when individuals are deleted on the basis of the phenotypes at *both* loci, an ascertainment bias may well occur. Consider, for example, a family of the CEPH type (Dausset et al., 1990), in which both parents are doubly heterozygous with known phase. Assume two codominant loci with alleles *A* and *B* at locus 1 and alleles *1* and *2* at locus 2, the mating being *A1/B2* × *A1/B2* (see Section 5.5 and Problem 5.2). All but one offspring type can be scored unambiguously for two recombination events in each offspring. The ambiguous type is the result of either two recombinations or two nonrecombinations and occurs with probability $\frac{1}{2}[r^2 + (1 - r)^2]$ (see Table 5.4). Not trusting maximum likelihood estimates except when known recombinations and nonrecombinations can be counted, rather than analyzing all the observations, researchers have often felt safer deleting ambiguous offspring from the analysis so that the recombination fraction can be estimated as the proportion of recombinants among all unambiguous meioses. This is not a good strategy, which is demonstrated below (Ott, 1978b).

When all offspring are analyzed, no bias exists, and expected lod scores $E_0[Z(r)]$ are as shown in Table 11.1. When only unambiguous offspring are to be analyzed (first three classes in Table 5.4), one must distinguish two cases:

1. Ambiguous offspring are replaced by unambiguous offspring so that, in the end, the same number of offspring are analyzed but a larger number of families has to be collected to find them.

2. Ambiguous offspring are lost to the analysis so that one has fewer individuals available to study.

The two cases will differ in the amount of linkage information furnished (calculated below), but the offspring types (see Table 5.4) will occur in the same proportions under the two ascertainment schemes. Disregarding ambiguous offspring from the analysis introduces an inconsistency in the θ estimate (the same for the two cases), which can be shown by computing the value, $\tilde{\theta}$, at which the expected lod score E is a maximum (see Problem 5.2). Deriving $dE/d\theta$ (note that r is a constant in the derivative with respect to θ), setting this derivative equal to zero, and solving for θ leads to the asymptotic estimate

$$\tilde{\theta} + b, \, b = r(1 - r)(1 - 2r/[1 + 2r(1 - r)]. \tag{11.1}$$

The asymptotic bias, b, is equal to 0 for $r = 0$ and $r = \frac{1}{2}$ and is positive

Table 11.1. Asymptotic Bias b of Recombination Fraction Estimates, and ELODs, $E_i[Z(\tilde\theta)]$, for Some Ascertainment Schemes in Phase-Known Double Intercross Families

		Ambiguous Offspring Are				
		Disregarded			Nonrecombinant	
r	E_0	b	E_1	E_2	b	E_3
0.001	.44	0.001	0.59	0.30	≈ 0	0.60
0.010	.41	0.010	0.52	0.26	≈ 0	0.55
0.020	.37	0.018	0.46	0.24	≈ 0	0.52
0.050	.30	0.039	0.34	0.19	-0.001	0.43
0.100	.21	0.061	0.22	0.13	-0.005	0.33
0.200	.10	0.073	0.09	0.06	-0.020	0.19
0.300	.04	0.059	0.03	0.02	-0.045	0.11
0.500	0	0	0	0	-0.125	0.03

Note: E_0 = unbiased ascertainment; E_1 = ambiguous offspring are supplanted by unambiguous offspring; E_2 = ambiguous offspring are lost for the analysis.

otherwise, with a maximum value of $b = 0.073$ at $r = 0.19$. The relative asymptotic bias, b/r, tends to 100% as $r \to 0$; that is, with a large number of observations, deleting ambiguous offspring will lead to an apparent recombination fraction estimate, which is approximately twice the true recombination rate. For larger values of r, the apparent recombination rate is no longer twice the true value, but the recombination fraction may still be overestimated considerably. For example, a true recombination rate of 5% will be observed as an estimate of 9%. It is thus invalid to delete ambiguous offspring from family data unless one corrects for this ascertainment.

To compute ELODs for the two cases distinguished above, one calculates the weighted average of the lod score for the different offspring types and evaluates it at $\theta = \hat\theta$. When discarded ambiguous offspring are replaced by the same number of unambiguous offspring (case 1 above), the probabilities in Table 5.4 for the first three classes must be scaled to sum to 1. The ELOD is then given by

$$E_1 = \log(4) + [(1 - r^2)\log(1 - \tilde\theta) \\ + r(2 - r)\log(\tilde\theta)]/[\tfrac{1}{2} + r(1 - r)], \tag{11.2}$$

where all logarithms are to the base 10. When ambiguous offspring are lost to the analysis (case 2 above), the proportion of available offspring and, thus, of available linkage information is equal to the sum of the probabilities of the first three offspring classes in Table 5.4. The "available" ELOD, E_2, is then calculated by multiplying E_1 by that sum. For small values of r, about half of all offspring are ambiguous; deleting them results in a drastic loss of linkage information (Table 11.1). When as many unambiguous offspring are collected as are ascertained in an unbiased manner, that ascertainment scheme yields more linkage information than does unbiased ascertainment (E_1 versus E_0), but (as shown above) this gain is purchased at the expense of an asymptotic bias.

To researchers who routinely analyze all of their data in an unbiased manner, the discussion in the previous paragraphs may appear somewhat academic. Its main purpose is to outline in detail how such problems can be investigated statistically. It shows, however, that well-intended selection may have undesirable properties. In this vein, one may consider yet another ascertainment strategy. Because, at least at small recombination rates, ambiguous offspring most likely are nonrecombinants, why not simply pretend that they are nonrecombinants? The effect of this scheme is again investigated by calculating the expected lod score,

$$E_3[Z(\theta)] = \log(4) + [1 + (1 - r)^2]\log(1-\theta)$$
$$+ r(2 - r)\log(\theta), \tag{11.3}$$

and evaluating it at $\theta = \tilde{\theta}$ (the derivation of $\tilde{\theta}$ is deferred to Problem 11.1). Indeed, the asymptotic bias, $b = \tilde{\theta} - r$, is very small for small to moderate recombination rates and the gain in ELOD is considerable, but the asymptotic bias becomes relatively large when r approaches ½ (Table 11.1). Furthermore, it is negative so that this ascertainment scheme tends to mimic linkage when none is present, that is, it leads to false-positive results. At $r = ½$, with $E_3 = 0.03$, 100 offspring will yield an expected lod score of 3, whose maximum occurs at $\tilde{\theta} = 0.375$. For known small recombination rates, this ascertainment scheme may be useful, but it cannot generally be recommended. It may appear counterintuitive that, at least for some recombination rates, a deliberately biased ascertainment scheme performs much better (E_3 versus E_2 in Table 11.1) than the "cautious" approach suggested by analyzing unambiguous offspring only.

As already pointed out by Morton (1955, p. 304), it is essential that data be published without regard for whether they indicate linkage or not. Naturally, investigators prefer reporting positive linkage findings. In principle, this might lead to a bias of the recombination fraction estimate in the direction of linkage. However, it is often only the initial report of a positive finding that is made because linkage has been observed. If subsequent reports on the same relation are made without regard to the linkage outcome, then in the long run no harm is done.

In the example covered above, inconsistencies resulting from focusing on known recombination events were derived in a detailed manner. A simple straightforward example follows. Consider a phase-unknown double backcross mating with two offspring, for example, one parent with genotypes (*a/a, 1/1*) and the other parent with (*A/a, 1/2*). Looking at all possible genotypes of two offspring from this mating, it becomes obvious that only two types of recombination events occur. Either the offspring are two recombinants or two nonrecombinants (depending on phase on the doubly heterozygous parent) (example: *Aa/11* and *Aa/11*), or one offspring is a recombinant and the other a nonrecombinant (example: *Aa/11* and *Aa/21*). It is only the second type that allows an unequivocal recognition of recombination events. Focusing on these always leads to an estimate of ½ for the recombination fraction, irrespective of the true recombination fraction. This clearly demonstrates that focusing on known recombination events (without appropriate ascertainment correction) is a bad strategy.

In marker typing, an error rate of one to several percent is often quoted (see Section 11.5). For tight linkage, the rate of typing error may be larger than the recombination rate, which is probably why many people scrutinize apparent recombinants but not nonrecombinants. This practice tends to lead to a downward bias in the recombination fraction. To scrutinize typing results in an unbiased manner, one should in principle review all observations, not just the apparent recombinants. These questions will be discussed more generally in Section 11.5.

Curtis and Sham (1995b) have pointed out a possible bias in the application of the transmission disequilibrium test (TDT; see Chapter 13). When one parent is missing, only the available parent is typed, and equivocal cases of transmitted versus nontransmitted alleles are discarded as uninformative, there is a tendency for alleles with high population frequency to appear preferentially transmitted, which may lead to false-positive results.

Interesting examples of a "bias" introduced by ascertainment occur in genetic counseling. In predictive testing for Huntington's disease, one would expect that half of probands will receive a positive result and half will receive a negative result. However, practice shows that a majority of counselees receive a negative (good) result. The main reason for this is statistical—an affected parent is often dead and is unequivocally informative for linkage and risk calculation when affected and unaffected children inherit different marker alleles from that parent. If so, the risk is close to zero while otherwise the risk is not strongly different from 50%. This case does not really reflect a bias—the average risk is still

50% but the risk distribution is skewed so that extreme risks occur only in the vicinity of 0 but not 1 (see Section 12.5).

11.2. Misclassification

Although recombination occurs at the genotypic level, observations (phenotypes) are often several steps removed from direct observation of genotypes, even for codominant loci. Discordance between a phenotype and the underlying genotype may be viewed as a misclassification whose probability of occurrence represents a general form of incomplete penetrance. In this section, a very simple model of misclassification in connecting phenotypes with genotypes will be introduced (Ott, 1977a). Two consequences of misclassification will be considered:

1. Loss of linkage information owing to misclassification, which in itself does not lead to a bias, and
2. The bias introduced by using a wrong value for the misclassification rate in the analysis, in particular, by disregarding misclassification although it exists.

Some real-life situations that may lead to misclassifications are discussed in Section 11.5.

Consider recombinants and nonrecombinants occurring with respective probabilities r and $1 - r$. Assume that with a small probability, s, a recombinant is misclassified as a nonrecombinant and, with the same misclassification probability, a nonrecombinant is mistakenly scored as a recombinant. Thus, an apparent recombinant is either a true recombinant, occurring with probability $r(1 - s)$, or a false recombinant, occurring with probability $(1 - r)s$. Therefore, apparent recombinants occur with probability

$$p = r(1 - s) + (1 - r)s = r + s(1 - 2r). \tag{11.4}$$

The proportion of apparent recombinants is a consistent estimator of p rather than of r. To obtain r from p, solving (11.4) for r yields $r = (p - s)/(1 - 2s)$. Replacing parameter values in this equation by their estimates leads to an approximate estimate of the recombination fraction corrected for misclassification. In a linkage analysis of family data, in which one cannot necessarily count (apparent) recombination events, the usual lod score analysis will automatically furnish a recombination fraction estimate if misclassification is allowed for via incomplete penetrance. For example, consider a dominant disease locus with two alleles, a disease allele D and a normal allele d. The misclassification probability, s, may then be used as shown in Table 11.2.

The presence of misclassification blurs our view of the genotypes and represents random noise. It reduces linkage information even when misclassification is allowed for in the analysis. For counts of recombinants and nonrecombinants, without the presence of misclassification, the ELOD is given by $E_0 = r \times \log(2r) + (1 - r) \times \log[2(1 - r)]$ [equation (5.3)]. If misclassification occurs and is allowed for based on equation (11.4), the ELOD is equal to

$$E_s = \log(2) + p \times \log[r + s(1 - 2r)] + (1 - p)\log[1 - r - s(1 - 2r)]. \tag{11.5}$$

For the simple model defined above, the relative informativeness for linkage in the presence of misclassification as opposed to one without misclassification is given by $R = E_s/E_0$. Table 11.3 shows relative ELODs for selected values of s and r. For example, with a misclassification rate of $s = 0.05$, at a recombination fraction of $r = 0.01$, the relative ELOD is approximately $R = \frac{3}{4}$. Therefore, to obtain as much linkage information under this level of misclassification as one would have with fully informative meioses, one must increase sample size by a factor of $1/R = 4/3$, or by approximately 33%.

An investigator may be unaware of the presence of misclassification and may in the analysis assume $s = 0$ although in reality, $s > 0$ (this is usually done in practice). This misspecification introduces the following statistical inconsistency. As shown in equation (11.4), the proportion of apparent recombinants consistently estimates $r + s(1 - 2r)$ rather than r. Hence, the asymptotic bias is given by $b = s(1 - 2r)$. No bias exists for $r = \frac{1}{2}$, but b increases with decreasing r and is largest for $r = 0$. For example, at $r = 0$, when misclassification is not allowed for in the analysis,

Table 11.2. General Misclassification Probability s, Incomplete Disease Penetrance $1 - s$, and Probability s of Occurrence of Phenocopies as Special Cases of Penetrances

Genotype	Misclassification		Incomplete Penetrance		Phenocopies	
	A	N	A	N	A	N
D/D	$1 - s$	s	$1 - s$	s	0	1
D/d	$1 - s$	s	$1 - s$	s	0	1
d/d	s	$1 - s$	0	1	s	$1 - s$

Note: Phenotypes: A = affected; N = unaffected.

Table 11.3. Relative ELOD of the Recombination Fraction Estimate in the Presence of Misclassification, s

s	Recombination Fraction, r						
	0.001	0.01	0.05	0.10	0.20	0.30	0.50[a]
0	1	1	1	1	1	1	1
0.01	0.92	0.94	0.95	0.95	0.96	0.96	0.96
0.05	0.72	0.74	0.77	0.78	0.80	0.80	0.81
0.10	0.53	0.55	0.58	0.60	0.62	0.63	0.64
0.20	0.28	0.29	0.31	0.33	0.34	0.35	0.36

[a] Limiting values.

the estimated recombination fraction will tend to be equal to s rather than 0. For the assumed mating type, the ELOD is the same whether or not misclassification is allowed for. In other family types this is not the case (see Section 11.5).

11.3. Misspecification of Penetrance

Incomplete disease penetrance (introduced in Section 7.1) may be viewed as a special form of misclassification in which only the genotypes susceptible to disease are subject to misclassification. The occurrence of phenocopies (sporadic cases) is a form of misclassification of nonsusceptible genotypes (see Table 11.2).

Relative efficiency in the presence of incomplete penetrance is covered in Section 7.2. Here, we will investigate the effect of assuming full penetrance while in reality it is incomplete (assuming absence of phenocopies). Applying the methods used previously, one finds that, in this case, the ELOD has its maximum at

$$\tilde{\theta} = r + s(\tfrac{1}{2} - r), \tag{11.6}$$

where $s = 1 - f$ (f = disease penetrance). The asymptotic bias in (11.6) is only half as large as in the case of disregarding misclassification under the model discussed in the previous section. This is plausible because, under the misclassification model of Section 11.2, no known recombination events can be recognized. With incomplete penetrance, however, some genotypes can unambiguously be identified from the phenotypes.

When full penetrance is assumed while in fact it is incomplete, the ELOD is somewhat smaller than when incomplete penetrance is properly built into the analysis. The corresponding calculations are easy to carry out but are not shown here. The more general case of a true penetrance,

$f < 1$, with a possibly different penetrance assumed in the analysis, requires somewhat more elaborate calculations but shows similar results (Clerget-Darpoux, Bonaïti-Pellié, and Hochez, 1986).

11.4. Misspecification of Heterogeneity

In a mixture of linked and unlinked families (see Section 9.4) with respective proportions α and $1 - \alpha$, joint maximum likelihood estimation of α and r (the recombination fraction in linked families) ensures consistent estimates, that is, the expected log likelihood is highest at the true parameter values (assuming the absence of any biases). However, owing to the correlation between $\hat{\alpha}$ and $\hat{\theta}$, a misspecification of α will lead to an asymptotic bias in the estimate of r. Assume the particular case that an investigator is unaware of the presence of families of the unlinked type, that is, he or she assumes $\alpha = 1$ in the analysis while in reality, $\alpha < 1$. The resulting asymptotic bias may be obtained by evaluating the point $\tilde{\theta}$ at which the expected lod score attains its maximum. For the example of families with $m = 3$ meioses used in Section 10.4, the expected lod score is given by

$$E[Z(\theta)] = \sum_{k=0}^{3} P(k;\alpha,r)Z_k(\theta), \tag{11.7}$$

where $P(k; \alpha, r)$ is the probability of observing k recombinants in a mixture of families as given by equation (10.18), and $Z_k(\theta)$ is the corresponding lod score when homogeneity is assumed in the analysis. For example, $Z_2(\theta) = \log[8\theta^2(1 - \theta)]$. To find that value of θ at which $E[Z(\theta)]$ [equation (11.7)] is maximized, one computes the first derivative, $dE/d\theta$ (note that r is a constant in this context), sets it equal to zero, and solves this equation for θ. The result turns out to be equal to

$$\tilde{\theta} = r\alpha + \tfrac{1}{2}(1 - \alpha) = r + (1 - \alpha)(\tfrac{1}{2} - r). \tag{11.8}$$

In other words, $\tilde{\theta}$ is the θ estimate one tends to obtain when α is falsely assumed to be equal to 1, that is, when heterogeneity is disregarded in the analysis although it exists. For example, with $\alpha = 0.80$ and $r = 0.05$, assuming homogeneity in the analysis will, in large samples, lead to an estimate of $\tilde{\theta} = 0.14$. Equation (11.8) also says that the asymptotic bias is largest for $r = 0$, in which case the apparent recombination rate tends to be equal to one-half the proportion of unlinked families, assuming families of equal size $m = 3$. Of course, no inconsistency occurs for $r = \tfrac{1}{2}$ because then the value of α clearly is 0.

If calculations analogous to the ones above are carried out with phase-unknown (rather than phase-known) double backcross families of size $m = 3$ each, a result analogous to (11.8) is found as

$$\tilde{\theta} = r\sqrt{\alpha} + \tfrac{1}{2}(1 - \sqrt{\alpha}). \tag{11.9}$$

For example, with $\alpha = 0.80$ and $r = 0.05$, one tends to find $\tilde{\theta} = 0.10$.

In the previous paragraphs, a particular case of misspecification of α was considered, namely, that α is taken to be equal to 1 in the analysis while in reality it is less than 1. One may be interested in the more general question: If α is the true value of the proportion of linked families and one assumes in the analysis a value α', what is then the asymptotic estimate $\tilde{\theta}$ of the recombination fraction? Calculations analogous to the ones above are no longer straightforward but, for given true parameter values, α and r, one may compute the expected lod score for α' and θ and numerically maximize it over θ. For $m = 3$ offspring of a phase-known double backcross mating, Table 11.4 shows the probability of occurrence of a family with k recombinants [equation (10.18)] and the corresponding lod score. Using a spreadsheet program, it is then easy to calculate the weighted average of the lod score and find its maximum over θ.

For a true value of $\alpha = 0.5$ and several true recombination rates r, Table 11.5 shows asymptotic estimates $\tilde{\theta}$ and the maximum of the expected lod score at $\tilde{\theta}$, when the analysis is carried out assuming a proportion α' of linked families. Owing to the positive correlation between the estimates for α and r, too high a value of α leads to an overestimate of r, and vice versa. As Table 11.5 demonstrates, the bias in $\tilde{\theta}$ is quite strong. In practice, one generally estimates α jointly with r. But in small samples, α estimates may be quite different from the true values, which in turn leads to biased estimates of r. Table 11.5 also shows that the maximum lod scores obtained under wrong α' values are somewhat smaller than those obtained under the true value of α. This result is analogous to results found for misspecifying penetrance or gene frequencies (Clerget-Darpoux et al., 1986).

Table 11.4. Probability $P(k; \alpha, r)$ of Occurrence of k Recombinants and Associated Lod Score $Z(\theta; \alpha')$ in a Family with m Meioses

k	$P(k; \alpha, r)$	$Z(\theta; \alpha')$
0	$\alpha(1 - r)^3 + (1 - \alpha)/8$	$\log[8\alpha'(1 - \theta)^3 + 1 - \alpha']$
1	$3[\alpha r(1 - r)^2 + (1 - \alpha)/8]$	$\log[8\alpha'\theta(1 - \theta)^2 + 1 - \alpha']$
2	$3[\alpha r^2(1 - r) + (1 - \alpha)/8]$	$\log[8\alpha'\theta^2(1 - \theta) + 1 - \alpha']$
3	$\alpha r^3 + (1 - \alpha)/8$	$\log[8\alpha'\theta^3 + 1 - \alpha']$

Note: α = true proportion; α' = proportion assumed in the analysis.

Table 11.5. Maximum Z of the Expected Lod Score and Value $\tilde{\theta}$ at which that Maximum Occurs, when a Proportion α' of Linked Families Is Assumed in the Analysis while True Parameter Values Are $\alpha = 0.5$ and r

	$r = 0.01$		$r = 0.05$		$r = 0.10$	
α'	$\tilde{\theta}$	Z	$\tilde{\theta}$	Z	$\tilde{\theta}$	Z
0.7	0.08	0.210	0.13	0.166	0.18	0.123
0.6	0.04	0.219	0.09	0.172	0.14	0.127
0.5	*0.01*	*0.222*	*0.05*	*0.174*	*0.10*	*0.129*
0.4	0	0.217	0.01	0.172	0.06	0.127
0.3	0	0.164	0	0.162	0.01	0.121

11.5. Pedigree and Genotyping Errors

Thus far, the effect of specific analysis errors has been investigated. In Section 11.2, effects of misclassification were treated in a theoretical manner. This section covers sources of errors in the gathering of family data.

On the basis of typing results for seven polymorphic enzyme markers in close to 2000 individuals, Lathrop et al. (1983) set up a mathematical model for two classes of errors: (1) pedigree error (nonpaternity and other misidentification of individuals and relationships) and (2) typing errors of marker systems. From the observed distribution of genetic marker inconsistencies in data from a South Pacific island population, they estimated the error of nonpaternity at 4%, and the overall system typing error at 1% (a newer investigation of nonpaternity rates is due to Sasse et al., 1994). A third error category, "field error," might be distinguished (e.g., mislabeling of blood samples) but was not separately taken into account in that study. Below, attention is focused on errors in marker typing. In most genotyping laboratories, the error rate appears to be somewhat smaller than 1%. However, in a comprehensive reanalysis of CEPH pedigrees for several markers on chromosome 5, an average error rate of 3% was found (Brzustowicz et al., 1993). Thus, it is important to distinguish phenotypes from underlying genotypes.

In simulation studies, misreading an allele as the next largest or next smallest on a Southern blot results in overestimation of the recombination fraction and a loss in expected lod score (Terwilliger, Weeks, and Ott, 1990). For detecting linkage with a locus of unknown map position, loss of linkage information is a much larger problem than a bias in $\hat{\theta}$, while the latter is more important for fine mapping. Of all typing errors generated in family data, a sizeable portion may go undetected because they do not lead to genetic inconsistencies, but they still result in the negative consequences mentioned above. For example, consider a small family with two parents and one offspring (the "trio" family type typically considered in analyses of haplotype relative risks). A computer simulation was carried out to evaluate effects of errors (Gordon et al., 1998). For a marker locus with n equally frequent alleles, genotypes for 100,000 such families were randomly generated. For each allele, with probability e (true error rate), an error was introduced by changing the given allele into a neighboring allele. The proportion of alleles leading to a mendelian inconsistency is then the apparent error rate, p. For systems with $n = 2$ and $n = 10$ equally frequent alleles, Figure 11.1 shows the apparent error rate as a function of the true error rate. Clearly, the same true error rate is associated with a much lower detection rate (apparent error rate) for 2-allele systems than for 10-allele systems. In practice, errors are not only detected as mendelian inconsistencies but also, for example, through occurrence of multiple crossovers within a short interval. Nonetheless, Figure 11.1 demonstrates that 2-allele systems are more vulnerable to undetected errors than 10-allele systems. For true error rates between 1% and 5%, these simulations also showed that in "trios," 75% of all errors remain undetected when the marker locus has only two alleles. For markers with higher polymorphism the rate of undetected errors drops but it still is close to 40% for a 10-allele marker.

Assuming that precautions have been taken to minimize the occur-

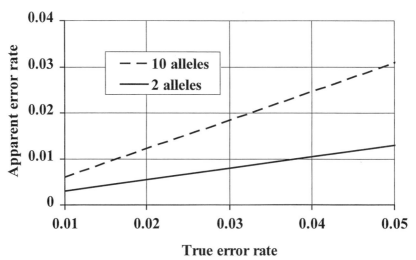

Figure 11.1. Apparent error rate as a function of the true error rate and number of alleles in marker system for families with two parents and one offspring.

rence of laboratory error, several recommendations for handling typing errors have been given. The main point is that errors should not simply be ignored. Generally, as suggested by the simple error model leading to equation (11.4), ignoring typing errors tends to overestimate map lengths (Shields et al., 1991; Buetow, 1991; Brzustowicz et al., 1993; Goldstein et al., 1997). Prior to a linkage analysis, it is beneficial to test for presence of errors and perhaps estimate the magnitude of the various errors, but this should be done on raw data, which have not been "cleaned up" before reaching the statistical geneticist (Lathrop et al., 1983).

1. Error rates may be incorporated in the analysis as a form of misclassification, for example, by allowing for a parameter such as s in the penetrances in Table 11.2 (Keats, Sherman, and Ott, 1990; Lincoln and Lander, 1992). Notice that marker systems are then no longer codominant, which dramatically increases computational effort. In practice, this way of allowing for errors is not generally a feasible solution.

2. In multipoint analysis, some typing errors simulate double recombinants (Keats et al., 1991), which at short distances are expected to be very rare. Scrutinizing apparent double recombinants occurring within 30 cM of each other is a common practice (the CRI-MAP program identifies individual recombinations on a chromosome) and indeed tends to identify a large proportion of them as errors (Kouri and Fain, 1990), but it also tends to bias recombination fraction estimates downwards. In two-point analysis, a bias in $\hat{\theta}$ is not serious for detecting linkage as errors are largely absorbed in the bias, but this is not the case for multipoint analysis.

3. Because marker errors tend to inflate map lengths, in a multipoint analysis one may remove one marker at a time and watch the resulting map length. Considerable shrinking of the map indicates that the marker removed is likely to contain errors.

4. Analogous approaches may successfully be taken by removing one family at a time (Brzustowicz et al., 1993).

5. In a pedigree, an individual's genotype may be predicted based on all available pedigree data and compared probabilistically with the observed genotype. Discrepancies are indicative of errors (Ott, 1993). Analogous, more general methods have been proposed by Stringham and Boehnke (1996).

As mentioned in Chapter 13, a well-known family type for nonparametric linkage analysis is a pair of affected siblings (ASP = affected sib pair). For diseases that tend to occur at high age only, parents are usually missing. It is then particularly important that the stated sibs are true sibs.

Whether or not parents are available, based on a large number of genotypes, the stated relationship between two individuals may be estimated and therefore verified or refuted (Göring and Ott, 1997; Boehnke and Cox, 1997). The program RELATIVE is available for this purpose (ftp://linkage.rockefeller.edu/software/relative/). Simply put, one may test whether two stated sibs are true sibs as follows. For the alleles received from each parent, one estimates the proportion of alleles shared IBD. In the absence of linkage, this proportion should fluctuate around 0.50. If it is significantly smaller than 0.50, the stated sibs are probably not true sibs. If markers are linked, then a likelihood analysis is more reliable than a simple allele sharing count (Göring and Ott, 1997). Also, if parents are unavailable, IBD status of sibs cannot be determined except when markers are highly polymorphic in which case IBS $\approx$ IBD.

11.6. Misspecification of Allele Frequencies

Equation (9.3) shows a lod score that depends on the frequency of a marker allele. In that case, as outlined in Section 9.1, the probability that a parent is informative for linkage is determined by the marker allele frequency. In unfortunate situations, wrong marker allele frequencies may lead to increased false-positive evidence for linkage. A dramatic example was shown in Ott (1992). Consider a 3-generation family, in which only the individuals in the last generation are genotyped but not individuals in generations 1 and 2. Assuming equal marker allele frequencies while in fact they are unequal leads to strong evidence for tight linkage even if no linkage exists. Much of the downward bias in the recombination fraction estimate can be avoided by using estimated marker allele frequencies. Even crude estimates will do, for example, based on the first sib in each sibship. Specific recommendations have been given by Freimer et al. (1993).

Generally, if all family members are genotyped, the lod score does not depend on marker allele frequencies. Otherwise, estimates of allele frequencies are required. These are often obtained from parents in CEPH reference families. However, for the analysis of specific diseases, families may be ascertained from ethnic groups with allele frequencies quite different from those in the CEPH families. One approach is then to count alleles in founder individuals (i.e., those that marry into the pedigree from the general population). However, founders often are not genotyped so that this avenue is rarely useful. A more sophisticated approach is to base such estimation on the pedigree likelihood (Boehnke, 1991). For example, one may estimate allele frequencies using the ILINK computer program.

Allele frequency estimation by the empirical Bayes method is outlined in Lange (1997, p. 44).

11.7. Other Model Misspecifications

Disregarding misclassifications amounts to a misspecification of the analysis model. Other model misspecifications are expected to lead to inconsistencies of various degrees (see below for an exception). For example, disregarding linkage disequilibrium (allelic association) in the analysis may result in an asymptotic bias (Clerget-Darpoux, 1982).

In linkage analyses, diseases are usually assumed to result from the action of a single gene, possibly modified by random environmental effects. Other models such as oligogenic or multifactorial models may be more realistic (see Section 11.3), but two-point analysis under a simple mode of inheritance seems to be quite robust for detecting linkage although not for estimating recombination fractions (Risch et al., 1989; Risch and Giuffra, 1992).

In multipoint analysis, effects of parameter misspecifications have not been studied much. One problem is that, in estimating the location of a new locus on a map of markers, that map is often assumed to be known without error, which is usually far from true. The limited work done on this subject suggests that it is better to have overestimates rather than underestimates of the interval lengths in maps on which a new locus should be placed (Ott and Lathrop, 1987b).

An example of a misspecification not leading to an inconsistency is the following. In phase-unknown double backcross matings with m offspring each (see Section 5.9), the phase probabilities are usually taken to be equal to ½ each, as one assumes independence of the phenotypes at the two loci under study (allelic association would lead to unequal phase probabilities). Consider now a true phase probability, $c \neq$ ½, while in the analysis the two phases are assumed to be equally frequent. Among the $m + 1$ possible phenotypes of the offspring, the kth phenotype occurs with a probability of $p_k = \binom{m}{k}[cr^k(1 - r)^{m - k} + (1 - c)(1 - r)^k r^{m - k}]$, where r is the true recombination fraction. Also, the $(m - k)$th phenotype occurs with probability $p_{m-k} = \binom{m}{k}[cr^{m - k}(1 - r)^k + (1 - c)(1 - r)^{m - k}r^k]$. Now, assuming equal phase probabilities in the analysis, the lod scores for the kth and $(m - k)$th phenotypes are the same. Hence, in the computation of the expected lod score, p_k and $p_{m - k}$ appear as their sum only, $p_k + p_{m - k}$. In this sum, however, c and $1 - c$ cancel so that the expected lod score does not contain c. Consequently, with assumed phase probabilities of ½ each in the analysis, the recombination fraction estimate is consistent, irrespective of the true value c of the phase probability.

11.8. Problems

Problem 11.1. Using the expected lod score function $E_3[Z(\theta)]$ given in equation (11.3), derive the asymptotic recombination fraction estimate $\tilde{\theta}$, that is, the value of θ at which E_3 attains its maximum. The relevant offspring class probabilities are given in Table 5.4.

Problem 11.2. Assume a phase-known double backcross mating and a misclassification scheme at one locus as shown on the left side of Table 11.2. With $s = 1\%$ misclassification, at $r = 0.001$, by what factor must the number of offspring be increased for the ELOD under misclassification to be the same as without misclassification?

12.

Linkage Analysis with Mendelian Disease Loci

An important aspect of the effort to obtain a dense map of markers spanning the human genome is the mapping of disease genes. The rationale in this "positional cloning" approach (Collins, 1995) is to find map locations for diseases with unknown biochemical defects and to elucidate the mechanism leading to disease via identification of the gene and its molecular sequence, thereby paving the way for finding a cure. Spectacular results have already been obtained for Duchenne muscular dystrophy (Monaco and Kunkel, 1988), cystic fibrosis (Kerem et al., 1989; Davies, 1990; Kerem et al., 1990), breast cancer (Hall et al., 1990; Cannon-Albright and Skolnick, 1996), Huntington disease (Gusella et al., 1983; J. K. White et al., 1997), and Alzheimer disease (Saunders et al., 1993; Levy-Lahad and Bird, 1996).

For the more common mendelian diseases such as cystic fibrosis, researchers often wonder what might have caused these diseases to persist for a long time. It appears reasonable to speculate about possible selective advantages of heterozygotes. However, population genetics theory shows that such frequencies are expected as consequence of normal random variation so that there is no need to postulate positive selection (Thompson and Neel, 1997).

This chapter focuses on mendelian diseases, that is, traits whose genetic basis is a single gene, at least within a given family pedigree. Thus, mode of inheritance is typically well recognized. Occurrence of multiple disease genes (at most one of them in one family) is covered in Chapter 10 (locus heterogeneity). Complex traits are discussed in Chapters 14 and 15. A reminder—when localizing a disease gene through a genomic screen, critical lod scores for significance must be raised above the conventional level of 3 for a genome-wide significance level of 0.05 (see Section 4.7).

12.1. Mode of Inheritance

In this section, specific characteristics of different mendelian modes of inheritance are discussed as they impact linkage analysis. Dominant and recessive inheritance patterns will be considered first, followed by some special cases.

Dominant Inheritance. Dominant traits such as Huntington disease typically occur clustered in large pedigrees, with affected individuals being found in many generations. Affected individuals generally carry only one disease allele and, with full penetrance, unaffecteds carry none. Thus, the trait genotype is known for each individual. For rare traits, only one of two parents is heterozygous for the disease allele and thus potentially informative for linkage. Owing to the small gene frequencies of most dominant traits, homozygotes for the disease allele are extremely rare. Some of the few observed cases exhibit the same phenotype as heterozygotes (Nordström and Thorburn, 1980; Holmgren et al., 1988).

Recessive Inheritance. Autosomal recessive traits are usually manifest only in a single sibship and are therefore harder to study than dominant traits. Both parents of affected individuals typically are heterozygous (unaffected) carriers of the disease allele and are thus potentially informative for linkage. On the other hand, although affected offspring are homozygous for the disease, unaffected offspring may or may not carry a disease allele. This uncertainty about their trait genotype has the effect that they provide much less information for linkage than do affected offspring (Cantor and Rotter, 1986; Leal and Ott, 1990). As shown in Table 12.1, an affected offspring provides approximately five times as

Table 12.1. Increase, δ, in Expected Lod Score at Given True Value r of the Recombination Fraction Due to Adding One Affected (δ_a) or One Unaffected (δ_u) Offspring, Given a Sibship of n Affected and No Unaffected Offspring, for Autosomal Recessive Disease and a Highly Polymorphic Marker

	$r = 0$			$r = 0.05$		
n	δ_a	δ_u	R	δ_a	δ_u	R
1	0.602	0.125	4.8	0.329	0.055	6.0
2	0.602	0.125	4.8	0.383	0.066	5.8
3	0.602	0.125	4.8	0.415	0.075	5.5

Source: Data from Leal and Ott (1990).
Note: R = ratio of ELOD for an affected over that for an unaffected offspring.

much linkage information as an unaffected offspring. With tight linkage, each affected offspring independently contributes 0.602 and each unaffected offspring contributes 0.125 towards the expected lod score. Consequently, when affected children die at a young age, it becomes very hard to carry out linkage analysis for such traits. Examples of autosomal recessive conditions are phenylketonuria and cystic fibrosis. Notice that autosomal recessive inheritance may be difficult to distinguish from germline mosaicism, because the occurrence of both is restricted to sibs (Edwards, 1989b).

For rare autosomal recessive traits, the parents of an affected individual tend to be related more often than in the general population because they have an increased probability of sharing two copies of the same ancestral disease allele (the two copies are said to be identical by descent, IBD). The two disease alleles in an affected child are then also IBD, and the two alleles of a marker locus tightly linked with the disease gene tend to be IBD as well. This situation was discussed by Smith (1953) and shown to depend critically on close linkage and a high degree of polymorphism of the marker. As pointed out by Lander and Botstein (1986b), a dense map of genetic markers will satisfy these conditions. These authors further showed that, under ideal conditions, a single affected child born of first cousins is roughly as informative as a nuclear family with three affected children (for a count of meioses and a formal characterization of homozygosity mapping, see Section 12.2). The term *homozygosity mapping* was introduced by Lander and Botstein (1986b) to denote the fact that an increased degree of homozygosity for marker alleles in affected children of related parents is indicative of linkage between the marker and the disease. To take full advantage of this homozygosity, it is prudent to carry out a regular linkage analysis with one of the available computer programs. If the program "knows" of the relationship between the parents (and perhaps other pedigree members), it will automatically make use of the increased informativeness inherent in the family. Figure 12.1 shows a pedigree suitable for homozygosity mapping as the parents of the affected offspring are first cousins (other relationships among the parents would also yield increased informativeness over unrelated parents).

Table 12.2 demonstrates that homozygosity mapping strongly depends on marker heterozygosity and trait prevalence. Lod scores in the first two columns of the body of Table 12.2 were obtained for the pedigree shown in Figure 12.1 while the second two columns refer to an analogous pedigree with two offspring both of which have marker genotype *1/1*. The marker locus has two alleles, with the *1* allele having frequency q. In this setting, in terms of heterozygosity, this 2-allele locus is equivalent to a highly

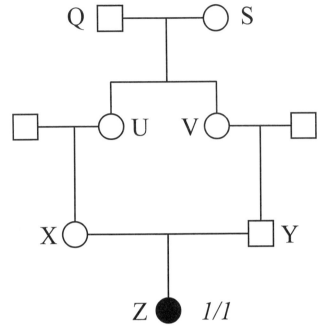

Figure 12.1. A family with a marriage among cousins demonstrating increased informativeness through homozygosity mapping.

polymorphic marker with n equally frequent alleles, where $n = 1/q$. For example, $n = 100$ for $q = 0.01$. The disease is assumed to be recessive with disease allele frequency of p such that trait prevalence is equal to p^2. As the lod scores in the left half of Table 12.2 show, informativeness drops off sharply with decreasing marker heterozygosity and increasing trait prevalence.

When parents are related, likelihood calculations tend to demand

Table 12.2. Lod Scores Obtained for a Family as Shown in Figure 12.1 with One or Two Affected Offspring, Each with the Same Homozygous Marker Genotype

	One Affected		Two Affecteds	
Marker	$p = 0.001$	$p = 0.10$	$p = 0.001$	$p = 0.10$
$q = 0.001$	1.19	0.88	1.79	1.48
$q = 0.010$	1.14	0.83	1.72	1.41
$q = 0.100$	0.80	0.53	1.29	1.02

Note: p = allele frequency of recessive disease; q = frequency of #1 marker allele.

much computer time, particularly for multipoint analysis. Several solutions have been proposed. For example, Kong (1991) presented a novel representation of the pedigree likelihood, and Kruglyak et al. (1995) developed a method to rapidly compute likelihoods in nuclear families and implemented it in a computer program, HOMOZ. In general, approaches have been developed that involve approximation by computer simulation rather than exact calculation of likelihoods. They tend to allow the processing of large complicated pedigrees and multiple loci (Irwin et al., 1994; Heath, 1997).

Because in some eastern countries marriages among first cousins are customary, families from these countries are particularly suitable for linkage analysis of recessive traits. If parental relationship is unknown, it may be estimated based on a large number (at least 50) of marker genotypes and the estimated relationship used in the linkage analysis as if it has been observed. However, this should only be done when evidence for the estimated relationship is supported by a likelihood ratio of at least 10:1 against the parents being unrelated (Mérette and Ott, 1996).

X-linked traits are most often recessive with full penetrance in (hemizygous) males. An exception is, for example, the fragile X syndrome, which is inherited as an X-linked recessive trait with incomplete penetrance in males (Sherman et al., 1985).

Special Inheritance Cases. In Chapter 15 of their book, Strachan and Read (1996) classify diseases according to mechanisms underlying them. For example, loss of function (usually recessive) is likely when various mechanisms (point mutations, deletions, etc.) lead to the same disease, whereas gain of function is likely when only a specific mutation in a gene is the cause for a trait. In some cases, a loss of function mutation and the corresponding 50% reduction in gene product lead to a dominant phenotype (heterozygote). This mechanism is called *haploinsufficiency.* For a list of corresponding diseases, see Fisher and Scambler (1994).

Although many Mendelian diseases are due to single base substitutions, some diseases, as mentioned in Section 1.1, are due to trinucleotide (for example, CAG) repeat expansions (Strachan and Read, 1996; Koob et al., 1998). Some of them are characterized by anticipation, that is, increasing severity or progressively earlier age at disease onset in successive generations.

Genes with protective effect are also known, for example, AIDS-resistance genes (Moore, 1997; Winkler et al., 1998). They show interesting geographical clines that permit conclusions on past epidemiologic events (O'Brien and Dean, 1997).

12.2. Number of Informative Meioses

As shown in Section 9.7, computer simulation methods may be applied to estimate the probability (power) to obtain a maximum lod score exceeding 3 in a lod score analysis of a given body of data. Several such simulations with different numbers of families allow determining the number of families required for given power and other test parameters. A simpler and often useful approach is to approximately determine the number of meioses required to localize the gene underlying a mendelian trait and how this number varies with complicating factors such as incomplete penetrance. This may be done as outlined in this section.

It was shown in Section 5.11 that approximately $n = 20$ known meioses (often called fully informative gametes, FIGs) are required for significant linkage. Various complicating factors may now translate this figure into a higher number of family members. Unknown phase in an informative parent adds one offspring (more for loose linkage) to a sibship (see Section 5.8). Marker heterozygosity determines the frequency with which a parent is potentially informative for linkage. As a rough adjustment for less than 100% marker informativeness, the number of families required is divided by the marker's heterozygosity. However, in a multipoint analysis, the "equivalent" heterozygosity of several markers jointly tends to be high so that this is not a major determinant of sample size.

Other factors reducing informativeness may be taken into account using the various tables of previous sections in which ELODs or variances have been calculated. With incomplete penetrance, n must be multiplied by the inverse of the relative ELOD (see Section 7.2). For example, with an average penetrance of 50%, a threefold number of offspring (meioses) is required (see Table 7.2). Heterogeneity also reduces informativeness and may be allowed for by further multiplying the number of meioses by the inverse of the relative efficiency (ratio of variances). As a rough guideline, Table 10.7 provides standard errors for θ estimates in a specific family type. As an example, when 20% of families are of the unlinked type ($\alpha = 0.80$), with $\theta = 0.05$, the number of offspring must be multiplied by the inverse of the ratio of the variances, that is, by $(0.075/0.042)^2 = 3.2$. Errors in marker typing may be allowed for under a simple misclassification model (see Section 11.2). Table 11.3 lists the corresponding relative ELODs. For example, with $\theta = 0.05$ and a misclassification rate of $s = 0.05$, the number of meioses must be increased by a factor of $1/0.77 = 1.3$. In summary, for example, the original number of 20 meioses is increased to $20 \times 3 \times 3.2 \times 1.3 \approx 250$ meioses by a penetrance of 50%, a proportion of linked families of 80%, and a misclassification rate of 5%.

In linkage analyses of autosomal recessive traits, an important practical question is, how much linkage information do unaffected offspring provide? Is it useful at all to carry out marker typing for unaffected offspring? This question may be answered by calculating the ELOD for given numbers of affected and unaffected offspring. Assume that the disease is rare and that the marker locus is highly polymorphic so that the parents have four different marker alleles. At the disease locus, each parent is heterozygous, *d/D,* where *d* is the disease allele and *D* is the normal allele. The joint genotype of parent 1 is *d1/D2* or *d2/D1* and that of parent 2 is *d3/D4* or *d4/D3.* Four different phase combinations can be distinguished among the parents, each occurring with prior probability of ¼. It is then straightforward although somewhat tedious to calculate the expected lod score, $E[Z(r)]$, where *r* is the true recombination fraction between disease and marker genes (Leal and Ott, 1990). The results shown in Table 12.1 suggest that an affected offspring provides approximately five times as much linkage information as an unaffected offspring. With tight linkage, each affected offspring independently contributes 0.602 and each unaffected contributes 0.125 towards the ELOD. For an ELOD of 3, for example, one needs 5 affected offspring or 24 unaffected offspring or a total of 3 affected and 10 unaffected offspring.

In Section 12.1, homozygosity mapping was mentioned as making use of the fact that parents are first cousins. For a very rare disease and a highly polymorphic marker, this method allows inferring phase-known meioses in parents and grandparents even though these individuals are not genotyped. In Figure 12.1, the only genotyped individual is *Z* who is affected. Owing to the low trait prevalence it is assumed that all other individuals are unaffected. Because the *1* allele is rare, it is highly likely that the two *1* alleles of individual *Z* are copies of a single *1* allele in one of the grandparents, that is, her two *1* alleles are identical by descent (IBD), and so are her two disease alleles. The following derivation is based on Smith (1953) who presented this situation in great detail. Assume that disease and marker loci are linked with recombination fraction θ and that the grandparental disease allele came from *Q.* Then, given that *Z* is homozygous for the disease allele, the two *1* alleles in *Z* originated from a single grandparental allele in *Q* or *S* if one of the following conditions holds:

1. All steps *QU, UX, XZ, QV, VY, VZ* are nonrecombinants
2. Steps *QU, QV* are both recombinants, all others nonrecombinants
3. *U* and *V* received the same *1* allele from *S, UX* and *VY* are recombinants, and *XZ* and *YZ* are nonrecombinants.

As mentioned by Smith (1953), written in terms of θ, the total probability of these three mutually exclusive events is given by

$$P = (1 - \theta)^6 + \theta^2(1 - \theta)^4 + \tfrac{1}{2}\theta^2(1 - \theta)^2. \tag{12.1}$$

From this expression, the lod score is obtained as $\log(16P)$. For $\theta = 0$, one has $P = 1$ so that the maximum lod score under tight linkage turns out to be $\log(16) = 1.20$. Although this lod score is the same as that for four phase-known nonrecombinants, this equivalence evidently no longer holds for $\theta > 0$.

Additional children do not derive the same benefits from this situation as does the first child. For each additional child, one can score two meioses, one in each parent, but meioses further up the pedigree have already been "used" by the first child. For example, parent X is a single child receiving a nonrecombinant haplotype, irrespective of the number of children she has herself. Thus, each additional child will at best contribute 0.60 towards the total lod score of the sibship.

If the pedigree "loop" in Figure 12.1 is expanded in the sense that additional generations are inserted between top and bottom generations, even higher lod scores may be obtained than those shown in Table 12.2 if the trait is rare enough and the marker is polymorphic enough.

12.3. Candidate Loci

Candidate loci are genes that, for some a priori reason, have been implicated as possible causes of a disease; for example, their function may be suggestive of their being involved in the disease etiology. Usually, candidate loci are the first loci with which linkage analysis is carried out in the attempt to map a given disease. Examples of successfully applied candidate loci are the nerve growth factor receptor and neurofibromatosis (Seizinger et al., 1987); a collagen gene, COL2A1 on chromosome 12, which was implicated as a candidate gene for familial osteoarthrosis (Palotie et al., 1989); and the prion protein PRIP on the tip of the short arm of chromosome 20, which was suspected to be the cause of Gerstmann–Sträussler syndrome (Hsiao et al., 1989). Sometimes, investigators feel that the prior probability of linkage is larger for candidate genes than just for any marker gene so that a lower critical lod score than 3 should be allowed as proof for linkage. A "regular" significance level such as 0.05 or 0.01 should then be applicable to testing for candidate genes. Based on equation (4.10), a critical lod score of 2 would then guarantee a p-value of no more than 0.01. Although this reasoning appears sound, the relatively poor record of the candidate gene approach suggests that the increase in prior probability of linkage is rather modest and does not warrant a strong deviation from the classical critical lod score level of 3.

In linkage analyses with candidate genes, one is often interested in knowing how many meioses one must investigate to *dis*prove that a particular candidate gene is the real disease-causing gene. Throughout this section, assume that you have phase-known matings such that recombinations and nonrecombinations can be scored in the offspring. Disproving a candidate gene then amounts to finding an obligate recombinant. Further assume that the true recombination fraction is equal to $r = \frac{1}{2}$. What number n_1 of recombination events does one have to inspect such that, with probability P, that number will contain at least one recombination? By the binomial formula, one has $P = 1 - (\frac{1}{2})^{n_1}$, or

$$n_1 = \log(1 - P)/\log(\frac{1}{2}).$$

For probabilities $P = 0.95$ and 0.99, one has $n_1 = 4$ and 7, respectively. Furthermore, as given by the mean of the geometric waiting time distribution (Elandt-Johnson, 1971), one will on average have to inspect two nonrecombinants before the first recombinant is found.

One may not want to reject a candidate gene based on only a single recombination but may want to see at least two recombinations before excluding a candidate gene. Under absence of linkage, the probability of finding two or more recombinations is given by $P = 1 - (\frac{1}{2})^{n_2}(1 + n_2)$. This equation cannot be solved directly for n_2, but the following equation provides an iterative solution:

$$n_2 = [\log(1 - P) - \log(1 + n_2)]/\log(\frac{1}{2}).$$

For $P = 0.95$ and 0.99, $n_2 = 8$ and 10, respectively. On average, under absence of linkage, four recombination events must be investigated before the second recombination is found (mean of negative binomial distribution; Elandt-Johnson, 1971).

As another criterion for excluding a candidate gene, one may want to require the observation of as many recombination events as necessary so the expected lod score at a given value of θ falls below the classical boundary of -2. As long as only nonrecombinants are seen, lod scores will be positive. So, this criterion can be applied only when at least one recombination has already been observed. The expected lod score is then equal to $-\infty$ at $\theta = 0$ and rises to perhaps positive values for larger θ values. At a given value of θ, assuming absence of linkage, the expected lod score for a single opportunity for recombination is equal to $\frac{1}{2}[\log 2 - 2\theta) + \log(2\theta)]$. The condition that the expected lod score should be equal to or less than -2 is thus given by the inequality $(n/2)\log[4\theta(1 - \theta)] \leq -2$ or

$$n \geq -4/\log[4\theta(1 - \theta)].$$

For $\theta = 0.01, 0.05$, and 0.10, the corresponding values of n are 3, 6, and 9, respectively. The preceding results suggest that fewer than ten meioses must be looked at for rejections of a candidate gene in the absence of linkage.

When nothing but nonrecombinants are being observed, one may wonder how many offspring must be investigated to be able to *prove* linkage to a candidate gene. In Table 5.10, it was shown that under a true recombination fraction of $r = 0.01$, $n = 16$ recombination events are required to obtain a maximum lod score of 3 with power of 90%. In other words, if one has a candidate gene, $n = 16$ recombination events provide good power to prove linkage ($r \ll \frac{1}{2}$). However, to show that one has a candidate gene requires more than that—one must show that the confidence interval for r is restricted to small values. Assume that one observes only nonrecombinants. The estimate of the recombination fraction is then zero and the $100(1 - \alpha)\%$ confidence interval ranges from 0 through $\theta = 1 - \alpha^{1/n}$ (see Section 3.6). Solving its upper bound for n leads to

$$n = \log(\alpha)/\log(1 - \theta),$$

which is the number of nonrecombinants required so that the $100(1 - \alpha)\%$ confidence interval for r extends from 0 through θ. For a short confidence interval, large numbers of observations are required. Specifically, for $\theta = 0.01, 0.05$, and 0.10, the respective numbers required are $n = 298, 59$, and 29.

12.4. Exclusion Mapping

In the search for a disease gene on the human genome, "negative" information is useful because it narrows the region of the genome possibly containing the gene. (Criteria for excluding candidate loci were discussed in the previous section.) Classically, values of θ between a disease and a marker locus are considered "excluded" (highly implausible) if the lod score is less than or equal to -2, corresponding to a likelihood ratio of $1 : 100$ or less. The same criterion is also applied to the multipoint lod score in linkage analysis of a disease versus a map of markers. After negative linkage analyses of a disease with a set of markers, there are thus regions of exclusion around the markers. When markers on a chromosome are rather closely spaced, the region of exclusion may eventually be continuous along the whole chromosome if the disease locus is not on that chromosome. The exclusion criterion of $Z \leq -2$ is quite stringent, so linkage analyses tend to furnish small regions of exclusion, which are unlikely to contain the disease locus (a small probability for the disease to be in the excluded region remains).

In this classical approach, the exclusion criterion is always the same no matter how many markers have been investigated. A different approach makes use of the fact that a gene excluded from one region must have a higher probability of being in another region of the genome (Edwards, 1987), provided that the phenotype used for mapping is indeed due to a single gene (or perhaps a small number of genes). Initially, one may assume that the disease has an equal prior probability of being in any interval of a given size. Each linkage analysis then modifies this prior density of disease location, resulting in a posterior density. A successful application of exclusion mapping is that of Marfan syndrome (Kainulainen et al., 1990).

For *heterogeneous traits,* exclusion mapping is somewhat problematic. Assume that a small proportion of the families investigated segregate a gene located on the map of markers under study but the overall lod score (summed over families assuming homogeneity) is smaller than -2 at each point on the map. If exclusion is based on the total lod score, a true disease location will be excluded. A possible solution is to estimate the proportion α of families in which the disease gene is linked to a given region of the genome (estimates will often be $\hat{\alpha} = 1$), jointly with the map position x of that gene. A disease gene should only then be excluded from a map only when the families appear to be homogeneous. Good evidence for heterogeneity, however, indicates that in some of the families there is a gene located on the map under study. For detecting linkage under heterogeneity, requirements for significance were discussed in Chapter 10. Applying the same stringent criteria for significance when excluding linkage tends to exclude true locations of disease genes. Hence, for exclusion mapping under heterogeneity, a better approach is to apply less stringent criteria, for example, to declare heterogeneity significant (thus allowing for the presence of a disease gene) with a p-value of 0.01 or a likelihood ratio of $100:1$. In practice, this means that one evaluates $Z(\hat{\alpha}, x)$ (the hlod) at each map position, x, where $\hat{\alpha}$ is determined by the maximum of the likelihood over α at the given x value. Only those points x are then excluded for which $Z(\hat{\alpha}, x) < +2$ (or $+1$) and $Z(x) < -2$, where $Z(x)$ is the lod score under homogeneity.

A partly nonparametric approach to exclusion mapping under possible heterogeneity via the exclusion of certain IBD probabilities (Hyer et al., 1991) is discussed in Section 13.5.

12.5. Genetic Risks

A genetic risk may be defined as the probability (usually conditional on observations of relatives) that an individual will develop a genetically inherited trait. For mendelian traits, the genetic risk is the conditional probability that an individual has the disease predisposing genotype, given his or her phenotype and other family information, notably phenotypes at marker loci. The *proband* or counselee is the individual for whom risk is calculated. Risks may be based on the marker genotype at a linked marker, on cytogenetic analysis or a direct molecular probe for disease alleles. This section focuses on the linkage aspect of risks. Many research and clinical laboratories perform tests for inherited diseases. An organization, *Helix,* provides a listing of such laboratories, which currently lists over 550 diseases and more than 300 laboratories world-wide (http://healthlinks.washington.edu/heli; telephone, 206–527–5742; fax, 206–527–5743).

For complex traits (mode of inheritance unknown), risks must largely be based on empirically obtained estimates of recurrence risks (Murphy and Chase, 1975; Vogel and Motulsky, 1986), but various statistical problems make empirical risk estimation difficult (Chakraborty, 1987). In this section, genetic risks are restricted to mendelian traits and risks will be calculated parametrically on the basis of a known model of disease inheritance.

As an introduction to the concept of genetic risk, consider the following application of Bayes theorem. In Duchenne muscular dystrophy (DMD, X-linked), female carriers of the disease gene are unaffected but their serum level of the enzyme creatine kinase (CK) is elevated. Denote a carrier by C and a noncarrier by N. If one distinguishes only between low (L) and high (H) CK values, and the 95th percentile of the normal range is taken as a cutoff point, then the probability is $P(H|N) = 0.05$ that a noncarrier woman has a high CK value. On the other hand, women carrying a DMD allele have elevated CK levels with probability $P(H|C) \approx \frac{2}{3}$ (Vogel and Motulsky, 1986). If a woman randomly drawn from the population shows an elevated CK value, what is her probability of being a carrier? By Bayes theorem,

$$P(C|H) = \frac{P(H|C)P(C)}{P(H|C)P(C) + P(H|N)PN}, \tag{12.2}$$

where $P(C) = 1 - P(N) = p$, say, is the proportion of carriers in the population, and $P(C|H)$ is the woman's risk of being a carrier given her elevated CK status. With the values for $P(H|C)$ and $P(H|N)$ given above, the risk (12.2) becomes $\frac{2}{3} p/[\frac{2}{3} p + 0.05(1 - p)] = p/(0.075 + 0.925p)$. Because $p \ll 0.075$, $0.925p$ is negligibly small and the woman's risk is approximately $13p$, that is, thirteen times the population prevalence.

For mendelian traits, in which no direct molecular or cytogenetic test for the disease gene is available, risks are usually determined via a closely linked marker. For single individuals, allowing for allelic association may improve accuracy of genotype predictions. For example, an unaffected individual has a probability of 0.0392 of being a carrier of the CF allele, but the analogous probability for an individual with the BB marker genotype is 0.199, approximately five times the population risk (Beaudet et al., 1989).

In family data, the risk to a proband may sometimes be calculated analytically. For example, consider the family shown in Figure 4.1, in which the linkage relationship between Charcot–Marie–Tooth disease (CMT1) and ABO blood type is investigated. The same family was also analyzed for CMT1 versus the Duffy blood group (FY) (Dyck et al., 1983). The father (individual 3.1) was doubly heterozygous with known phase, *Db/da*, where D is the disease allele and a and b are the relevant two Duffy alleles. He had passed the disease allele and the Duffy b allele to each of his four offspring, so these were all nonrecombinants. Assume now that a newly born child (not shown in Figure 4.1) has received the Duffy allele a from his father. What is this proband's risk of having inherited the disease allele D from the father? Given that the father passes an a allele to the proband, he transmits a D allele with probability θ and a d allele with probability $1 - \theta$. Hence, the risk to the proband is equal to the recombination fraction, $R = \theta$. Usually, the recombination fraction is not known with certainty but only as a more or less precise estimate around which one constructs a confidence or support interval for the true recombination fraction. In this case, obviously, the risk estimate is as precise as the recombination fraction estimate, so the support interval for θ also applies to the risk R.

There has been some debate as to whether it is meaningful to compute support intervals for genetic risks, R (Edwards, 1989). R is a probability just as, for example, the proportion α of the linked family type in a mixture of linked and unlinked families (see Section 10.4), and for this and other proportions it is customary to compute support or confidence intervals. There is thus no reason why support intervals should not also be constructed for genetic risks. Knowing the support interval for a genetic risk will enable a genetic counselor to see how much faith he or she should have in the point estimate of R. Of course, because it is often difficult to convey even the notion of a risk to a counselee, the concept of a support interval for the true risk is even more difficult to grasp and may best be avoided in genetic counseling sessions. Methods for constructing risk support intervals have been developed and implemented in computer programs (Leal and Ott, 1994, 1995).

Calculating genetic risks in pedigree data is related to the pedigree likelihood (Elston and Stewart, 1971). The risk that the ith individual has a particular genotype g_i is given by the conditional probability, $P(g_i|x) = P(x, g_i)/P(x)$, where $P(x) = \Sigma_j P(x, g_j)$ is the pedigree likelihood, and $P(x, g_i)$ is that likelihood when the ith individual has the specific genotype g_i. Genetic risks may be calculated in exactly this manner by carrying out two likelihood calculations using the LIPED program. In other computer programs, however, particular procedures are implemented for directly calculating genetic risks. For example, in the MLINK program of the LINKAGE package, this is achieved by "peeling" the likelihood onto the proband (the individual for whom a risk is to be calculated), such that the proband is the last individual in the recursive likelihood calculations.

Kinship L, shown in Figure 4.1, is one of a number of pedigrees forming a mixture of linked and unlinked families with respect to CMT1 and the Duffy locus (see Section 10.4). In such a situation, one may calculate a risk R_L assuming a proband's family is of the linked type and a risk R_U given that the family is of the unlinked type (generally one may have more than two types). When $R_L \approx R_U$ one not need to go any further. If the two risks are quite different, one will in many cases recognize from the linkage analysis which of the risks is the more plausible figure. A more rigorous solution consists of calculating the overall risk as a weighted average of R_L and R_U (Weeks and Ott, 1989). As an example, if the mixture analysis (e.g., furnished by the HOMOG program) yields an estimate $\hat{\theta} = 0.05$ for the recombination fraction in the linked families, the risk for the hypothetical new offspring in family L is $R_L = 0.05$ when the family is of the linked type and $R_U = 0.50$ when it is of the unlinked type. The overall risk estimate is

$$R_w = wR_L + (1 - w)R_U, \tag{12.3}$$

where w is the conditional probability that the proband's family is of the linked type. The estimated value of w may be obtained from equation (10.11) or the HOMOG program. For the given family, for example, at $\theta = 0.05$ and $\alpha = 0.65$, one finds $w = 0.92$ so that $R_w = 0.92 \times 0.05 + 0.08 \times 0.50 = 0.086$. A support interval for R_w would be based on the support interval for the estimates of α and θ. Each pair (α, θ) inside the support region is associated with a value of R_w. Scanning a large number of pairs (α, θ) will yield a range of R_w values whose endpoints define the desired support interval (Leal and Ott, 1994).

For X-linked lethal recessive traits, the prior probability that a woman with no information about her male relatives carries a disease allele is equal to $q = 4\mu$ (Murphy and Chase, 1975), where μ is the mutation rate. This implies that a woman with one affected son has posterior probability ⅔ of being a carrier and ⅓ of not carrying the disease allele (Murphy and Chase, 1975). This result is sometimes phrased as "one third of all cases are new mutations" while, of course, only ⅓ of the *isolated* cases are new mutations. Also, under equilibrium, the gene frequency is equal to 3μ (Haldane, 1935). In most computer programs, q depends on the population frequency p of the disease allele, $q = 2p(1 - p)$. Therefore, in these programs, one should not use p as the gene frequency but rather use p to set the appropriate prior carrier probability. In other words, one should choose p such that $2p(1 - p) = q$ or $p \approx \frac{1}{2}q = 2\mu$, with the mutation rate generally being in the order of $\mu = 10^{-5} = 0.00001$ (e.g., for DMD) (Cavalli-Sforza and Bodmer, 1971).

Often, one is interested in knowing what risks might be expected before marker typing is carried out. In simple situations, hand calculations can provide the answer (Ott et al., 1990b). A more complicated example in which all possible risks can be enumerated and evaluated by computer is demonstrated in Section 9.4. In most applications, however, risk distributions before marker typing must be approximated by computer simulation (Sandkuyl and Ott, 1989). Briefly, given the disease status for family members at some mendelian disease locus and parameter values such as recombination fraction and gene frequencies, marker genotypes are randomly generated, which is repeated for many replicates. For each replicate, the risk to the proband is computed as if the marker genotypes had actually been observed. The resulting distribution of risks can then be represented as a histogram and risks R may be classified into informative and uninformative, where, for example, risks $R > 0.90$ and $R < 0.10$ may be called informative. The proportion of informative risks may be taken as a measure for the probability of successful counseling of the family at hand.

One might expect that theoretical risk distributions obtained before marker typing should be symmetric about 50%. Experience with testing for Huntington disease (autosomal dominant) shows, however, that in many cases the risk distribution is strongly skewed towards low risk figures. Three major reasons account for this skewness:

1. Probands are often already far past the age of onset, yet are still unaffected. Hence, their risk of carrying the disease allele is less than 50%.

2. Genetic testing is carried out as so-called nondisclosure or nondisclosing testing (Folstein, 1989), in which the proband has a risk of 50% or ≈ 0, depending on whether the relevant gene marker was obtained from the affected or unaffected grandparent. Nondisclosure testing of a proband child is either voluntary (the unaffected parent at risk, who is

potentially a carrier of the disease gene, does not want to be tested) or the consequence of insufficient information (parent at risk is uninformative for linkage).

3. Consider a mother at risk and two offspring. Of these, one is affected and the other (the proband) is unaffected. The mother is not tested and is thus not known a priori to be heterozygous. To recognize unequivocally that she is heterozygous for the marker and thus informative for linkage, one must know that the two children have received two different marker alleles from the mother. With close linkage, this situation leads either to a low risk to the proband (when the mother is heterozygous) or to a risk in the neighborhood of 50% (when the mother is not known to be heterozygous). An example may be found in Ott et al. (1990b).

The phenomenon mentioned in the last point above is easily demonstrated based on the family shown in Figure 12.2. One parent is affected with a dominant trait (penetrance age dependent, full penetrance at high age), both parents unavailable for marker typing. One offspring (proband, P) is affected, the other offspring (counselee, C) is below the age of risk. A marker is tightly linked with the disease locus and has two equally frequent alleles, 1 and 2. Table 12.3 shows all possible offspring genotypes and associated risks (probability of carrying the disease allele) computed with the MLINK program, in which the disease allele frequency was taken to be 0.001. Relative likelihoods are calculated as outlined in Section 9.4. There are only four possible risks: 0.001, 0.334, 0.600, and 0.667

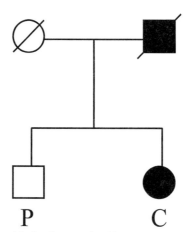

Figure 12.2. A family with dominant trait of late onset, one affected child (proband, P) and one young child (counselee, C). Both parents were unavailable for marker genotyping.

Table 12.3. All Possible Risks to Counselee in Pedigree Shown in Figure 12.2

Genotype		Risk for Heterozygous Genotype	Relative Likelihood
P	C		
1/1	1/1	0.667	22.8416
1/1	1/2	0.334	15.2278
1/1	2/2	0.001	2.5380
1/2	1/1	0.334	15.2278
1/2	1/2	0.600	50.7592
1/2	1/2	0.334	15.2278
2/2	1/1	0.001	2.5380
2/2	1/2	0.334	15.2278
2/2	2/2	0.667	22.8416

with the respective probabilities 0.031, 0.375, 0.313, and 0.281. The risk distribution (Figure 12.3) is obviously very skewed towards low values yet the average risk is 0.5 as it should be.

The population-genetic consequences of genetic testing and selective abortion were long ago well investigated (Crow, 1966; Motulsky, Fraser, and Felsenstein, 1971). Prospects for extensive screening of all newborns for many disease genes were discussed by Vogel and Motulsky (1986, p. 628–629). The possibility of predicting one's genetic fate at birth, envisioned more than 60 years ago by Haldane (reprinted 1985), may well have a strong influence on society.

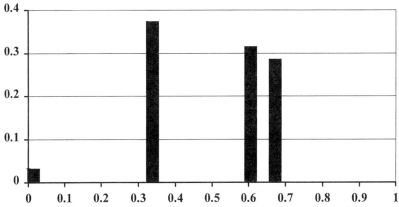

Figure 12.3. Risk distribution for counselee in Figure 12.2 based on results shown in Table 12.3.

12.6. Irregular Segregation

In most linkage analyses, regular mendelian inheritance is taken for granted. Sometimes, however, unusual inheritance patterns cast doubt on the mode of inheritance assumed. This section briefly points out some of these irregular segregation patterns and discusses their effect on linkage analysis. Recognition of many cases of special segregation has become possible only with the advent of molecular genetic techniques.

For a parent with marker genotype *1/2*, one expects half of the children to receive the *1* allele and half to receive the *2* allele. Deviations from such mendelian ratios are called *segregation distortion,* or *gametic drive* if due to lethality of gametes (Strickberger, 1985). Segregation distortion has no effect on the estimate of the recombination fraction but should make investigators alert to possible errors in the data such as sample mix-ups.

As mentioned in Section 1.2, for some conditions, disease alleles are preferentially received from the father or from the mother, which represents a form of *genomic imprinting.* Imprinted genes have unusual characteristics (Hurst et al., 1996) and some imprinted genomic regions are conserved between mice and humans (Dao et al., 1998). As long as one recognizes unequivocally which parent passed the disease allele(s) to the children, this is analogous to skewed segregation and has no negative effect on linkage analysis. Similarly, for some disorders, new mutations tend to originate preferentially in a male or a female. Other forms of imprinting result in different disease phenotypes depending on parental origin of the disease allele. Well-known cases include Prader–Willi and Angelman syndromes (Cassidy and Schwartz, 1998).

Uniparental disomy represents a problem for linkage analysis—both chromosomes of a pair were received from the same parent (Engel, 1980). This can usually be recognized with molecular genetics techniques (e.g., Gelb et al., 1998). Obviously, such phenomena if unrecognized can lead linkage analysis astray.

Another serious problem in linkage analysis is *mosaicism.* Consider a mother with a number of offspring, two of whom are affected with a dominant disease. Explaining the two affecteds as two independent mutations is unsatisfactory as it has very low probability. A more plausible interpretation is germ line mosaicism, also called gonadal mosaicism (Murphy and Chase, 1975; Edwards, 1989b; Zlotogora, 1998), which postulates that one mutation has occurred during the formation of the germ cells so that a germ line mosaic produces mutant and nonmutant gametes. Mosaicism has long been considered as a potential factor in linkage analysis (Bell and Haldane, 1937), but only in the past 10 years or so has it become possible to clearly document the rather widespread occurrence of germ line mosaicism and similar phenomena. Unrecognized mosaicism may be confused with genetic heterogeneity, and this can have a devastating effect on linkage analysis. Also, it may lead to wrong estimates of genetic risks. Linkage programs currently do not routinely allow for germ line mosaicism. Its deleterious effect may be reduced by allowing for a rather high mutation rate, but the safest solution is to trace the origin of each chromosome as best as one can.

12.7. Problem

Problem 12.1. In Section 12.2, 70% of obligate carriers of the X-linked recessive Duchenne muscular dystrophy (DMD) gene are said to have CK values above the 95th percentile of the normal range. Taking that 95th percentile as a cutoff point to distinguish between low and high CK values, set up the penetrance model for the various male and female DMD phenotypes, assuming that genotypes cannot be identified by DNA analysis. *Note*: disregard female homozygous carriers.

Additional problems on risk calculation are found in Chapter 13 in connection with linkage disequilibrium.

13.

Nonparametric Methods

In parametric (lod score) linkage analysis, mode of inheritance of the loci must be specified exactly. For some conditions, however, several modes of inheritance appear plausible. This problem is addressed in Section 15.4. Here, I briefly discuss particular types of linkage and linkage disequilibrium analysis, which require no assumptions about mode of inheritance of the trait studied. Nonparametric methods are also covered in our handbook (Terwilliger and Ott, 1994). Power calculations with nonparametric methods are covered in Section 15.5.

Although most of this chapter is devoted to affected sib pair and linkage disequilibrium methods, a few special methods should be mentioned. The AGFAP method (Thomson, 1983; Risch, 1983) compares the observed distribution of HLA genotypes in a sample of affected individuals with the distribution expected for specific genetic models for the trait. In this manner, mode of inheritance for the trait may be estimated. Thus, this method falls into the category of segregation analysis. The MASC method (Clerget-Darpoux et al., 1988) combines segregation and association analysis and is expected to perform better than regular association (linkage disequilibrium) analysis.

13.1. Sets of Relatives

Special analysis methods have been developed for pairs of (or sets of more than two) relatives. The best known of these approaches is the affected sib pair (ASP) method.

The sib-pair method of Penrose (1935) is based on the relative frequencies of pairs of sibs to be alike or unlike for two traits whose linkage is to be investigated. It thus analyzes single-sibship data. For two phenotypes at each of two loci, the sib pairs are tabulated in a 2×2 table such that rows refer to locus *1* and columns to locus *2*. Each sib pair contributes

272

one entry to the table. When the two sibs are alike with respect to their phenotype at the first locus, the pair is entered in the first row; otherwise, it is entered in the second row. Analogously, a sib pair is entered in the first column when the sibs are alike at the second locus and in the second column when they are unlike. It can be shown (see Section 5.8) that, in the presence of linkage, the upper left and lower right hand cells of the table will preferentially be filled, so that linkage can be tested for by a chi-square analysis of the table. Because parental phenotypes are disregarded, many uninformative matings fill the table with useless data so that power of this sib pair analysis is rather low. Nonetheless, it was by this method that the first autosomal linkage was found in humans, that between the Lutheran and Secretor blood groups (Mohr, 1954). In the 1930s and 1940s, Penrose's sib-pair method evidently was *the* linkage analysis method and was applied to numerous traits such as presence of cross eyes, ability to curl the tongue, occurrence of warts, and so on (Kloepfer, 1946).

The modern form of the sib-pair method focuses on *affected* siblings (some also on affected–unaffected pairs) (for an overview, see Knapp, 1997). These ASP methods rest on the hypothesis that a marker locus is closely linked to a disease locus so that the disease gene is transmitted to different offspring always with the same marker allele, that is, the one in coupling with the disease allele. Attention is, thus, focused on affected offspring who are known to have received a disease gene. This elegantly circumvents problems of incomplete penetrance but hinges on the assumption of absence of nongenetic cases—occurrence of phenocopies can severely reduce power of ASP methods (Bishop and Williamson, 1990). The relevant observation in these methods is how frequently two affected offspring share copies of the same parental marker allele—such copies are said to be inherited identical by descent (IBD) (Fishman et al., 1978; Suarez, 1978). For example, consider a sufficiently polymorphic marker so that the parents show four different marker alleles. The number of alleles shared IBD among two affected sibs is 0, 1, or 2. If inheritance is according to the mendelian laws, these numbers occur in the expected proportions of $1:2:1$. However, if the marker is close to a disease gene, then one or both parents presumably have a disease allele in coupling with one of the marker alleles, which is then likely to be passed to both affected offspring. Thus, with linkage, one expects a deviation towards higher numbers of alleles shared IBD. One may distinguish between methods for single markers versus all markers on a chromosome, and affected sib pairs versus more than two affecteds in a sibship versus affected relatives other than siblings. Knapp (1997) provides a brief overview of today's affected sib pair methods. Note that all calculations are done on marker inheritance—the only connection to disease is through ascertainment of *affected* siblings.

A detailed treatment of gene identity by descent for various pairs of relatives may be found in Chapter 2 of Thompson (1986). Let k_0, k_1, and k_2 denote the probabilities that a pair of individuals shares 0, 1, or 2 alleles as copies of an ancestral allele (IBD). Thompson (1986) showed that for any degree of relationship between two noninbred individuals, $4k_2k_0 \leq k_1^2$.

Single Marker, Sib Pairs. Increased IBD sharing may be measured and tested for by various methods. Consider the probabilities, z_0, z_1, and z_2, that an ASP shares 0, 1, or 2 alleles IBD. These probabilities may be estimated by the corresponding observed frequencies, $\hat{z}_i$, $i = 0, 1, 2$, of ASPs sharing i alleles IBD. Under no linkage between trait and a marker, one expects $z_0 = \frac{1}{4}$, $z_1 = \frac{1}{2}$, and $z_2 = \frac{1}{4}$. For a fully penetrant recessive disease without phenocopies and tightly linked to a marker, $z_0 = z_1 = 0$ and $z_2 = 1$ whereas for a dominant trait, $z_0 = 0$ and $z_1 = z_2 = \frac{1}{2}$. For dominant traits, only one of the two parents is informative for linkage. Therefore, IBD sharing methods treating both parents the same are inherently more powerful for recessive than for dominant genes and, consequently, tend to find more recessive-like than dominant-like genes. One way to test for a deviation from random IBD sharing is to carry out a goodness of fit test for observed proportions, $\hat{z}_i$, $i = 0, 1, 2$, in ASPs. The resulting test has 2 df. For example, assumed that parents 1 and 2 have the respective genotypes *1/2* and *3/4,* and two affected offspring have genotypes *1/3* and *1/4.* Thus, the sibs share one allele from parent 1 (the #1 allele) and none from parent 2. The total number of alleles shared by this ASP is 1. If parent 1 has genotype *1/1,* it cannot be decided whether alleles received from this parent by the two offspring are shared or not—this parent is uninformative for linkage. Only the heterozygous parent can be scored (see mean test below).

The three IBD probabilities provide information not only on IBD sharing but also on mode of inheritance. Thus, power of the goodness of fit test must be lower than tests focusing on deviations from IBD sharing. On the other hand, one of the dfs in this test may be used to test for mode of inheritance or for heterogeneity, but the latter test has good power only for tight linkage and numbers of ASPs of at least 100 (Chakravarti, et al., 1987). Other tests involving 2 dfs have been described, for example, by Risch (1990b) and Holmans (1993) ("possible triangle method").

Tests involving only a single df tend to be more powerful than those with 2 dfs. Various tests have been proposed. Schaid and Nick (1990) represent such tests as weighted sums of observed proportions, $\hat{z}_i$, $i = 0$,

1, 2. Feingold and Siegmund (1997) compare properties of different statistics for ASP data and compute sample sizes under different models. Whittemore and Tu (1998) provide lucid overviews of these approaches and propose an optimal weighting scheme resulting in what they call the "minmax test." This test is more powerful than, for example, Holmans' (1993) possible triangle method. The test statistic (Whittemore and Tu, 1998; simplified) is given by

$$X = 1.04476(1.58 - 2.58\hat{z}_0 - 1.87\hat{z}_1)\sqrt{n}, \tag{13.1}$$

where $\hat{z}_0$ and $\hat{z}_1$ are the respective observed proportions of sib pairs with 0 and 1 alleles shared IBD, n is the total number of ASPs, and X follows a standard normal distribution under no linkage, with large values being significant (e.g., $X = 3.719$ has an associated significance level of 0.0001). With $\hat{z}_0 = \frac{1}{4}$ and $\hat{z}_1 = \frac{1}{2}$, equation (13.1) furnishes $X = 0$ as it should. As indicated below, different 1-df tests are optimal for different alternatives (modes of inheritance). A suboptimal test incurs a penalty in terms of loss of power vis-à-vis the optimal test. The minmax test is characterized by a maximum penalty, which is lower than that of any other 1-df test (Whittemore and Tu, 1998).

A 1-df test in common use is the *mean test,* which tests the mean number of shared alleles, $2\hat{z}_2 + \hat{z}_1$, and against the expected null value of 1. This test does best for dominant traits (called additive model in Whittemore and Tu, 1998), in which case it is more powerful than the minmax test. Two-df tests rely on both parents being informative for linkage, that is, the unit of observation is a sib pair. In practice, some parents may be unavailable or uninformative and then, for some sib pairs, only one parent can be scored. In this situation, it is simpler to score parents rather than sib pairs so that more data will be available for the mean test than for the minmax test. That is, each heterozygous parent is scored as to the number of alleles that the two offspring share from this parent—there are only two possibilities, 0 or 1, for each parent. On such a per parent (rather than per sibship) basis, the mean number of alleles shared IBD without linkage is $\frac{1}{2}$. For example, in the assumed nuclear family considered above, parental genotypes are *1/2* and *3/4,* with affected offspring genotypes of *1/3* and *1/4.* For parent 1, the *#1* allele is shared by the two sibs, so this furnishes an entry to the count of alleles shared. Parent 2, on the other hand, transmits two different alleles to the two offspring, so no allele is shared for this parent. Let $\hat{p}_1$ denote the observed proportion of parents for which sib pairs share an allele IBD. To test this against the null expectation of $\frac{1}{2}$, one forms the normal deviate,

$$X = (2\hat{p}_1 - 1)\sqrt{n}, \tag{13.2}$$

where n is the number of parents scored. An example for the minmax and mean test is given in Problem 13.2 and Solution 13.2. The mean test appears to have good power against many alternatives (Blackwelder and Elston, 1985).

Another 1-df test, the *proportion test,* compares the observed proportion $\hat{z}_2$ of ASPs sharing two alleles IBD with the null expected value of ¼. This test does best for recessive traits (Whittemore and Tu, 1998). The test statistic is

$$X = (4\hat{z}_2 - 1)\sqrt{n/3},\tag{13.3}$$

with n = number of sib pairs. Any of the normal deviates, X, mentioned above, may be translated into a lod score, $Z = X^2/4.6$. Even though such a transformation does not add any information to the results, it may be better interpretable by linkage analysts.

Several other nonparametric methods for linkage analysis have been described. For example, Haseman and Elston (1972) based inference on the regression of the squared sib-pair trait difference on the estimated proportion of alleles IBD, where the trait may be quantitative or qualitative. This method is implemented in the S.A.G.E. program package (http://darwin.cwru.edu/pub/sage.html).

Using the mean test, Davies et al. (1994) and Hashimoto et al. (1994) carried out genome-wide linkage analysis (a so-called genome screen) for type 1 diabetes. Based on 282 ASP families and roughly 300 markers, Davies et al. (1994) found strong evidence for a locus (IDDM1) in the HLA region on chromosome 6p, and some evidence for a locus (IDDM2) near the insulin gene on chromosome 11p15. There was nonsignificant evidence for a few other genes.

Single Marker, Multiple Affected Siblings. For sibships comprising more than two affected members, one may form all possible pairs of affected sibs and treat them as if they were independent (Hodge, 1984; Suarez and Van Eerdewegh, 1984). However, although the resulting test statistic asymptotically has the correct properties, these are only realized with several hundred sibships. Therefore, various weighting schemes have been proposed that take into account sibship size. Collins and Morton (1995) provided a lucid description of this problem. They proposed to use all possible pairs and estimate the significance level by computer simulation.

Davis and Weeks (1997) investigated a large number of different nonparametric linkage tests and their implementations in computer programs and evaluated their performance under some two-locus disease models. Their paper is a useful source of information on various approaches for nonparametric linkage analysis. Among the many computer programs implementing tests for multiple affected siblings, the SIBPAIR program in Joseph Terwilliger's ANALYZE package (ftp://linkage.cpmc.columbia.edu/software/) uses an emulation of the lod score method described in Satsangi et al. (1996) and appears to do quite well.

Single Marker, Affected Relatives Not Necessarily Sibs. Pairs of relatives other than siblings are suitable for nonparametric linkage analysis (Risch, 1990b). An extension from ASPs to sets of affected relatives was developed by Weeks and Lange (1988; 1990) in the affected pedigree member (APM) method. It is based on identity by state (IBS, now also called identity in state [IIS]), rather than IBD. That is, it only checks whether alleles look the same rather than that they are copies of an ancestral allele. Figure 13.1 makes the two concepts plausible by examples. For three pairs of parents with two offspring each, with all individuals genotyped at a marker locus, identities for the 5 allele among the two offspring are examined. In the leftmost family, the two 5 alleles in the offspring are clearly copies of the 5 allele in the mother (i.e., they are IBD). In the middle family, the son's 5 allele must come from the mother and the daughter's 5 allele is from the father. Thus, if parents are unrelated, the two 5 alleles in son and daughter are IBS, not IBD. Finally, in the rightmost family, as the mother is homozygous 5/5, identity status cannot be ascertained. In principle, IBS should include the term IBD, that is,

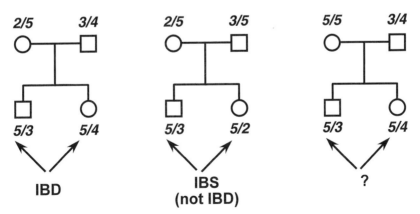

Figure 13.1. Nuclear families demonstrating identity by descent (IBD) and identity by state (IBS) for allele #5.

two alleles that look the same may or may not be IBD. However, IBS and IBD are often used as describing two mutually exclusive situations—two alleles are either IBD or IBS, where IBS specifically means "not IBD."

An improved version of the APM method, *SimIBD*, is based on IBD rather than IBS (Davis et al., 1996) and has dramatically increased power over the APM method. This method has been implemented in computer programs available at http://watson.hgen.pitt.edu/.

Multiple Markers. An early approach to nonparametric gene mapping was developed by Lalouel (1977). It combines pair-wise recombination data using Guttman multidimensional scaling. More recently, Fulker and Cardon (1994) described a multipoint extension to the Haseman–Elston (1972) approach. It estimates the position of a hypothesized gene locus in an interval flanked by two markers.

Procedures have been developed that take information from all markers on a chromosome into account. The MAPMAKER/SIBS program (Kruglyak and Lander, 1995) carries out multipoint affected sib-pair analysis for quantitative and qualitative trait loci. A nice feature of it is "information-content mapping," which measures the fraction of the total inheritance information extracted by the available marker data and points out regions in which typing additional markers is most useful. More than two affected siblings are handled in one of two ways, either by looking at all possible pairs or by forming independent pairs, sib 1 versus each of the remaining sibs in turn. A similar approach, developed by Dr. Neil Risch (Schwab et al., 1995), was implemented in the ASPEX program, which is available at ftp://lahmed.stanford.edu/pub/aspex/.

As mentioned in Section 9.3, the GENEHUNTER program (Kruglyak et al., 1996; Kong and Cox, 1997) carries out parametric and nonparametric linkage analysis. For the nonparametric analysis, IBD sharing information for the set of all affected relatives in a family is captured in a statistic developed by Whittemore and Halpern (1994). A nice example analysis with pictures of families suitable for GENEHUNTER may be found in Gulcher et al. (1997).

One of the most widely applied sampling techniques is the ascertainment of phenotypically extreme individuals. This has paid off, for example, in the search for breast cancer genes, where families with extremely early age at onset show the strongest evidence for linkage (Hall et al., 1990). In sib-pair analysis, it has been recommended that siblings concordant for extreme values, or extremely *dis*cordant pairs, provide substantial power (Risch and Zhang, 1995). However, more detailed analyses have shown that such a blanket statement is not generally correct and that, depending on mode of inheritance of the trait, power to detect linkage or

LD can actually decrease by sampling extreme sib pairs (Allison et al., 1998). In addition, when extremely high values may be characteristic for a certain disease, it does not necessarily follow that extremely low values represent strong evidence for normality. For example, extremely high BMI (body mass index = body weight divided by the square of body height, kg/m^2) values indicate severe obesity, which is thought to have a genetic component. Extremely low values, on the other hand, are also indicative of disease (e.g., bulimia).

13.2. Equivalence between ASP and Lod Score Analysis

Certain forms of ASP analysis show a striking resemblance to parametric linkage analysis and are, in a sense, equivalent to lod score analysis (Hyer et al., 1991). Specifically, Knapp et al. (1994a) considered the following assumed mode of inheritance (unrelated to the real inheritance mode of the trait) and lod score analysis procedure for the trait under study: recessive inheritance, full penetrance, no phenocopies, parental phenotypes disregarded, nuclear families. They proved that the maximum lod score obtained under the assumed mode of inheritance is a monotone transformation of the observed total number of marker alleles shared IBD in the ASPs. That is, the ASP mean test is equivalent to the lod score test in the sense that, for suitable critical values, when one test is significant so is the other.

As mentioned in the previous section ("multiple affected siblings"), this equivalence may be exploited to carry out an ASP analysis with lod score programs. In particular, such an approach lends itself to handle more than two affected siblings in an elegant way. However, it is not easily extended to multiple marker loci.

An elegant approach to nonparametric analysis, emulated by lod score analysis, in large pedigrees is due to Joseph Terwilliger (Trembath et al., 1997). The test statistic consists of 3 components, (a) linkage within sibships, (b) linkage between sibships, and (c) association between pedigrees, which may be interpreted as linkage within a population and between pedigrees. The first component is evaluated by an assumed recessive inheritance model within sibships of a large pedigree as noted above. For the second component, it is noted that more distantly related individuals share at most one allele IBD. With suitable modifications to pedigrees, this component may be emulated by a dominant mode of inheritance.

13.3. Exclusion Analysis

In lod score analysis, as outlined in Sections 4.4 and 12.4, it is straightforward to "exclude" some values of the recombination fraction or portions of the genome as being incompatible with observed data. This works because the known mode of inheritance imposes rigorous constraints on what parameter values are plausible. For example, if two affected siblings have marker genotypes *1/2* and *3/4*, this implies at least one recombination unless phenocopies are present, in which case small values of the recombination fraction are not excluded. On the other hand, in nonparametric linkage analysis all calculations are done on the basis of marker inheritance so that there is no basis for excluding disease genes except when specific assumptions are made regarding mode of inheritance of the trait studied.

For 2-allele mendelian modes of inheritance, associated IBD sharing probabilities may be computed (e.g., appendix D in Feingold and Siegmund, 1997). Hyer et al. (1991) made use of such analogies in an exclusion analysis of diabetes susceptibility genes from a candidate region of chromosome 11. These authors carried out a primary analysis in a nonparametric manner by estimating two identity-by-descent probabilities, p_1 and p_2, that is, the respective probabilities that two siblings share one or two alleles IBD. The likelihood $L(p_1, p_2)$ can then be pictured as the height above the point (p_1, p_2) in a plane with coordinates p_1 and p_2, and a support region for the true IBD probabilities is easily constructed. Next, they considered a large number of parametric models and for each model derived its prediction of the two IBD probabilities. Depending on whether or not the predicted pair of values (p_1, p_2) was inside the support region, the parametric models could be divided into those that were compatible with the observations and those that could be rejected.

What is often assumed about a disease locus at a given genomic position is its "strength," which may be measured by the value of λ_s, that is, the (locus-specific) recurrence risk to a sibling divided by the population prevalence (see Section 15.2). For a given value of λ_s, power to detect or exclude such a locus can be computed (Hauser et al., 1996). This is generally done with Risch's (1990b) lod score statistic, which is made dependent on a given value, say, $\lambda_s = 2.0$, and genomic position. Wherever the lod score is strongly negative, those positions are considered excluded from harboring a locus with given or larger value of λ_s.

13.4. Linkage Disequilibrium

This section discusses a phenomenon called linkage disequilibrium (LD) that has long been recognized but has recently gained importance in human genetics as a potential tool for fine mapping. By way of introduction, association of phenotypes is first briefly discussed.

Association. An *association* is said to exist between two phenotypes when they occur together in the same individual more often than expected by chance. For example, assume that in the population, p_1 is the proportion of individuals with stomach ulcer and p_2 is the proportion of individuals with the A blood type. If these two characteristics occur independently of each other one expects a proportion $p_1 \times p_2$ of individuals to have both stomach ulcer and the A blood type. One finds, however, that the A blood type is clearly associated with cancer of the stomach; that is, it is more frequent among individuals with stomach cancer than in the general population (Vogel and Motulsky, 1986).

To investigate whether phenotypes are associated, one usually collects two groups of individuals, for example, patients (in this case with stomach ulcers) and a control sample. In each group the proportion of interest is then determined (in this case the proportion of individuals with the A blood type). The usual chi-square test for 2×2 tables is then applied to determine significance. The strength of an association is often measured by the relative incidence or *relative risk,*

$$R = \frac{n_1/(n_1 + n_3)}{n_2/(n_2 + n_4)} = \frac{n_1(n_2 + n_4)}{n_2(n_1 + n_3)},$$
(13.4)

where n_1 is the number of patients with the characteristic, n_2 is the number of control individuals with the characteristic, and n_3 and n_4 are the corresponding numbers without the characteristic. If one of the two phenotypes refers to disease with the two levels *affected* and *unaffected,* and the other "phenotype" or factor refers to genotypes that do or do not confer susceptibility to disease, then the relative risk (13.4) is equivalent to the penetrance ratio, which plays an important role in linkage analysis (Ott, 1994). Often, the odds ratio,

$$R_1 = \frac{n_1 n_4}{n_2 n_3}$$
(13.5)

is used as an approximation to the relative risk and is referred to as *approximate relative risk* or simply as relative risk (Armitage and Berry, 1987). For example, the odds ratio for the association between blood type A and stomach ulcer is $R_1 = 1.2$ and is highly significant (Vogel and Motulsky, 1986). Well-known procedures exist for evaluating significance and heterogeneity among a set of 2×2 tables, some of which are implemented in the RelRisk program (one of my Linkage Utility programs).

Another measure for the strength of an association is the correlation coefficient,

$$\rho = \frac{[n \times n_1 - (n_1 + n_2)(n_1 + n_3)]}{\sqrt{[(n_1 + n_2)(n_3 + n_4)(n_1 + n_3)(n_2 + n_4)]}} \tag{13.6}$$

where $n = n_1 + n_2 + n_3 + n_4$. Note that $n\rho^2$ is identical with the usual formula for the chi-square statistic in a 2×2 table with cells containing n_1, n_2, n_3, and n_4 observations.

Definition of Linkage Disequilibrium. Consider a gene on a chromosome and a genetic marker at a short distance from the gene. The marker has two alleles, *1* and *2*, with approximately equal frequencies, while the gene is not polymorphic so that everybody has genotype $+/+$ at the gene locus. At this stage, there are two equally frequent haplotypes in the population, $+1$ and $+2$.

Now, imagine that a mutation occurs, $+ \rightarrow T$, and this happens to take place on a chromosome carrying a *1* marker allele (for any marker with multiple alleles, this is expected to occur in coupling with the allele that has highest population frequency). At this point, the population contains three haplotypes, the two common ones considered above, $+1$ and $+2$, and a new one, *T1*. The population is assumed to grow so that eventually recombinations occur between the two loci and slowly a fourth haplotype, *T2*, emerges. There is then a marked difference between two classes of haplotypes, those carrying a $+$ allele and those carrying a T allele. The former contains marker alleles *1* and *2* in approximately equal frequencies. However, haplotypes carrying a T allele contain far more *1* alleles than *2* alleles (originally only *1* alleles). This situation is referred to as *linkage disequilibrium* (LD). As outlined in more detail below, if T is a mutant allele at a disease locus, there must be a marked difference of marker allele frequencies between affected and unaffected individuals.

More formally, let p_1 be the frequency of the *1* allele so that the *2* allele, or all alleles other than *1*, have combined frequency $1 - p_1$. Also, let p_T denote the frequency of the *T* allele, with $1 - p_T$ being the frequency of the $+$ allele. If alleles at the two loci occur independently of each other in haplotypes, then the frequency of the *T1* haplotype is given by $P_{T1} = p_T p_1$. However, with LD as introduced above, the T and *1* alleles appear positively associated so that the *T1* haplotype has frequency

$$P_{T1} = p_T p_1 + D, \qquad D = P_{T1} - p_T p_1, \tag{13.7}$$

where D is referred to as the disequilibrium parameter. The equilibrium state is characterized by $D = 0$ and is called gametic phase equilibrium or linkage equilibrium, and values $D > 0$ are referred to as positive disequilibrium or association. For simplicity, only one disequilibrium parameter is considered here. With multiple alleles, several disequilibrium parameters must be distinguished (Elandt-Johnson, 1971), and gametic disequilibria at multiple loci require consideration of higher-order disequilibrium parameters (Weir, 1996).

Denote the probabilities of the four possible haplotype classes by P_{T1}, P_{T2}, P_{+1}, and P_{+2}, where T and $+$ refer to the two alleles at the disease locus and *1* and *2* to the two marker alleles. Then the disequilibrium parameter can also be written as

$$D = P_{T1}P_{+2} - P_{T2}P_{+1}. \tag{13.8}$$

Above, LD was introduced as occurring between two loci on the same chromosome. However, the two loci could also have been assumed to reside on different chromosomes (see Section 1.4), which demonstrates that the derivation of LD is independent of the assumption of linkage. It is important to note that the presence of LD does not necessarily imply linkage between the loci considered (see below). Although the term linkage disequilibrium originally just referred to an association of alleles at different loci, it has become customary among human geneticists to take linkage disequilibrium to mean association among alleles due to close linkage. For this reason, Edwards (1980) proposed the neutral term *allelic association* for a deviation from gametic phase equilibrium, without any implication as to the nature of the deviation.

Decay of Linkage Disequilibrium Over Time. As all haplotype and allele frequencies must stay in the range between 0 and 1, D can take only a limited range of values (Hartl, 1988):

$$\left. \begin{array}{l} D_{\min} = \max(-p_T p_1, \ -p_+ p_2) = \min(p_T p_1, p_+ p_2) \\ D_{\max} = \min(p_T p_2, p_+ p_1) \end{array} \right\} \tag{13.9}$$

Because of these bounds, the strength of an allelic association is often indicated as the standardized disequilibrium,

$$D' = D/D_{\max} \text{ or } D' = D/D_{\min}, \tag{13.10}$$

depending on whether D is positive or negative (Lewontin, 1964). The 2BY2 program (one of my Linkage Utility programs) computes all these values and carries out Fisher's exact test for association. Zapata et al. (1997) derived the large sample variance of the estimate of D'.

As recombination occurs between two loci, an existing LD between them gradually breaks down. Specifically, an existing disequilibrium D is reduced by a factor of $1 - r$ in each generation, where r is the recombination fraction between the two loci (Hartl, 1988). Hence, after t generations, the disequilibrium D is changed to a value

$$D_t = (1 - r)^t D. \tag{13.11}$$

The half-life of a disequilibrium value, that is, the number of generations it takes for D to fall to one half of its value, is obtained by setting $D_t/D = \frac{1}{2}$ and solving (13.11) for t, which yields

$$t = \log(\frac{1}{2})/\log(1 - r). \tag{13.12}$$

Decay of D is most rapid when two loci are unlinked ($r = \frac{1}{2}$). Note that HWE at each locus occurs after one generation of random mating but this is not true for the two loci jointly (i.e., D does not vanish after one generation). Figure 13.2 graphically shows the decay of D' with time.

For tightly linked loci, appreciable allelic association may exist for a long time in the population, which is the basis for "disequilibrium mapping" discussed below. Consider a disease for which it is assumed that all disease alleles go back to a single original mutation t generations ago. If one has determined a value of D' between disease and a marker locus and is willing to assume that the marker has not changed in past generations, it is of interest to estimate t from the given value of D'. Solving equation (13.11) yields the desired result as

$$t = \log(D')/\log(1 - r). \tag{13.13}$$

To use this formula, a good estimate of the recombination fraction between the two loci is required. More thorough methods for estimating the age of mutant disease alleles have been developed, for example, by Guo and Xiong (1997) and Slatkin and Rannala (1997).

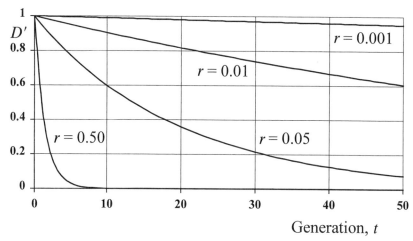

Figure 13.2. Decay of disequilibrium, D', over time for different values of the recombination fraction, r.

Causes of Linkage Disequilibrium. Thus far, LD was depicted as a consequence of tight linkage between two loci. However, as listed below, other factors can also create LD. To verify linkage between loci showing allelic association, the most direct procedure would be to carry out a linkage analysis in which haplotype frequencies instead of allele frequencies are specified (most computer programs can accommodate allelic association). Allelic association, as long as it is not due to an interaction among loci, is relevant only for individuals marrying into a pedigree but not for other family members, whose genotypes are determined by the genotypes of their parents. A well-known example of allelic association due to tight linkage are the MN and Ss blood groups. Each of the two loci is in HWE, but linkage disequilibrium is present and equal to $D = 0.07$, which is one half of its maximum value (Hartl, 1988). Below is a (partial) list of mechanisms that potentially lead to phenotypic associations and, in particular, linkage disequilibrium.

1. *Clustered sampling* can lead to association. For investigations of an association, one usually collects unrelated individuals and carries out a chi-square test. Assume now that in the population no association exists between two phenotypes. In the absence of a sufficient number of unrelated individuals affected with a rare trait, investigators sometimes collect related individuals for the patient group. However, the presence of relatives amounts to a deviation from the null hypothesis of independence of the observations, which the chi-square test may detect. In other words, the lack of independence among individuals tends to inflate chi-square, but the effect is entirely due to clustered sampling. For tests of Hardy–Weinberg equilibrium, Sing and Rothman (1975) showed that the average value of chi-square is inflated by a factor of $1 + \rho(n - 1)$, where ρ is the average correlation between any two of the n individuals sampled. Cohen (1976) obtained a similar result for chi-square tests in contingency tables.

2. *Interaction* between the two loci, either on the phenotypic level or on the allelic level (epistasis), will lead to an association of phenotypes. The association between ABO blood types and stomach ulcer mentioned above is thought to be due to some form of interaction, for example, a protective effect of the O blood type. In linkage analysis, phenotypic interactions are usually assumed to be absent. One way of allowing for phenotypic interactions in linkage analysis is to make the penetrances at one locus depend on the phenotypes at the other locus (Ott and Falk, 1982).

3. *Admixture* is a potentially strong factor leading to spurious allelic association. This generally occurs when individuals from two source populations form a new population, where the source populations have different allele frequencies but each may be in equilibrium. The resulting

mixed populations will then exhibit LD (see Problem 13.6). As an analogy, consider two variables measured on each individual in two groups. In each group, the two variables are uncorrelated. If the variable means are higher in one group than in the other, an analysis carried out on all individuals from the two groups combined will show a strong correlation between the two variables. Of course, analyzing stratified data in an unstratified manner is well known to possibly lead to paradoxical (spurious) results. It can be shown, for example, that the relative risk in each of two portions of a population can be larger than 1 while for the total population it is smaller than 1 (see example 12.5 in Armitage and Berry, 1987). This phenomenon is known as Simpson's paradox (Louis, 1982).

Testing for Linkage Disequilibrium. One of the main differences between LD and genetic linkage is that identity of alleles plays an important role in LD but not in linkage. Thus, alleles must be identified unambiguously for a LD analysis, for example, allele #5 must always be the same allele in all individuals. In linkage analysis, this is only necessary for individuals within a given family unless allele frequencies matter.

For genetic marker loci, haplotype frequencies may be estimated on the basis of a *random sample* of individuals and their genotypes (Hill, 1974). Consider alleles A and a at locus 1 and alleles B and b at locus 2. For many individuals (two-locus genotypes), a direct count of haplotypes will be possible. For example, the genotype *AB/aB* contains the known haplotypes *AB* and *aB*. Which haplotypes are contained in a double heterozygote, however, depends on the gametic phase. Because that is generally unknown, phase must be estimated. An elegant iterative estimation procedure (a form of the EM algorithm; Dempster et al., 1977) is based on the gene counting technique (Ceppellini et al., 1955; Smith, 1957; Ott, 1977b) and works as follows. Assuming preliminary values for the haplotype frequencies, one determines the probabilities of the two phases and uses these as weights in counting haplotypes from each assumed phase. The obtained count yields improved estimates for the haplotype frequencies with which the phase probabilities are again determined, and so on. This procedure furnishes maximum likelihood estimates and has been implemented in computer programs. For example, the ASSOCIATE program, one of the Linkage Utility programs (see Section 9.5), allows estimation of disequilibrium and other interactions between two loci with any number of alleles. Also, the EH program estimates haplotype frequencies for a sample of controls or for a case-control sample (Xie and Ott, 1993). A description of this method may also be found in Slatkin and Excoffier (1996). For data with missing observations or large numbers of alleles, programs such as Haplo (ftp://paella.med.yale.edu/pub/haplo/) or Arlequin (http://acasun1.unige.ch/arlequin/) are appropriate.

Estimates of haplotype frequencies involving disease genes are usually based on a sample of families segregating the disease. Care must be taken to adjust estimated frequencies for ascertainment biases (Chakravarti et al., 1984). As an example, consider the data for cystic fibrosis (CF) reported by Beaudet et al. (1989), which are based on close linkage of the CF locus to two DNA probes, XV-2c and KM-19 (not on direct recognition of the mutant gene). Each marker has two alleles, with the resulting four haplotypes being coded *A* through *D*. Because of tight linkage among these and other markers analyzed, it was possible in most cases to recognize phase in the doubly heterozygous parents of affected offspring. This allowed a count of marker haplotypes in coupling with either a disease allele or a normal allele at the CF locus.

The result of such a count of CF haplotypes is shown in Table 13.1. Preliminary counts are adjusted to proportions reflecting the population frequencies of the *CF* and *NL* (normal) alleles. For example, the population frequency of the *A-CF* haplotype is estimated as $0.02 \times 17/252 = 0.0013$. Also shown in Table 13.1 are the corresponding frequencies expected under the assumption of linkage equilibrium. For example, the haplotype *B-CF* is observed with population frequency of 0.0173 but would be expected with a frequency of only $0.1543 \times 0.02 = 0.0031$.

Testing for LD amounts to showing that haplotypes *A* through *D* occur in significantly different proportions on *CF* and normal chromosomes. Thus, a simple chi-square test of homogeneity may be carried out. For the data in Table 13.1, this leads to $\chi^2 = 269.5$ on 3 df, which is highly significant. Analogously, if samples of affected and unaffected

Table 13.1. Counts of Marker Haplotypes *A* through *D* on *CF* and Normal (*NL*) Chromosomes

Marker Haplotype	Chromosome Count		Estimated Haplotype Frequency			Expected under Equilibrium	
	CF	*NL*	*CF*	*NL*	SUM	*CF*	*NL*
A	17	74	0.00135	0.290	0.29135	0.0058	0.2855
B	218	35	0.01730	0.137	0.15430	0.0031	0.1512
C	7	110	0.00056	0.431	0.43156	0.0086	0.4230
D	10	31	0.00079	0.122	0.12279	0.0025	0.1203
Sum	252	250	0.02	0.98	1	0.02	0.98

Source: Data from Beaudet et al. (1989).

individuals have been collected, a simple test for LD is to compare allele frequencies among affecteds and unaffecteds.

Power to detect disequilibrium depends on various factors. Analytical investigations have shown that negative LD is more difficult to detect than positive LD. Also, for a rare allele at one locus with positive disequilibrium to a rare allele at another locus, power decreases with increasing allele frequency at the other locus (Thompson et al., 1988).

Which markers are more powerful for detecting disequilibrium, those with small or large numbers of alleles? The answer is not immediately obvious. For a small number of alleles, the test has only a small number of df, which is generally a good thing. On the other hand, larger numbers of alleles tend to be associated with lower allele frequencies, which should help detecting LD. For the situation that a single founder in a population is responsible for a mutation at a disease locus, it turns out that power increases with increasing number of alleles at a marker (Ott and Rabinowitz, 1997).

More specialized tests for LD than those considered here are based on small families and are discussed in the next section.

Measures of Linkage Disequilibrium. Although testing for LD is relatively straightforward, it is not very clear how one should measure the strength of LD, which is important for LD mapping discussed below. In addition to D (13.8), D' (13.10), and ρ (13.6) discussed above, various other statistics have been proposed. Under idealized conditions (single initial disease mutation, no recurrent mutations at disease and marker loci), D' has optimal properties because its magnitude, on average, depends only on the genetic distance between the marker and disease loci (Guo, 1997). A very commonly used statistic is

$$\rho^2 = D^2/(p_T \, p_+ \, p_1 \, p_2), \tag{13.14}$$

which is identical to χ^2/n and is often denoted by Δ^2. However, even under idealized conditions, its expectation depends not only on genetic distance but also on marker allele frequencies (Guo, 1997). In more realistic situations (initial incomplete LD, recurrent mutations), all measures for LD perform rather poorly and no measure performs well in all cases (Guo, 1997).

Another quantity often used to express the strength of LD is the empirical significance level (p-value) in the chi-square test for association. However, because this is strictly a monotonic function of ρ^2 (13.14), it can be expected to perform suboptimally as well.

Disequilibrium Mapping. With tight linkage between a disease and marker loci, one rarely finds recombinants, which would allow assigning the disease locus to one of the intervals between markers. In this situation, the presence of allelic association is sometimes used to localize a disease gene more accurately, the idea being that the disease gene is closest to that marker showing the highest degree of allelic association with it (Edwards, 1980). In effect, this approach makes use of the effects of ''historical'' recombination events even though these can no longer be directly observed. It has been applied to homogeneous diseases such as cystic fibrosis and Huntington disease (Sneel et al., 1989), but estimates of map location based on allelic association are generally imprecise and may not really represent an improvement over linkage analysis (Weir, 1989). Furthermore, this method must be unreliable when several disease-causing mutations occurred at different times because the disequilibrium depends on the recombination fraction and on the number of generations passed since a single mutation occurred. Also, selection at the disease locus may influence gene frequencies at nearby markers (Weir, 1989). On the other hand, LD tends to exist only over very short regions so that strong disequilibrium generally indicates very short distance. For populations with histories of striking recent expansions, LD is expected up to ½ cM between any two loci (Thompson and Neel, 1997). In large outbred populations, however, LD should be detectable only for markers within about 0.1 cM $\approx$ 100 kb of DNA (Bodmer, 1986).

With a single original disease mutation, a genomic segment of a certain length around that mutation is expected to be passed unchanged from one generation to the next. Therefore, distant relatives should share such extended haplotypes. Indeed, based on a surprisingly small number of probands, methods for detecting such shared segments can successfully be applied to rare mendelian disorders (Houwen et al., 1994; Durham and Feingold, 1997).

LD mapping appears unsuitable as a general screening tool, at least with today's maps, except to follow up indications of linkage in given genomic regions (Lander and Botstein, 1986b). However, it represents a promising screening technique in special populations. Two such population types are suitable: (1) a population originating from a small number of founder individuals with subsequent rapid expansion (often showing founder effects); and (2) an ancient small population having remained stable over a long time (Terwilliger et al., 1998). In the latter type, genetic drift creates LD over time whereas in the former, an originally strong LD decays over time. Examples for the first population type are the Finns, and of the second type the Saami (Lapland) (see Figure 13.3). Interestingly,

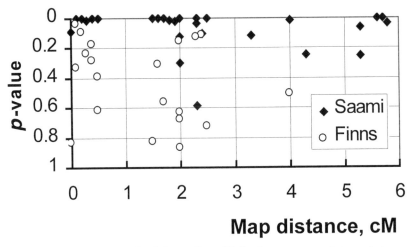

Figure 13.3. *P*-value (test for linkage disequilibrium) versus map distance between pairs of marker loci. (Data from Laan and Pääbo, 1997.)

even though in populations of type 2, LD extends over wider genomic regions, shared segment methods are not expected to work (Terwilliger et al., 1998). Table 13.2 summarizes the relevant population characteristics. Other examples of populations suitable for LD mapping are found in Sardinia, Iceland, and South Africa (Afrikaans-speaking residents). Note, however, that more is not always better. When disequilibrium extends over a wide genomic region, although this is most useful for initially localizing disease genes, it essentially precludes fine mapping.

With specific assumptions, Risch and Merikangas (1996) have argued that LD mapping could be a suitable screening tool in general populations and is more powerful for detecting loci of small effects (see Section 15.2) than ASP analysis. However, these assumptions are quite restrictive. For

Table 13.2. Comparison of Two Types of Special Populations Suitable for Disequilibrium Mapping

Population		Linkage Disequilibrium		
Type	Size	Extent	Pattern	Example
1	Expanding	Few cM	Single haplotype	Finns
2	Constant	Many cM	Random	Saami

Source: Based on Terwilliger et al., 1998.

example, a single disease allele was assumed to be associated with a marker allele. Experience has shown that in a large proportion of diseases multiple disease alleles exist. Although this severely dilutes power for LD analysis, it has no negative effect on ASP (linkage) analysis.

Although plotting an estimated LD parameter for each marker across the genome is a useful approach, some multipoint methods have been developed (e.g., Lazzeroni, 1998) and are expected to be more powerful than single-locus approaches. A somewhat more technical aspect of LD mapping is the use of DNA pools that allows a rapid first pass through large numbers of marker loci (Barcellos et al., 1997).

In genome-wide analysis for many markers, results for contiguous markers are much less correlated in LD analysis than in linkage analysis. With moderately dense maps, results are essentially independent for different markers so that the multiple testing problem is most severe and appropriate corrections are called for (see Section 4.7). If distant relatives are used, theoretical results for appropriate p-values have been obtained (Durham and Feingold, 1997) but in many cases, the safest approach is to approximate the empirical p-value by computer simulation. That is, genome screens are carried out with marker genotypes generated on the computer, perhaps taking into account an approximate suitable ancestry of the probands studied. Then the p-value is approximated by the proportion of replicates in which the test statistic is at least as large as the one observed in the actual data.

It is not completely clear which of the various statistics should be used in a marker-by-marker LD analysis over regions of the genome. Results quoted above suggest that D' should have good properties, but multipoint methods appear preferable over analyses evaluating LD to one marker at a time. Nonetheless, the latter approach has furnished some interesting results. For example, while genome screens for Tourette syndrome (TS) in outbred populations have been largely unsuccessful (Barr and Sandor, 1998), a pilot case-control LD study in a special population has yielded strong evidence for susceptibility genes on chromosomes 11 and 21 (locus-specific $p < 0.00001$ each) (Simonic et al., 1998).

A molecular genetic method, genomic mismatch scanning (GMS), for LD mapping is based on hybridization rather than genotyping. Originally developed for *Escherichia coli*, it has been adapted to detect regions of DNA sharing among distant relatives (Cheung and Nelson, 1998). The feasibility of this approach was demonstrated by the localization of an autosomal recessive disease gene to a 2-MB region on chromosome 11 (Cheung et al., 1998).

13.5. Haplotype Relative Risk and Related Methods

Several multifactorial diseases (see Chapter 15) such as insulin-dependent diabetes and multiple sclerosis are associated with specific HLA alleles or haplotypes (Lechler, 1994). These associations are usually measured as a relative risk on the basis of two samples, a disease and a control sample. One of the problems with case-control studies is that control individuals may not be well matched to cases, particularly for ethnic origin. Differences in allele frequencies between cases and controls will be interpreted as evidence for LD even though they may just be the result of differences in ethnic origin. Family-based cases and "internal" controls are able to overcome this problem.

As a general approach to LD analysis, it has been suggested that family-based controls should replace population-based controls in the following sense (Rubinstein et al., 1981; Falk and Rubinstein, 1987; Thomson et al., 1989). Consider an affected offspring and his or her parents, all being genotyped for a genetic marker. At the marker locus, a specific allele, *H,* is singled out for evaluation of LD with disease, while all other marker alleles are lumped together into *h.* Those alleles transmitted to the offspring are designated as belonging to a contrived "disease sample" and alleles not transmitted belong to a contrived "control sample." In analogy to Woolf's (1955) relative risk method, Falk and Rubinstein (1987) took the two marker alleles (one from each parent) transmitted to an affected offspring to form a "disease genotype" and the nontransmitted alleles a "control genotype." With this, they computed a so-called haplotype relative risk (HRR) statistic, that is, a relative risk with numbers of contrived disease genotypes and control genotypes. The associated significance for a deviation from HRR = 1 was assessed with chi-square in the usual manner.

Statistical properties of this HRR method were rigorously derived from the conditional distribution of parental marker genotypes given ascertainment of one affected offspring, where for analysis purposes a recessive mode of inheritance was assumed (Ott, 1989a). The resulting expressions for the joint distributions of transmitted and nontransmitted marker alleles per parent are shown in Table 13.3. They demonstrate two important properties of the HRR approach:

1. Transmitted and nontransmitted parental marker alleles are statistically independent only when $\theta\delta = 0$, that is, when either $\theta = 0$ or $\delta = 0$, where δ = disequilibrium between the *H* and disease alleles, and θ = recombination fraction between disease and marker loci. Thus, the chi-square test of the null hypothesis, $\delta = 0$, of no LD is valid while estimates of the HRR are not unless $\theta = 0$.

2. This approach is sensitive to $\delta \neq 0$ (i.e., to detecting LD) only when $\theta \neq \frac{1}{2}$, that is, when there is linkage. In other words, only that form of allelic association is detected that is due to linkage. This is quite different in case-control studies in which any type of LD is detected.

Rather than focusing on contrived genotypes, it is more powerful to work directly with alleles (or haplotypes at the HLA locus). Table 13.3 (Ott, 1989a) formed the basis for several important statistical tests, including the TDT (see next paragraph). Probably the most important of these tests is the haplotype-based haplotype relative risk (HHRR) test (Terwilliger and Ott, 1992b). This is a test of the hypothesis, $(A + B) = (A + C)$ (i.e., of homogeneity in the marker allele distributions between transmitted and nontransmitted alleles). Figure 2 in Terwilliger and Ott (1992b) shows power curves for different values of the recombination fraction, θ, between disease and marker locus. Not unexpectedly, the test is most powerful for $\theta = 0$. For $\theta = \frac{1}{2}$ (Figure 2 in Terwilliger and Ott, 1992b), the test has some minimal power because the test statistic implicitly depends on the assumption of Hardy–Weinberg equilibrium, and LD represents a deviation from HWE, which the test detects although with very low power.

This HHRR test may easily be applied to any number of marker alleles. All one needs to do is compile histograms of transmitted and nontransmitted alleles, which leads to a $2 \times m$ contingency table with m columns corresponding to the total number m of alleles and two rows corresponding to transmitted and nontransmitted alleles. Homogeneity of this table is then tested in a chi-square test, for example, with the CONTING program. An alternative procedure is to test one allele at a time, allele i versus all other alleles "not i." Because of multiple testing

Table 13.3. Probabilities of Transmitted and Nontransmitted Marker Alleles for One Parent and an Offspring Affected with a Recessive Trait

	Not Transmitted		
Transmitted	H	h	Sum
H	$A = (q + \delta/p)q$	$B = (q + \delta/p)(1 - q)$ $- \theta\delta/p$	$q + (1 - \theta)\delta/p$
h	$C = (1 - q - \delta/p)$ $+ \theta\delta/p$	$D = (1 - q - \delta/p)$ $(1 - q)$	$1 - q - (1 - \theta)\delta/p$
Sum	$q + \theta\delta/p$	$1 - q - \theta\delta/p$	1

Note: q = frequency of H allele, p = frequency of recessive disease allele, δ = disequilibrium between disease allele and H allele.

Source: Based on Ott, 1989a.

($m - 1$ tests), the smallest p-value obtained must then be adjusted by application of formula (4.13) with $g = m - 1$, which is approximately equivalent to multiplication with $m - 1$. It is not obvious which of the two procedures is more powerful. This presumably depends on the mode of inheritance of the trait but there may not be much of a difference in performance between the two approaches.

Terwilliger and Ott (1992b) also investigated the McNemar test as applied to Table 13.3; that is, the test of $B = C$ or of $B - C = (1 - 2\theta)\delta/p = 0$, which focuses on heterozygous parents and does not depend on HWE. Spielman et al. (1993) developed this test into a test for linkage, called transmission/disequilibrium test (TDT), which is powerful only in the presence of LD. This allowed the use of multiple affected siblings, which was a major step forward for sampling designs with family-based controls. The genotype of each (heterozygous) parent may be viewed as a matched pair of alleles, one transmitted and the other not. The McNemar statistic for matched pairs does not require independence of parental alleles and is insensitive to population stratification. However, as Bickeböller and Clerget-Darpoux (1995) have argued, such stratification can lead to dependencies between parental genotypes, which violate assumptions underlying the TDT. Examples of extreme population stratification can be shown to lead to high frequencies of false-positive results of the T_{mhet} statistic (Lazzeroni and Lange, 1998), although in reality less extreme patterns of ethnic stratification may not be a matter of concern. Many authors have contributed to further developments in this area. Here, only a few highlights can be given. Overviews may be found in Spielman and Ewens (1996) and Kaplan et al. (1997). In terms of *efficiency,* family-based association tests (one offspring and two parents) are inferior to case-control designs. Each trio is scored for two transmissions and two nontransmissions while three individuals in a case-control design give six informative alleles so that the latter provides 3/2 as much information as the former (Morton and Collins, 1998).

Curtis and Sham (1995b) made the interesting observation that the TDT tends to furnish an excess of false-positive results when one of the parents is missing. They recommended that in those cases the whole family trio be discarded when a marker has only two alleles. For markers with more than two alleles, single parent–child pairs may be included when the child is heterozygous and has a genotype different from that of the parent. As shown by Génin and Clerget-Darpoux (1996), power to detect LD is increased when parents are related, which may be an important consideration in the planning of association studies. Although the TDT was developed for a qualitative trait (affected–unaffected phenotype), analogous tests have been developed for quantitative traits (Allison, 1997), also for multiple alleles and multiple sibs in a family (Rabinowitz, 1997).

Several authors have extended the original TDT to multiple alleles. Simulation analyses show (Kaplan et al., 1997) that one of the most powerful extensions is that due to Spielman and Ewens (1996). The associated test statistic focuses on heterozygous parents with possibly multiple affected offspring and reads

$$T_{mhet} = \frac{m-1}{m} \sum_{i=1}^{m} \frac{(b_i - c_i)^2}{b_i + c_i}, \tag{13.15}$$

where b_i = total number of times that the ith allele is transmitted to affected offspring, c_i = total number of times that it is not, and m = total number of alleles. Note that $n_{ii} = 0$ in Spielman and Ewens (1996) is zero when attention is restricted to heterozygous parents. Under no linkage, T_{mhet} has a limiting chi-square distribution with m df and defaults to the usual formula for the TDT (not shown here) in the case of two alleles.

A major problem with disease of late onset is that parents may no longer be available for genotyping. In ASP analysis, one often resorts to weighted averages of test statistics, weighted by expected parental genotype probabilities as computed from population allele frequencies. For the TDT, Spielman and Ewens (1998) developed a statistic, S-TDT, that compares affected with unaffected siblings and does not reconstruct parental genotypes through estimates of allele frequencies.

Researchers are naturally wondering what is more appropriate to use, the case-control or HHRR/TDT design? Statistically, a family-based design is preferable over case-control sampling because it largely eliminates potential problems with population stratification. However, there is also a cost question: Case-control sampling requires two individuals to be genotyped per sampling unit (one case and one control), while the HRR design requires three individuals (a trio). On the other hand, for many traits, phenotyping is as expensive as genotyping—a psychiatric interview may take two or more hours per proband. Case-control sampling then requires phenotyping two individuals whereas the HRR requires only one because parental phenotypes are ignored.

13.6. Problems

Problem 13.1. Show formally that the IBD sharing probabilities are $z_0 = 0$ and $z_1 = z_2 = \frac{1}{2}$ for a fully informative marker tightly linked with a dominant trait (Section 13.1).

Problem 13.2. In an ASP study on IDDM (type 1 diabetes) versus the FGF3 locus on chromosome $11q13$, observed proportions of ASPs sharing 0, 1, and 2 alleles were $20/119 = 0.168$, $59/119 = 0.496$, and $40/119 = 0.336$, respectively (Hashimoto et al., 1994). The total number of ASPs scored was $n = 119$. What is the empirical significance level (*p*-value) in a test for increased IBD sharing? *Hint*: Use equation (13.1) to obtain a normal deviate, then use a table or the NORPROB utility program to calculate the *p*-value. Compare this result with the one obtained for all parents scored, where the proportion of parents for which sib pairs shared an allele was $173/301 = 0.575$, and evaluate this number with equation (13.2).

Problem 13.3. Consider two (unaffected) parents who had a child affected with cystic fibrosis, who has passed away. The wife is pregnant again, and marker typing with haplotypes *A* through *D* (Table 12.2) has been carried out. The father is *BC,* the mother *AB,* and the fetus is *BB.* What is the risk to the fetus of being affected with cystic fibrosis (1) without knowledge of marker types and (2) with the given marker types? For simplicity, assume zero recombination among the loci.

Problem 13.4. Consider a healthy male, who had a sister with cystic fibrosis. Sister and parents are no longer alive. (1) What is his risk of being a carrier for the disease allele? (2) He was tested for the most common disease-causing mutation (ΔF_{508}) and turned out to be negative. That mutation is known to occur on 75% of the CF chromosomes, and 25% of chromosomes carrying a CF gene do not show the mutation. What is now his risk of carrying a cystic fibrosis gene?

Problem 13.5. Assume two loci with two alleles each. For what allele frequencies is the linkage disequilibrium parameter *D* highest and what is this maximum value?

Problem 13.6. Consider to loci with alleles *A* and *a* at locus 1 and alleles *B* and *b* at locus 2, with allele frequencies being different in two different populations. Allele frequencies are as follows. *Population 1*: $p_A = 0.6$, $p_a = 0.4$, $p_B = 0.3$, $p_b = 0.7$. *Population 2*: $q_A = 0.2$, $q_a = 0.8$, $q_B = 0.9$, $q_b = 0.1$. In each population, there is linkage equilibrium at each locus. Assume that the two populations mix in equal proportions. What is the resulting linkage disequilibrium, *D* and *D'*? Notice that what is being mixed are haplotypes (gametes), not alleles.

14.

Two-Locus Inheritance

Parametric linkage analysis requires specification of an inheritance model but for some conditions, called complex traits (covered in Chapter 15), an appropriate mode of inheritance is unknown. For this reason, nonparametric analysis methods have been introduced as they do not require specification of an inheritance model. Their performance does, however, depend on the true state of nature. For example, as mentioned in Chapter 13, affected sib-pair (ASP) and linkage disequilibrium (LD) analysis are more powerful for recessive than dominant traits because they treat both parents as being equally informative.

Even when a trait is governed by multiple disease genes, for practical reasons analysis is generally carried out under the implicit assumption of a single disease gene. As an introduction to Chapter 15 on complex traits, it is of interest to study properties of inheritance models that postulate two genes underlying a disease.

Two-locus inheritance appears to be quite frequent in nature. Strickberger (1985) provides 12 examples in animals and plants, where two gene loci are jointly responsible for a phenotype. Figure 14.1 lists three of these. Each locus has two alleles, A and a for locus 1, B and b for locus 2. A few examples of two-locus inheritance in humans are as follows: Two structural genes on different chromosomes are required for encoding the major subunit of human red cell glucose-6-phosphate dehydrogenase (Kanno et al., 1989). Risk to thrombosis is conferred by protein C deficiency and modified by APC resistance due to a mutation in the FV gene (Koeleman et al., 1994). Thus, interaction of two loci in the same pathway causes risk to thrombosis. For the dominantly inherited disease, familial adenomatous polyposis, Dobbie et al. (1997) demonstrated the existence of a strong modifier gene in the mouse and showed evidence for a homologous gene location in humans.

	BB	Bb	bb
Flower color in the sweet pea			
A>a purple dominant over white			
B>b color dominant over colorless			
1 = purple, 0 = white			

Flower color in the sweet pea
A>a purple dominant over white
B>b color dominant over colorless
  1 = purple, 0 = white

	BB	Bb	bb
AA	1	1	0
Aa	1	1	0
aa	0	0	0

Shape of seed capsules of
shepherd's purse (Bursa)
  1 = ovoid, 0 = triangular

	BB	Bb	bb
AA	0	0	0
Aa	0	0	0
aa	0	0	1

Feather color in fowl
  1 = color, 0 = white

	BB	Bb	bb
AA	0	0	0
Aa	0	0	0
aa	1	1	0

Figure 14.1. Examples of two-locus inheritance in nature. (Based on Table 11–1 in Strickberger, 1985.)

14.1. Two-Locus Models

Early on, authors investigated two-locus inheritance models. For published pedigrees segregating various diseases, Hogben (1932) contemplated different modes of transmission, for example, two recessive genes or two dominant genes, and analytically derived various properties of two-locus models. Mittmann (1938) emulated the effects of multiple genes as a second locus in a two-locus disease model. Defrise-Gussenhoven (1962) carried out an analytical study of five types of two-locus models and computed various statistics characterizing these models. Newer references will be mentioned below.

In two-locus and multilocus disease models, each locus can in principle have multiple alleles. For simplicity, however, most authors restrict the number of alleles to two per locus. Here, the two alleles at each disease locus are labeled *n* and *d,* where *d* is the susceptibility allele with population frequency generally smaller than 0.50. Also, unless noted otherwise, the two disease loci are assumed unlinked.

Table 14.1 shows three broad classes of two-locus models. The model labeled ''epistasis'' shows two dominant (''dom'') loci interacting epistatically. Because penetrances may be represented as products of marginal

Table 14.1. Examples of Two-Locus Disease Models: Penetrances for Given Genotypes

| | Genotype at Locus 2 | | | | | | | | |
| | Epistasis | | | Heterogeneity | | | Threshold | | |
Locus 2	*nn*	*nd*	*dd*	*nn*	*nd*	*dd*	*nn*	*nd*	*dd*
nn	0	0	0	0	0	f	0	0	0
nd	0	f	f	0	0	f	0	0	f
dd	0	f	f	f	f	f	0	f	f

"penetrance factors" (Risch, 1990a), such a model is also called multiplicative. The particular one shown on the left side in Table 14.1 is a "dom *and* dom" model—it is not sufficient to have a particular genotype at one locus to be susceptible, this depends on both, genotypes at locus 1 *and* 2. In contrast, in a heterogeneity type model, susceptibility is conferred by a genotype at locus 1 *or* 2. The particular model shown in Table 14.1 is a "rec *or* rec" model (an approximately additive model). Finally, in a threshold model it is the number of *d* alleles that is critical irrespective of which locus they come from. In this case, an individual is susceptible whenever the number of *d* alleles is 3 or higher. This model is analogous to the polygenic threshold model.

As an example, Neuman and Rice (1992) determined two-locus models for schizophrenia and bipolar disease that are compatible with trait prevalence and recurrence risks in relatives of probands (see Section 15.2). Their best-fitting model for schizophrenia is the threshold model in Table 14.1 with $f = 0.35$ and allele frequencies of $p_1 = 0.354$ and $p_2 = 0.101$ for loci 1 and 2, respectively. These parameters predict a trait prevalence of 0.01. As these authors noted, two-locus models exhibit unusual properties that deviate from those of mendelian models. Consider, for example, the threshold model in Table 14.1 with $f = 1$ (full penetrance) and the mating shown in Figure 14.2. One parent is unaffected (he has only one *d* allele) and one is affected (she has three *d* alleles). Each of the parents potentially passes one of two haplotypes to the four children, who represent the four possible offspring genotypes (given this mating) occurring with probabilities of ¼ each. Now consider each locus separately. Among all offspring of such a mating, heterozygotes *nd* are affected with probability 0.50; that is, locus 1 appears dominant with incomplete penetrance (homozygotes *dd* do not occur). The informative parent is the one who is affected. For locus 2, only homozygous offspring are affected and that with probability 0.50. Thus, locus 2 appears recessive with incomplete penetrance.

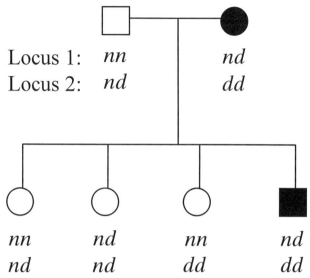

Figure 14.2. Mating with assumed genotypes at loci jointly underlying a two-locus threshold trait and all possible offspring genotypes.

The informative parent is the one who is unaffected. Thus, the two loci exhibit different mendelian modes of inheritance even though the two-locus inheritance is symmetric with respect to the penetrance pattern.

With multiple disease loci, in analogy to analysis of variance, one can distinguish between main and interaction effects. For example, Frankel and Schork (1996) considered a two-locus model with $p(n) = p(d) = 0.5$ at each locus. Among the nine joint genotypes, only those three in the main diagonal have positive penetrances. Let genotypes be written as an ordered pair with the locus 1 genotype preceding the locus 2 genotype. Then, genotypes (*nn, dd*) and (*dd, nn*) have penetrance of 0.5 each, and genotype (*nd, nd*) has a penetrance of 1. For this model, the marginal penetrances are all equal to 0.25, which Frankel and Schork (1996) interpret as absence of main effects. In the following paragraph, main and interaction effects at the level of allele sharing are considered. Note, that for Frankel and Schork's (1996) model, both main and interaction effects for allele sharing exist so that such loci should be detectable by linkage analysis.

A theoretically interesting two-locus model is shown in Table 14.2. Locus 1 has a mode of inheritance that depends on the genotype at locus 2: It is dominant (given *dd* at locus 2) or recessive (*nn* or *nd* at locus 2). Thus, locus 2 may be viewed as a modifier locus. With assumed allele

Table 14.2. A Two-Locus Model Predicting Average Numbers of 1.89 and 1.05 of Alleles Shared at Loci 1 and 2, Respectively

		Locus 2		
Locus 1		*nn*	*nd*	*dd*
nn		0	0	0
nd		0	0	1
dd		1	1	1

frequencies, $p(d) = 0.04$ at locus 1 and $p(d) = 0.05$ at locus 2, this model predicts a population prevalence of 0.002. What makes this model particularly interesting are the predicted IBD sharing probabilities for an ASP (these probabilities were obtained numerically by a computer program, IBD, written for this purpose by my student Harald Göring). For locus 1, as Table 14.3 shows, the marginal sharing probabilities deviate strongly from the random values of 0.25, 0.50, and 0.25 expected for an unselected pair of siblings (irrespective of their phenotypes). The average number of alleles shared by an ASP is 1.89, which is much higher than the value of 1 expected at random. Thus, this locus should be easy to detect in a linkage analysis. On the other hand, the marginal allele sharing probabilities of 0.24, 0.47, and 0.29 for locus 2 deviate little from their random values, and the average number of alleles shared is 1.05, only slightly in excess of 1. Obviously, this locus is hard to detect by standard ASP methods. However, for a subset of data, namely those with IBD = 0 at locus 1, the sharing probabilities at locus 2 are 0.103, 0.282, and 0.615, with an average of 1.51 alleles shared per sibship (right side of Table 14.3). Thus, conditioning on locus 1 helps find locus 2, but note that ASPs with IBD = 0 have a probability of occurrence of only 0.4% among all sib pairs affected with the trait. Also, conditioning on ASPs

Table 14.3. IBD Sharing Probabilities for Two-Locus Model in Table 14.2

	Joint Probabilities				Probability Given Sharing at Locus 1				
	IBD Sharing at Locus 2				IBD Sharing at Locus 2				
Locus 1	0	1	2	Sum	0	1	2	Sum	Average IBD
0	.0004	.0011	.0024	.0039	.103	.282	.615	1	1.51
1	.0194	.0412	.0452	.1058	.183	.390	.427	1	1.24
2	.2155	.4335	.2413	.8903	.242	.487	.271	1	1.05
Sum	.2353	.4758	.2889	1					

with IBD = 2 at locus 1 decreases informativeness—average number of alleles shared is 1.03, which is less than the value of 1.05 for unselected ASPs at locus 1.

I have looked at various two-locus models and their associated IBD sharing probabilities. It appears doubtful that a two-locus model exists that predicts, at the IBD sharing level, no main effects and only interaction effects, but this has not been investigated in depth.

14.2. Parametric Analysis under Mendelian Inheritance

Many authors have investigated this question: If a trait is under the control of two disease loci, what are the properties of linkage analysis carried out under single-locus (mendelian) disease models? This question will be covered more generally in Chapter 15 for complex traits.

In many papers addressing this question, computer simulation was carried out under two-locus models followed by analysis under single-locus models. After computer programs became available for analysis under two-locus models (TLINKAGE and MENDEL; Spence et al., 1993), investigators were able to properly compare analysis under ''correct'' (two-locus) and ''incorrect'' (single-locus) model assumptions. For example, Schork et al. (1993) generated two-locus family data in a computer simulation, where each of the two unlinked disease loci was within 5 cM of a marker locus. Analysis was carried out under the generating two-locus model with estimation of parameters such as penetrances, and under different single-locus models. The best single-locus model in terms of maximum expected lod score achieved was a heterogeneity model in which three proportions of families were estimated, one with linkage to marker 1, one with linkage to marker 2, and one without linkage to either locus (analysis with HOMOG3R program). That is, analysis was carried out with the *hlod* (see Section 10.4). Performance depended much on the particular two-locus model studied. In one case, the expected lod score under the best single-locus model was almost as high as under the two-locus model but in the other two cases, there was a loss of expected lod score of over 30%. Thus, it depends on the nature of the trait whether single-locus analysis captures much of the linkage information or not. Generally, if a trait is governed by two underlying disease loci, it appears preferable to work with two-locus analysis models.

One of the consequences of working under a wrong analysis model was that in most analyses, recombination fractions were overestimated. This observation, made previously by different authors, is in line with a general trend; that is, errors in the analysis tend to lead to an upward bias in the recombination fraction estimate. As a consequence of this, a disease locus somewhere within a map of markers tends to have its map position estimated outside the marker map (Risch and Giuffra, 1992); it is ''driven out'' of the map because its estimated position tends to be away from any marker. Indeed, this is a picture often seen: A lod score curve with its maximum attained beyond the last marker in a map. Thus, multipoint analysis should be delayed as long as possible for a trait presumed to be due to multiple disease loci.

For diseases under the control of two genes, Dizier et al. (1996) investigated power to detect linkage by the lod score method. They showed that an initial segregation analysis with strong evidence for a major gene does not guarantee that such a gene will be found. Thus, segregation analysis does not appear to be useful. Furthermore, in many cases they found an increase in power with the ASP method when compared with lod score analysis in which true or estimated parameter values were used. Because ASP analysis is equivalent to lod score analysis with full penetrance and no phenocopies, the conclusion from this observation is that the use of estimated parameters in lod score analysis may not be useful for two-locus traits. This appears plausible because lod score analysis works under wrong assumptions anyway; it may not make sense to stick to quasi-realistic assumptions by estimating model parameters under single-gene models. Thus, what is needed are *robust* rather than ''realistic'' analysis models. That ASP analysis does well seems to suggest that strong analysis models (i.e., those with large penetrance ratios between genetic and nongenetic cases) should be the universal models of choice in lod score analysis. For example, penetrances of 0.008, 0.80, and 0.80 for genotypes *nn, nd,* and *dd* at a dominant locus correspond to a penetrance ratio of 100. Unfortunately, there are two-locus models (not shown here) for which weak single-locus models do better than strong models. But if in doubt, because of the analogy between ASP and lod score analysis, a strong single-locus analysis model appears reasonable for the analysis of two-locus (or multilocus) traits. Durner et al. (1996) discussed such questions and provided practical guidelines.

For a specific pair of unlinked loci (or chromosomal regions), Mac-Lean et al. (1993) proposed to investigate the correlation of lod scores at two given loci. Although this is an interesting idea and results are expected to demonstrate interaction or heterogeneity among loci, the method does not seem to have furnished practically useful results.

One might consider genome screens under two-locus models. In principle, with m markers, $m(m - 1)/2$ two-locus analyses could be carried out, one for each pair of markers. A more economical way to proceed would be to focus on markers that have provided positive lod scores under single-locus analysis. For each such marker at a time, a two-locus analysis (e.g., with the TLINKAGE programs) would be carried out by fixing one disease locus at that marker and letting the other disease locus move across the genome. Determining what two-locus analysis model to use may not be immediately clear. One possibility would be to use a threshold model such as the one shown on the right side of Table 14.1. Thus far, very few, if any, two-locus genome screens seem to have been carried out. There is also a question of the appropriate lod score threshold for significance. One might be tempted to think that the critical lod score has been established by Lander and Kruglyak (1995) to be somewhere between 3 and 4 for as many loci considered. However, these authors considered a "unilineal" genomic search, and looking at all possible pairs of markers involves many more tests than a simple genome screen. This is discussed further in the next section.

14.3. Two-Locus Affected Sib-Pair Analysis

In recent years, much work has been done on nonparametric two-locus analysis, mostly in the form of some type of ASP analysis for two markers jointly. For example, for two disease loci, each tightly linked with a marker locus, Knapp et al. (1994b) introduced an extension of the mean test for two marker loci and demonstrated its superiority over single-locus analysis under various two-locus modes of inheritance. Dupuis et al. (1995) compared three methods for genome-wide searching for disease loci: (1) single-locus search, (2) simultaneous search (searching for linkage at all pairs of markers), and (3) conditional search (detecting multiple loci sequentially by conditioning appropriately on already detected loci). To detect at least one of the two disease loci, these authors found that single-locus search and simultaneous search perform approximately the same. The simultaneous search technique suffers from the large number of tests done and the corresponding penalty imposed by correction for multiple testing: For m markers in the genome, single-locus search requires m tests while simultaneous search requires $m(m - 1)/2$ tests. These observations explain the apparent discrepancy to the findings of Knapp et al. (1994b). Finally, conditional search is most useful in connection with loci that have already been found (see discussion of Table 14.3). But performance of this method critically depends on the type of interaction between the two disease loci.

Tiwari and Elston (1997) extended the Haseman-Elston (1972) sib-pair method to joint analysis at two loci. Presumably, properties in genome-wide application to many (pairs of) markers would be similar to those of single-locus search and simultaneous search described in the previous paragraph.

14.4. Problems

Problem 14.1. For each of the three models in Table 14.1, compute the population prevalence, K, as an expression in f and p, where f = probability of being affected for given genotypes. Assume that the susceptibility allele has the same frequency, $p = p(d)$, at each locus.

Problem 14.2. For Neuman and Rice's (1992) two-locus model of schizophrenia (threshold model as in Table 14.1 with $f = 0.35$, $p_1 = 0.354$, $p_2 = 0.101$), compute appropriate single-locus modes of inheritance for each locus. *Hint:* compute marginal penetrances as follows. For each genotype at locus 1, compute the probability of being affected as a weighted sum of penetrances over the genotypes at locus 2, weighted by the locus 2 genotype probabilities. Proceed analogously for locus 2.

15.

Complex Traits

A *complex system* is characterized by one's inability to predict the properties of the whole from the properties of its parts. Such systems are said to have "emergent properties"—living organisms are prime examples of complex systems (Root-Bernstein and Dillon, 1997). In neural networks (see Section 15.4), even though the actions of each element are easily understood, the complexity of interactions among nodes in the whole network can attain emergent properties (Hopfield, 1982). Many phenotypes (e.g., of lipid metabolism) are evidently regulated by an extremely complicated mesh of genetic and environmental influences (Sing et al., 1996). Last but not least, the DNA sequence has been shown to exhibit complexity (Li, 1997). The scientific approach, of course, has been reductionist in which one tries to understand component elements of these systems, resulting in a concentration on molecular genetics as the central object of biological science (Stewart, 1992).

In human genetics, a *complex trait* is a genetic condition whose *mode of inheritance* does not follow any of the known mendelian laws. Also, the phenotype definition is often somewhat ambiguous in the following way. For mendelian traits such as cystic fibrosis or Huntington disease, based on the known mode of inheritance or detection of a susceptibility locus, it is relatively straightforward to remedy any uncertainties about which aspects of the phenotype are genetically controlled and which are not. For complex traits, this avenue is unavailable so that phenotype definition is quite arbitrary. Of course, for example, psychiatrists know very well how they define schizophrenia and there is high inter-rater reliability, but the question is whether this diagnosis is genetically relevant or whether the hypothesized underlying genes act on a wider or more narrowly defined phenotype. This problem will be discussed further in Section 15.3.

What is considered a complex trait now may no longer be a complex trait 5 years from now. A case in point is breast cancer. Before the discovery of the BRCA1 gene (Hall et al., 1990), the mode of inheritance of breast cancer was quite unclear and I doubt that many people considered single genes to play a clear-cut role in this common disease. Another telling example is Hirschsprung disease. At one time considered a typical polygenic threshold trait, it is now known to be due to multiple genes with complicated interactions (Angrist et al., 1998). In experimental animals, many complex gene interactions have been disentangled, for example, QTLs in the mouse that influence susceptibility to lung cancer (Fijneman et al., 1996).

This chapter is intended to outline a number of current statistical approaches for the localization of complex trait genes on the human gene map. Weeks and Lathrop (1995) provided a lucid overview of the statistical aspects of this field. Moldin (1997b) described the status and difficulties in the search for schizophrenia genes. Various approaches are also outlined in a book edited by Haines and Pericak-Vance (1998).

15.1. Genetic Basis and Heritability

Genes and Environment. Regarding the transmission of a disease, one of the first questions to be asked is: "Is it genetic?" The main clue for an etiologic involvement of genes stems from the observation that the disease "runs in families." However, one must be aware that a concentration of disease cases among family members is not specific for genetic factors—infection is another possible cause for familiality of disease (for an overview, see Ott, 1990a). A case in point is *kuru,* the first human degenerative neurologic disease shown to be caused by a virus. The account given here is based on the booklet by Lindenbaum (1979). A newer reference is Zigas (1990).

Kuru occurs only among some native tribes in Papua New Guinea. It is characterized by loss of balance, incoordination of movements, and tremor, and usually progresses to complete motor incapacity and death in about a year. Because it seemed to run in families, it was thought to be determined by a single autosomal gene that was dominant in females but recessive in males (Bennett et al., 1959). The estimated risk of kuru in female relatives of kuru victims was 51%, compared with a population prevalence of close to 1%. Hadlow (1959) pointed out the similarities between kuru and scrapie, a degenerative disease of the central nervous system in sheep, which was transmissible by inoculation. Gajdusek et al. (1966) then injected the brains of chimpanzees with brain material from individuals who had died of kuru. They reported that, after incubation periods of up to 4 years, the chimpanzees developed a clinical syndrome very similar to human kuru (Carleton Gajdusek received the Nobel prize in medicine in 1976 for his pioneering work on kuru). Hence, kuru appeared to be a disease like scrapie, caused by a slow-acting infectious agent. The disease evidently had reached epidemic proportions as a result of cannibalism; women and children particularly used to eat the corpses of relatives. Indeed, after government and missionary intervention led to the abandonment of cannibalism, the incidence of kuru dramatically declined. It is interesting to note an analogy to Gerstmann–Sträussler syndrome and Creutzfeld–Jacob syndrome in humans and scrapie and mad cow disease in animals, all of which belong to a class of slow, transmissible, lethal brain diseases caused by an unusual pathogen called a prion (Prusiner, 1997). In 1997, Stanley Prusiner received the Nobel prize for Medicine for his pioneering work on prions.

It is often difficult to distinguish between genetic and cultural inheritance. For example, it is hard to determine whether food preferences are transmitted genetically or culturally (Cavalli-Sforza, 1990). For other cases such as myopia, causation by a single autosomal dominant gene (MIM no. 16070) is generally accepted. However, the visual image received by the eye plays an important part in regulating the eye's growth: if in early development the retina does not receive a visual image, the eye overgrows and becomes myopic (Judge, 1990).

The relative influences of inheritance and environment are often not easy to tease apart. Transmission of an infectious disease is usually thought of as being due to environmental factors, but different individuals may react to infection differently depending on their genotypes. An interesting finding in this regard is the existence of a dominant gene for poliovirus sensitivity on chromosome 19 (Miller et al., 1974; Siddique et al., 1988). Another example are the AIDS-resistance genes (Moore, 1997; Winkler et al., 1998) mentioned in Section 12.1.

A well-known method for establishing genetic involvement in disease etiology is to compare the phenotypic concordance rate for a disease among monozygotic (MZ) twins with that among dizygotic (DZ) or fraternal twins (Vogel and Motulsky, 1986; Plomin et al., 1994), where concordance of a trait is the proportion of affected twins that have affected co-twins (Hartl and Clark, 1989). Whereas MZ twins are genetically identical, DZ twins on average share 50% of their genes. Hence, a disease, which is at least partially determined by genes, is expected to show a higher frequency (recurrence rate) in an MZ co-twin than in a DZ co-twin of an affected individual. However, for behavioral and psychiatric traits, comparisons of concordance rates between MZ and DZ twins must be interpreted with caution (Kendler, 1983). As long as twins share the same family environment, effects of this environment contribute to the similarity of both MZ and DZ twins so that environmental and genetic influences are confounded. Investigating twins reared apart is thus important for separating genetic effects from those due to common family environment.

Heritability. Genetic involvement in disease causation does not mean that a single gene is predisposing individuals to become affected. Various other genetic mechanisms could be acting. Depending on the number of genes involved, one distinguishes mendelian (one gene), two-locus, oligogenic (few genes), and polygenic (large number) inheritance. Under each of these, the resulting phenotype could be quantitative or qualitative. In the latter case, one generally assumes there is an underlying quantity called *liability*. If it exceeds a certain threshold then an individual is affected (polygenic threshold trait). It is useful to have a measure of the extent to which genetic factors play a role. One such measure is the heritability, another is the lambda-ratio discussed in Section 15.2.

For an analytical method of determining the relative "influence" of genes, one must work with a mathematical model (Hartl and Clark, 1989). Usually, various effects of genes and environment are taken to be additive and mutually independent so that the (quantitative) phenotype is just the sum of these factors. The variance of the phenotype is then simply the sum of the variances of the postulated components. For a qualitative phenotype, an unobservable underlying quantitative trait (liability) is assumed that leads to disease when it exceeds some threshold. Among genetic factors, one distinguishes additive effects (due to alleles) and dominance effects (due to interaction among alleles in a genotype). Heritability in the narrow sense is the proportion of the additive genetic variance, and heritability in the wide sense is the proportion of the variance due to all genetic factors. The next two paragraphs outline a few methods for calculating heritability. The reader interested in more detail than is given here should consult one of the textbooks covering this topic (e.g., Hartl and Clark, 1989).

For *twin data,* an estimate of the broad-sense heritability is

$$h^2 = 2(\rho_{MZ} - \rho_{DZ}),$$ (15.1)

where ρ is the correlation coefficient of the quantitative phenotype in MZ and DZ twins, respectively. For example, Herskind et al. (1996) carried out a careful epidemiologic study on age at death for various birth cohorts of MZ and DZ twins. A total of 2872 twin pairs was investigated and resulted in an estimate of heritability of 0.26 for longevity in males and 0.23 in females. Thus, longevity appears only moderately heritable. Interestingly, these authors found no evidence for an impact of shared family environment. An explanation for the low heritability of traits such as fertility and longevity is strong selection pressure on these fitness traits, which leads to low inter-individual genetic variation. Based on evidence in another study, exclusion of violent deaths is not expected to change these heritability estimates much.

For many diseases, the phenotype is qualitative (affected–unaffected). Then one usually works with a polygenic threshold model and determines correlations and heritability for the underlying liability. One may proceed with data on concordance; that is, the proportion of affected twins that have an affected co-twin. From such concordance rates and the population prevalence of the trait, the relevant correlations on the liability scale can be obtained (e.g., Figure 24 in Hartl and Clark, 1989) so that expression (15.1) may be used. For example, with more detailed model fitting, Kendler et al. (1995) estimated heritability of liability of 64% for affective illness using narrow diagnostic criteria (largely additive genetic effects), and of 83% using broad criteria (increase largely due to dominance genetic effects).

For *parent–offspring* data, the narrow-sense heritability is obtained as

$$h^2 = 2\rho_{po},\tag{15.2}$$

with ρ_{po} being the correlation coefficient between parent and offspring values.

For sets of *sibships* (no parents), wide-sense heritability of a quantitative trait is obtained from the int*ra*class correlation coefficient, ρ_I, as $h^2 = 2\rho_I$ (Fisher, 1970; Snedecor and Cochran, 1967), which is a different thing than the regular int*er*class (product-moment) correlation. The intraclass correlation coefficient may be estimated through a one-way analysis of variance (ANOVA) as follows. Let n be the number of siblings per sibship (class). In a one-way ANOVA, one determines the mean squares, s_b^2 and s_w^2, between and within classes, respectively. Then the estimate of the intraclass correlation coefficient is given by

$$r_I = \frac{s_b^2 - s_w^2}{s_b^2 + (n-1)s_w^2}\tag{15.3}$$

(expression [10.20.1] in Snedecor and Cochran, 1967), and heritability is estimated as $2r_I$. For sibships of unequal sizes, using the average sibship size for n in (15.3) will yield an approximate heritability estimate. Significance levels of heritability estimates depend on the significance levels of the quantities from which heritability is constructed (correlation coefficients, concordances, or ANOVA). It should be noted that heritability may also be estimated under more complicated inheritance models, for example, by variance components techniques (see Section 15.4).

With $n = 2$ (sib pairs), the intraclass correlation coefficient can be computed directly. Denote the observations of the i-th pair as (x_i, x_i'). Then, the intraclass correlation coefficient is estimated directly by

$$r_I = \frac{2\Sigma(x_i - \bar{x})(x_i' - \bar{x})}{\Sigma(x_i - \bar{x})^2 + \Sigma(x_i' - \bar{x})^2} \tag{15.4}$$

where the mean, $\bar{x}$, is obtained from all values (two per pair) and the sums extend over all pairs (Fisher, 1970). The intraclass correlation coefficient so obtained will be very close to the one furnished by the ANOVA. Another convenient approach is to use each pair twice, once as (x_i, x_i') and once as (x_i', x_i), except when x_i and x_i' are the same, in which case the pair is used only once (Snedecor and Cochran, 1967). With such data, the ordinary product moment (interclass) correlation coefficient will yield essentially the same result as (15.4).

Heritability is often estimated from *prevalence data* in the general population and in offspring of affected individuals (the latter is also called offspring recurrence risk; see next section). Under a polygenic threshold model (Figure 23 in Hartl, 1988), the liability has a normal distribution and the proportion, B_p, of affected individuals in the population are those whose liability exceeds some threshold, t. The trait may have a higher prevalence, B_o, among offspring or other first-degree relatives of affected individuals, which defines the distribution of liability among these relatives (note that $\lambda_o = B_o/B_p$ is discussed in the next section). Heritability of liability is computed from such data as

$$h^2 = \frac{2B_p[t - X(B_o)]}{f(t)} \tag{15.5}$$

where $X(B_o)$ indicates the normal deviate (threshold) such that the upper tail probability of the normal distribution is B_o [a statistician would write $X(B_o) = \Phi^{-1}(1 - B_o)$, where Φ^{-1} is the inverse of the normal distribution function], $t = X(B_p)$ is the threshold, and $f(t) = [\exp(-\frac{1}{2}t^2)]/\sqrt{(2\pi)}$ is the density of the normal curve at the threshold. For any upper tail probability, B, $X(B)$ may be computed with the NORINV program (option 1), which also furnishes the normal density at X. For example, schizophrenia has a prevalence of $B_o = 0.094$ among children of probands. With a population frequency of $B_p = 0.01$ as often quoted, calculation of heritability is done in the following steps: For $B_p = 0.01$, the NORINV program yields $t = X(B_p) = 2.3263$ and $f(t) = 0.02665$. For $B_o = 0.094$, NORINV furnishes $X(B_o) = 1.3165$. Finally, application of formula (15.5) leads to $h^2 = 2 \times 0.01 \times (2.3263 - 1.3165)/0.02665 = 76\%$. Based on disease prevalence data in various types of relatives of probands, McGue et al. (1986) carried out a path analysis and obtained a presumably more accurate estimate of 74% for the heritability of schizophrenia. As another example, Commuzzie and Allison (1998) quote heritabilities between 40% and 70% for various components of obesity such as body mass index (BMI) and skinfold thickness.

For any heritability estimates based on correlations among relatives, readers should be aware that ascertainment must be taken into account whenever individuals have been collected because of extreme phenotypes, and this is the norm rather than the exception. Often families are collected because one of the members, the proband, has an extreme phenotype (e.g., a cholesterol level exceeding the 95th percentile of normal values). In such a situation, correlation coefficient estimates for pairs of siblings are biased, not only between proband and one of his sibs, but also between non-proband sibs. Statistically, these observations may be viewed as multivariate normal variables with a common correlation coefficient, ρ, for each pair of siblings. One of these variables, x_1, say, is truncated so that only those values above a given threshold, $x_1 > h$, are observed. Such truncation can strongly alter the correlation coefficient between variables (Johnson and Kotz, 1972; Ott, 1979c). For simplicity, consider the phenotypes of three siblings, x_1, x_2, and x_3, ascertained such that $x_1 > h$, where h is set to reflect, for example, the 95th percentile. The correlation coefficient between the proband and one of his sibs is then given by

$$\rho_{12} = \rho\sqrt{\frac{v(h)}{1 - \rho^2[1 - v(h)]}}, \tag{15.6}$$

where ρ is the original correlation coefficient among siblings (untruncated) and

$$v(h) = 1 + \frac{z(h)}{1 - \Phi(h)}\left[h - \frac{z(h)}{1 - \Phi(h)}\right]$$

is the variance of the phenotype, x_1, as a function of the truncation point, h; $z(h)$ is the normal density at h; and $\Phi(h)$ is the normal distribution function at h (modified after equation [64] in Johnson and Kotz, 1972). Similarly, the correlation coefficient between two siblings who are themselves sibs of a common proband is given by

$$\rho_{23} = \rho\frac{1 - \rho[1 - v(h)]}{1 - \rho^2[1 - v(h)]} \tag{15.7}$$

(modified after equation [69.2] in Johnson and Kotz, 1972, with errors corrected). For different values of truncation points (formulated in terms of resulting percentiles) and original (true) correlation coefficients, Table 15.1 shows correlation coefficients resulting from truncation of x_1. They are strongly underestimated between sibs 1 and 2. They are also underestimated, although not as dramatically, between sibs 2 and 3 whose phenotypic values are not truncated. For example, consider that a large number of non-proband sib pairs that have been ascertained on the basis of a proband with a trait value above the 95th percentile. Assume that the correlation coefficient for the pairs is determined as 0.30. This would lead to an estimate of heritability of 60%. However, as a consequence of truncation of the probands' phenotypes, the true correlation is $\rho = 0.40$ so that the heritability estimate should be 80% instead of 60%. Table 15.1 may profitably be used to correct correlation coefficients that are biased due to truncation. Values do not differ much in the 90th to 99th percentile range. Thus, Figure 15.1 may be a useful guide in a wide number of cases as it graphically shows the values for the 95th percentile in Table 15.1.

The concept of heritability is sometimes misunderstood. For example, the fact that a trait has heritability of 80% may be interpreted to mean that genes play an overwhelming role. However, it must not be overlooked that some of the variation is not explained by genes, that is, the trait may be influenced (cured or modified in the case of a disease) by nongenetic intervention. Also, heritability estimates are always relative to a given environment in which the trait is observed. Different heritabilities may be obtained in different environments.

Number of Disease Genes. Many traits are due to a small number of genes and it is of interest to estimate their number. For planned crosses

Table 15.1. Correlation Coefficient among Observations, x_1, x_2, and x_3, on Unselected Siblings (ρ, True Correlation) and after Ascertainment of Proband's Value x_1, Exceeding the Given Percentile

ρ	80th Percentile		90th Percentile		95th Percentile		99th Percentile	
	ρ_{12}	ρ_{23}	ρ_{12}	ρ_{23}	ρ_{12}	ρ_{23}	ρ_{12}	ρ_{23}
.1	.047	.093	.041	.092	.037	.092	.033	.092
.2	.095	.174	.084	.172	.076	.171	.065	.170
.3	.145	.247	.128	.243	.116	.241	.102	.239
.4	.200	.314	.176	.308	.160	.304	.140	.300
.5	.261	.379	.231	.369	.210	.363	.184	.356

Note: ρ_{12} = resulting correlation between the proband and a sibling (equation [15.5]); ρ_{23} = correlation coefficient between two siblings of the proband (equation [15.6]).

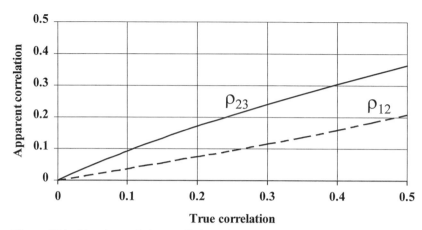

Figure 15.1. Biased correlation coefficients for quantitative observations in siblings when the observation on sib 1 is truncated so that only values above the 95th percentile are ascertained, while observations on sib 2 and sib 3 are not themselves truncated.

in experimental organisms, a method suggested by Sewall Wright (see Hartl and Clark, 1989, p. 485) is based on the variance, σ^2, of a quantitative phenotype in the F_2 generation when the parental generation is homozygous at each locus. Then, the number n of loci is estimated as

$$n = D^2/(8\sigma^2),\tag{15.8}$$

where D is the phenotypic difference between the two parental inbred lines. The assumptions underlying this expression are that all loci contribute equally to the phenotype and σ^2 is the genetic variance. However, the estimate of n (15.8) turns out to have a large variance (is imprecise) and tends to severely underestimate the number of loci (Zeng et al., 1990).

For human data, Hogben (1932) investigated different mating types (affected–unaffected, unaffected–unaffected) and compiled the proportion of affected offspring from published papers. For a number of diseases, he then tested observed values for agreement with the numbers expected under different two-locus models.

More recently, Risch et al. (1993) investigated diabetes in planned crosses in the nonobese diabetic mouse. These authors concluded that at least nine loci are responsible for diabetes in this mouse, with three of them conferring a protective effect. The significance of this study is that human diabetes can be expected to be due to a similar number of genes.

A method for estimating the number of genes involved in human diseases is based on the ratio between the recurrence risk to relatives and population prevalence and is discussed in the next section.

15.2. Recurrence Risk in Relatives versus Population Prevalence

Concordance rates discussed in the previous section are not easy to establish and require careful epidemiologic studies. A quantity closely related to the concordance rate is the recurrence risk to a relative, that is, the probability that a relative of a proband is affected. These recurrence risks are often scaled by the population prevalence, which is the recurrence risk to an unrelated person. Risch (1990a) defined the risk ratio, λ, as the recurrence risk divided by the population prevalence, and distinguished such ratios of risks to offspring, λ_o, to siblings, λ_s, to an MZ twin, λ_M, and so on. As shown by Risch (1990b) and outlined below, there is a close connection between these risk ratios and IBD sharing probabilities for different pairs of relatives. Bishop and Williamson (1990), on the other hand, looked at identity by *state* relations among pairs of individuals with different degree of relationship and their power to detect linkage. I summarized results in these papers in an easy to understand manner (Ott, 1990b).

A number of authors (e.g., Penrose, 1953; Edwards, 1960) proposed to use properties of λ risk ratios to distinguish between monogenic and polygenic threshold inheritance. More specifically, Gottesman and Shields (1982) suggested that the drop-off rate of recurrence risk by degree of relationship is indicative of mode of inheritance. Risch (1990a) evaluated this drop-off rate under a variety of models. He showed that for monogenic diseases, $\lambda - 1$ decreases by a factor of 2 with each degree of relationship. For example, if a monogenic trait is 20 times more prevalent among offspring of a proband than in the general population ($\lambda - 1 = 19$), then it will be 5.75 times more prevalent ($\lambda - 1 = 4.75$) among cousins (third-degree relatives) of the proband. These results also hold when multiple disease loci are responsible for susceptibility to the trait as long as these loci do not interact epistatically (see Chapter 14). Faster drop-off of λ with decreasing relationship is not compatible with mendelian inheritance and is interpreted as evidence for multiple loci interacting epistatically to cause disease. Fitting published recurrence risk data for schizophrenia to recurrence risks expected under various epistatic multilocus models, Risch (1990a) concluded that 2 to 3 loci acting on a polygenic background, with $\lambda = 2$ for each locus, are reasonable assumptions. Clearly, values of λ this small characterize loci that by themselves have only a small effect on the trait and must be difficult to detect by linkage or disequilibrium analysis (see Problem 15.1). With a population prevalence of 1%, observed risk ratios for schizophrenia are $\lambda_o = 9.4$ and $\lambda_s = 7.3$ (McGue et al., 1986).

Locus-specific risk ratios may be obtained from allele-sharing data observed at a given marker locus, which is assumed tightly linked with a disease locus. This allows determining the contribution of single loci to the overall genetic contribution as measured by λ_o or λ_s. The following relationships hold (formulas [8] through [10] in Risch, 1990b with $\theta = 0$):

$$
\left.
\begin{aligned}
z_0 &= 1/(4\lambda_s) \\
z_1 &= \lambda_o/(2\lambda_s) \\
z_2 &= \lambda_M/(4\lambda_s) = 1 - (2\lambda_o + 1)/(4\lambda_s),
\end{aligned}
\right\} \tag{15.9}
$$

where z_i = probability that an affected sib pair shares i alleles IBD. The far right-hand side of the last line in (15.9) was obtained through the substitution $\lambda_M = 4\lambda_s - 2\lambda_o - 1$ (formula [5] in Risch, 1990a). For example, based on line 1 in (15.9), Davies et al. (1994) estimated $\lambda_s = 0.25/z_0$ for IDDM1 and IDDM2 of 3.1 and 1.3, respectively, while the overall sib risk ratio for type 1 diabetes is 15. This shows that the only loci clearly established thus far account for only a fraction of the genetic contribution to diabetes. Previously, Rotter and Landaw (1984) proposed an alternative method for determining the relative contribution of a single locus to a complex trait. They defined a ''coefficient of genetic contribution'' as the ratio, (concordance rate of IBD = 2 siblings minus concordance rate of IBD = 0 siblings) divided by (MZ twin concordance rate minus concordance rate of IBD = 0 siblings). In terms of this coefficient, Rotter and Landaw (1984) estimated that the contribution of HLA toward IDDM amounts to 60%. This is much higher than the result based on the λ values and is more in line with the impression of diabetes researchers that HLA is the major contributor to disease (Dr. Graeme Bell, personal communication).

Note that the average IBD sharing *per parent* (expected to be ½ without linkage) is obtained from (15.9) as $z_1/2 + z_2$, which is identical with p_1 in expression (13.2). Thus, one obtains from (15.9)

$$
p_1 = (\lambda_M + \lambda_o)/(\lambda_M + 2\lambda_o + 1) = 1 - (\lambda_o + 1)/(4\lambda_s), \tag{15.10}
$$

which expresses the average number of alleles shared IBD per parent given that a trait exhibits an MZ twin ratio λ_M and an offspring risk ratio λ_o, or an offspring risk ratio λ_o and a sib risk ratio λ_s. For example, with a population prevalence of 0.01 for schizophrenia and the risk ratios $\lambda_M = 44.3$ and $\lambda_o = 9.4$ (McGue et al., 1986), if a single locus were responsible for schizophrenia, it would be expected to show an IBD allele sharing proportion of $p_1 = 0.84$, which is quite a bit higher than the value of 0.50 expected by chance. Of course, if multiple loci contribute to schizophrenia, each is expected to lead to a smaller excess IBD sharing proportion. If in (15.10), λ_s and λ_o rather than λ_M and λ_o are used, a different value is obtained for IBD sharing. This must be due to the inherent imprecision of these estimates. As noted above, more reliable estimates are based on the joint analysis of λ values for different types of relatives.

Among the large number of possible multi-locus inheritance models for a trait, the multiplicative model has mathematically appealing properties. This model represents epistatic interaction among multiple loci and is characterized by multi-locus penetrances, which are the products of the corresponding marginal penetrances or penetrance factors (Risch, 1990a). For such models, the overall risk ratio for a trait is just the product of the risk ratios for the component loci. For example, let λ_i denote the locus-specific risk ratio at the ith locus for some type of relative (offspring, sib, MZ twin, etc.). Then, the overall risk ratio is given by $\Pi_i\lambda_i = \lambda_1 \times \lambda_2 \times \ldots$. For instance, assume that the overall observed sib risk ratio for a given trait is 15. If one makes the hypothetical assumption that 10 loci equally contribute to the trait in an epistatic manner, the locus-specific sib risk ratio is expected to be $(15)^{1/10} = (15)^{0.1} = 1.31$. At each such locus, one would expect the proportion of sib pairs sharing no alleles IBD to be reduced to $1/(4 \times 1.31) = 0.19$ from the value of 0.25 expected without linkage.

For a single-locus inheritance model with given values of penetrances and allele frequencies, it may be of interest to find, for example, the sib risk ratio, λ_s. A convenient way to do this is by a numerical approach, which was suggested to me by Dr. Lodewijk Sandkuijl. Because most linkage programs can carry out risk calculations, one simply creates a "family" consisting of two siblings, one affected (the proband) and the other of phenotype "unknown," with parents also being "unknown." The program is then used to carry out a risk calculation for the second sib. A worked example is given in Problem 15.3.

Risk ratios, λ, may be taken to characterize component loci of a trait and indicate their "strength" in terms of their contribution to trait susceptibility. Power calculations mentioned in Section 15.5 are often carried out as a function of the λ_o or λ_s value of a locus.

15.3. Disease Phenotype

Thus far, diseases have been assumed to be dichotomous traits. In many cases, however, such a dichotomy is arrived at after observing several variables on an individual, on the basis of which a rule is applied as to who is affected and who is unaffected. As pointed out in the introduction to this chapter, such rules may or may not be genetically relevant.

Ideally, one would use all variables jointly in a linkage analysis of a multivariate phenotype, in which the observations form a mixture of two (presumably overlapping) multivariate distributions whose two mean vectors correspond to genetically susceptible and non-susceptible individuals. One may also try to reduce the dimensionality of the phenotypes (given by the number of variables) to a one-dimensional quantity, for example, using discriminant or principal components analysis. One method, based on sib pairs, incorporates multiple variable measurements on each individual and estimates the linear function that results in the strongest correlation between the squared pair differences in these measurements and identity by descent at a marker locus (Amos et al., 1990). Instead of principal components analysis, which maximizes the variance for each component, one may want to perform an analogous type of analysis that maximizes heritability for each component (Ott and Rabinowitz, 1999). Specialized methods for looking at the genetic contributions of quantitative variables in such settings of pleiotropy have also been developed (Comuzzie et al., 1997).

Although multivariate methods are statistically appealing, forming two classes (affected/unaffected) has its advantages. It obviates the need for parameter estimation, although dichotomization generally entails a great loss of information (Cohen, 1990). As it is often unclear how to define the genetically most relevant class boundaries, investigators tend to try several alternative classification schemes, for example, by applying various degrees of stringency in their criteria for affectedness. If each such scheme is used to carry out a linkage analysis and if the overall maximum lod score under any classification scheme is reported, computer simulation may have to be used to assess the empirical significance level associated with such a maximum lod score (see Section 9.7).

The appropriate phenotype definition may depend on the purpose of a linkage analysis. For example, the gene underlying the fragile X syndrome (Martin–Bell syndrome; Vogel and Motulsky, 1986) potentially causes two distinct phenotypes: (1) mental retardation and other clinical features and (2) cytologic abnormalities (secondary restrictions in X chromosome, fragile X phenotype) (Sherman et al., 1985). For gene mapping and carrier detection, one would like to make as much use as possible of the phenotype for recognizing the underlying genotype. For that reason, one would call someone affected when that person either is mentally retarded *or* shows cytologic abnormalities. In genetic counseling, on the other hand, one may only be interested to know whether the proband is mentally retarded or not. The cytologic status is then a covariate that should not be part of the phenotype. In that case, "affected" is taken to mean only "mentally retarded," with two penetrance classes defined by the presence or absence of cytologic abnormalities. In cancer genetics, a variable often used to refine the phenotype is loss of heterozygosity (LOH). Use of such data can improve the power to localize tumor suppressor genes (Rohde et al., 1995).

One possible avenue to finding genetically relevant phenotypes would be to work with component phenotypes (sub-phenotypes) rather than a global definition of "affected." Linkage analysis would then be carried out with each of the component phenotypes, or these would be screened for being associated with high heritability. The following example demonstrates the usefulness of working with component phenotypes. Hypertension in humans is defined as systolic blood pressure ≥ 140 mm Hg or diastolic blood pressure ≥ 90 mm Hg (NIH, 1997). In the Lyon hypertensive rat, Dubay et al. (1993) found that diastolic pressure and pulse pressure (systolic minus diastolic pressure) are under the control of two different genes. Thus, if a similar situation exists in humans, it would be more difficult to find one of these genes if the global definition of "affected" were applied. Instead, looking at each component should be much more promising. As an example, Grigorenko et al. (1997) investigated five component phenotypes of dyslexia and for some of them found strong evidence of genetic linkage.

In discussing the application of principles of complex systems to behavioral traits, McClearn (1993) also took issue with phenotype definition and concluded that "multiple indicator variables will be required to tap the information about a system." He proposed the derivation of composite measures that are maximally heritable but also warned that many researchers may regard these measures with suspicion and will be more comfortable with traditional single variables (e.g., affected–unaffected). For example, Brzustowicz et al. (1997) found strong evidence for linkage for certain symptom–scale scores while no evidence for linkage was obtained with the classical disease definition.

It was pointed out previously that for many conditions, earlier disease onset is indicative of stronger genetic involvement. Similarly, *severity of disease* may be indicative of genetic loading. In this situation, researchers often carry out multiple analyses, one for each classification scheme, where classification schemes can be ordered by severity of disease. An alternative approach is to introduce a measure c for disease severity and combine different classification schemes into a single analysis. This measure may also be thought of as reflecting the certainty that an individual is truly affected (Ott, 1991a). It may be derived from Rice et al.'s (1987) estimated probability that an observed case is a true case. One may then form classes of c values, for example, class 1 with $c = 1$ (very severely affected), class 2 with $0.90 < c < 1$ (severely affected), and so on. Now, assume a monogenic analysis model with penetrance f for the most extreme "affected" phenotype (and penetrance $1 - f$ for most extremely unaffected), given a susceptible genotype. An individual with, for example, 60% severity will have penetrance for "affected" status of $0.6 \times f + 0.4 \times (1 - f)$, and one minus this quantity as the penetrance for "unaffected." That is, the penetrance is a weighted average of the penetrances for the extreme classes. Individuals midway between the extremes ($c = \frac{1}{2}$) will receive a penetrance of $\frac{1}{2}$ irrespective of the genotype, which is equivalent to the "unknown" phenotype. Although this scheme may appear arbitrary and subjective, it does not suffer from the shortcomings of multiple analyses carried out with multiple diagnostic schemes.

A theoretical underpinning for the above procedure of handling severity classes may be found in the framework of misdiagnosis. For example, one distinguishes two levels of phenotypes, true, but hidden, phenotypes A (affected) and U (unaffected), and corresponding apparent phenotypes A^* and U^* (a similar approach was taken by Lathrop et al. [1983] in their investigation of pedigree errors). Given a genotype g conferring disease susceptibility, the penetrance for true affecteds is $f = P(A|g)$. Through misclassification, the hidden phenotype A is seen only with probability $c = P(A^*|A)$ and mistaken for phenotype U with probability $1 - c = P(U^*|A)$. Analogously, $c = P(U^*|U)$ and $1 - c = P(A^*|U)$. Then, the penetrance for the apparent phenotype "affected" becomes $P(A^*|g) = cf + (1 - c)(1 - f)$, with penetrance for "apparently unaffected" = $1 - P(A^*|g)$ (cf. Section 11.2 on misclassification).

15.4. Current Approaches

This section is intended as a brief outline of current approaches to localizing genes for complex traits on the human gene map. The material will cover such topics as genetic basis, sampling strategies, and analysis strategies.

One of the first steps in the endeavor to localize susceptibility genes for a complex trait is to determine that there is an appreciable genetic basis for it. Methods for doing so and some potential pitfalls are outlined in Section 15.1. Previously, it was considered essential that a (complex) segregation analysis be carried out demonstrating the presence of single major genes. However, this is no longer considered necessary, partly because segregation analyses tend to be very sensitive to mode of ascertainment, which it is almost impossible to allow for correctly (Greenberg, 1986).

Several inheritance models have been discussed in this chapter and in Chapter 14. Which of these models might be realistic for a given trait is difficult to answer. Animal models for human traits often provide valuable insight. For example, as mentioned in Section 15.1, Risch et al. (1993) concluded from studies in the NOD mouse that at least nine genes are responsible for diabetes in the NOD mouse and, presumably, also in humans.

General sampling strategies and ascertainment biases are discussed in Section 11.1. For complex traits, some special considerations apply (Comuzzie and Allison, 1998). For example, population isolates offer distinct advantages over large outbred populations. For one thing, they tend to exhibit stronger disequilibrium, which makes disequilibrium mapping (see Section 13.4) a promising search technique. Also, because of founder effects, the number of genes underlying a trait is presumably smaller in such populations. The potential downside is that important genes in population isolates may be unimportant in other populations.

Whether one samples large pedigrees, affected sibs, trios of parents and an affected offspring, or still another set of relatives depends very much on the trait studied and the type of analysis contemplated. Large families are ideal for mendelian traits and also for studying allele-sharing (IBD) relations across generations. On the other hand, there is presumably a smaller number of genes segregating in smaller sets of families so that within-family heterogeneity will be reduced. In their computer simulation on localizing genes for oligogenic threshold traits by affected sib pair analysis, Suarez et al. (1994) found that those nuclear families contributing most to linkage informativeness were the ones with unaffected parents, presumably because affected parents tend to be homozygous at susceptibility genes. Thus, nuclear families are usually ascertained such that at most one of the two parents is affected.

Suarez et al. (1994) also demonstrated that on the order of 5 to 10 times as many families are required to replicate a linkage claim than to originally find linkage if criteria for significance are the same at the two stages. With multiple susceptibility genes contributing to a trait, some genes will by chance be most prevalent in a given data set, and these are the genes that will most likely be detected in an initial search. In a replication study focusing on the specific genes previously identified, it is unlikely that these will again be most frequent in the new data set

(Lernmark and Ott, 1998). On the other hand, a replication does not carry the burden of multiple testing (or only to a minor degree) as does a genome screen (Lander and Kruglyak, 1995). Thus, the significance level in a replication study of a previously *significant* finding may be set anywhere from 0.01 to 0.05. A critical lod score of 1 corresponds to an asymptotic significance level of 0.016, which appears suitable. If several markers are tested in the replication study, somewhat more stringent criteria ($p = 0.01$) should be applied (Lander and Kruglyak, 1995).

Researchers trying to characterize a gene by molecular methods are often faced with the following dilemma. An initial linkage finding was quite strong (e.g., $Z_{max} \approx 4$). However, it was pointed out to them that without a replication, this result should not be trusted. Indeed, a replication of the original finding failed (approximately the same number of families in replication than original study). What should they do? One consequence from the observation that a multiple of families are required for replication than for initial detection is that the failure of the replication was to be expected if the replication and original study each comprised about the same number of families. Because the original finding was quite strong, it is better to stick with those data and perhaps add some more families and markers, unless a replication with drastically increased numbers of families is planned.

Implicitly or explicitly, many parametric linkage analyses are carried out under single-gene models; that is, for a complex trait, under a "wrong" model. This aspect of linkage analysis is discussed in detail in Section 14.2. Single-locus analysis is profitably carried out under heterogeneity with the *hlod* (Sections 10.4 and 14.2). There is then a question as to which single-locus model to choose. As discussed earlier in this chapter and in Chapter 14, it is not reasonable to strive for an analysis under a "realistic" model because it can at best be quasi-realistic. Single-locus analysis is unrealistic for complex traits but is presumably quite robust. It has been recommended to carry out (at least) two parametric (lod score) analyses, one under a recessive and one under a dominant analysis model. This is based on the observation that lod scores are very sensitive to misspecification of dominant versus recessive inheritance but not to penetrance and allele frequency (Clerget-Darpoux et al., 1986). That is, an analysis under a recessive model may miss a dominant gene, and vice versa. At least, wrong analysis models have been shown not to lead to false-positive evidence of linkage (Williamson and Amos, 1990). This result has sometimes falsely been interpreted to mean that maximizing the lod score over model parameters will not inflate the lod score, but such a conclusion is fallacious. In fact, maximizing lods over diagnostic schemes *or* over penetrance values will tend to inflate the lod score, but the effect is much stronger when diagnostic classes are varied than when penetrance values are varied (Weeks et al., 1990). The technique of estimating parameter values by maximizing the lod score (the so-called mod score approach) has some merit (Clerget-Darpoux et al., 1986; Hodge and Elston, 1994). But interpreting the value of the maximized lod score is difficult unless allowance is made for multiple testing, for example, through adjusting the number of *df* in chi-square tests. As a way out of this dilemma, Curtis and Sham (1995a) recommended that the likelihoods under linkage and non-linkage be independently maximized over a limited set of transmission models, ranging from mendelian dominant to null effect and from null effect to mendelian recessive. Their approach, implemented in the MFLINK program, has attractive statistical properties.

Because of the known bias of the recombination fraction estimate in most parametric analysis types (e.g., Risch and Giuffra, 1992), multipoint analysis should be deferred as long as possible. Only two-point analysis (trait versus one marker at a time) should be carried out until good evidence for linkage has been obtained. Of course, there is no problem with nonparametric multipoint linkage as this refers to multipoint analysis of marker loci. In fact, one of the most common analysis methods are nonparametric genome screens carried out by the Genehunter or Aspex programs.

For complex traits, many researchers prefer nonparametric over parametric analysis. However, as pointed out in Chapter 13, nonparametric methods generally favor recessive over dominant genes. As outlined in Section 8.5, variance components methods have been developed and implemented in computer programs (e.g., SOLAR), which allow decomposing the variance of quantitative traits into components due to major genes, polygenes, random effects, and so forth (Amos, 1994; Almasy and Blangero, 1998). A particular type of analysis, based on Monte Carlo (computer simulation) methods, allows the joint estimation of inheritance models and recombination fractions (Heath, 1997; 1998). It has been implemented in the LOKI program mentioned in Section 9.3. There are several additional sophisticated methods that have been developed but go beyond the framework of this book, for example, those based on descent graphs (Thompson, 1996; Sobel and Lange, 1996).

Some investigators stratify their families by risk variables. Such stratification has been shown to be valuable, for example, in breast cancer, where most linkage information was furnished by families with early mean age at disease onset (Hall et al., 1990). In genome screens for type 1 diabetes, sib pairs have been stratified by IBD allele sharing status at

HLA (Davies et al., 1994; Mein et al., 1998). But it is unclear whether stratification was useful in those cases when adjustments are made for multiple comparisons (Lernmark and Ott, 1998). Clearly, in the presence of strong heterogeneity at one locus due to different genotypes at another locus or different values at some variable such as age at disease onset, stratification is expected to be useful as it reduces heterogeneity. However, it comes at a price. To see this, consider the hypothetical situation that 150 ASPs have been collected and genotyped for some marker. For each of the 300 parents, it was tested whether the same ($x = 1$) or a different allele ($x = 0$) was transmitted to the two offspring. It was believed that the data were heterogeneous due to the effect of some other variable, u, which might be onset age. Therefore, the parents were ordered by their u value and stratified into five ordered classes of equal size.

It is now of interest to find out what happens if in reality the u variable has no effect. How much of a penalty does one have to pay for stratification if there is no gain from it? I investigated this question with a small computer simulation. The effect of the disease next to the marker locus was measured by the expected value of the number of alleles shared IBD received from each parent. Values of $E(x) = 0.52$ through 0.66 in steps of 0.02 were assumed. For each value, 10,000 replicates of 300 parents were generated. In each replicate, an empirical significance level was computed in two ways: (1) Without stratification, equation (13.2) was applied and the resulting normal deviate converted into an empirical significance level, p. (2) With stratification, an analogous test was carried out for each of the five classes of the u variable. The smallest resulting p-value was picked and formula (4.13) applied to it with $g = 5$, which resulted in a value, p_s, adjusted for multiple testing. The p-values, p and p_s, were averaged over the 10,000 replicates and graphed. As Figure 15.2 shows, for a given IBD sharing probability, p_s is always higher (less significant) on average than p. In any given case, p_s may or may not exceed p. For example, at an IBD sharing probability of 0.54, p_s is smaller (more sigificant) than p in 25% of all replicates, and this proportion decreases to 4% at IBD sharing probability 0.60. To look at the situation in another way, a significance level of 0.05 is produced by a trait gene with IBD sharing probability of ~0.57 when no stratification is applied. But with (useless) stratification, the gene must show much stronger IBD sharing of 0.60 to produce the same significance. Evidently, stratification must have a very strong effect for it to be beneficial in linkage analysis. Details may be found in Leal et al. (1999).

For many genes underlying a complex trait, each with small effect, Risch and Merikangas (1996) postulated that disequilibrium mapping is

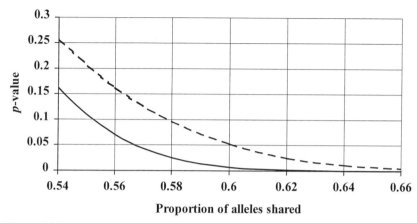

Figure 15.2. Effects of random stratification in analysis of 150 ASPs (300 parents): p-value achieved by linkage test to detect a given proportion of alleles shared for undivided data set (solid line) and after stratification in five classes, with minimum p-value over classes adjusted for multiple testing (broken line) (based on computer simulation with 10,000 replicates per data point).

more powerful than linkage analysis through ASPs. This is discussed in Section 13.4. The new SNP markers are introduced partly with the specific purpose to carry out LD mapping in dense marker maps.

Because complex traits are due to multiple underlying genes, it might be a good idea to carry out analyses under the assumption of more than a single disease gene. As discussed in Chapter 14, two-locus analyses might be carried out either in a parametric or nonparametric fashion. One would then investigate pairs of marker loci instead of single loci. However, for genome-wide application, this does not offer any benefits above those of single-locus search.

A novel method is based on the results of ASP analysis. At a given marker locus, IBD sharing results are recorded for each parent (IBD = 0 for no sharing, IBD = 1 for sharing). Thus, the data have a very simple structure. They consist of a matrix with as many rows as there are parents and as many columns as the number of marker loci. Neural networks were developed and applied to such data with the aim to identify sets of marker loci that jointly exhibit a deviation from random IBD sharing (Lucek et al., 1998). Details are provided by Lucek et al. (1999).

15.5. Power Considerations

In parametric linkage analysis, power calculations amount to determining the probability that a lod score threshold will be exceeded for a given set of families and given parameter values such as the recombination fraction(s) between trait locus and nearest marker(s). Such calculations are usually carried out with the SIMLINK or SLINK program. For complex traits, one would have to work with an assumed inheritance model as it was done, for example, by Suarez et al. (1994). It is then more convenient to compute power for nonparametric analysis types, for example, ASP and LD analysis. It is then not necessary to model trait inheritance. But some assumptions regarding the strength of linkage or disequilibrium must of course be made. These assumptions are usually made relative to a particular locus in the genome, where this locus presumably is one of several that are responsible for the trait under study.

In ASP analysis, one may simply assume some expected allele sharing probability as it was done for the construction of Figure 15.2 discussed above. For example, one might postulate an IBD sharing probability of $p = 0.56$ (per parent) and want to compute the power of n parents ($n/2$ ASPs) to detect this locus. Under the null hypothesis of no effect of this locus, one has $p = 0.50$. A given number, n, of parents, leads to a binomial situation in that a parent does (IBD sharing) or does not (no IBD sharing) pass the same allele to the two offspring. Assume that k parents lead to IBD sharing in the offspring. The empirical significance level associated with this result may be obtained from formula (13.2) with $\hat{p}_1 = k/n$, or one may use the BINOM program with $p = 0.50$ to compute the probability, $P(x \geq k)$, where x is the random variable with binomial distribution $B(p, n)$. For example, let $n = 300$ and $k = 180$. In the BINOM program, one chooses the B option and enters $n = 300$ and $p = 0.50$. Then, the upper tail probability, $P(x \geq k)$, is obtained by entering $k_1 = 180$ and $k_2 = 300$. The program furnishes 0.00032, which is the exact p-value associated with the observation $k = 180$. To compute power for a given significance level, say, 0.001, one must first find that critical number, k_1, with associated probability $P(x \geq k_1) \leq 0.001$. Entering trial values of k_1 (with $k_2 = 300$) leads to the result $k_1 = 174$. Now, the power associated with this critical limit, given a postulated allele sharing probability of $p = 0.56$, is obtained from BINOM as follows: Enter $n = 300$ and $p = 0.56$. Then enter $k_1 = 174$ and $k_2 = 300$, which produces a power of 0.26. Similarly, one finds a power of 0.78 for an allele sharing probability of $p = 0.60$, and a power of 0.99 for $p = 0.65$. For given values of recurrence risk ratios, equation (15.10) may be used to compute an allele sharing probability predicted by these λ values. Then the procedure outlined in this paragraph is applied.

Power to detect a given locus is often computed relative to some recurrence risk ratio, λ_s, for sibs. For example, Risch (1990b, Figure 1) computed power curves for different numbers of ASPs under the following assumptions: Fully informative marker, complete linkage between marker and trait locus, and a lod score exceeding 3. For an observed proportion, n_0, of sib pairs sharing no alleles IBD, the lod score was defined as

$$T = n_0 \log_{10} \frac{4n_0}{N} + (N - n_0) \log_{10} \frac{N - n_0}{0.75 \, N} \tag{15.11}$$

where N refers to the number of ASPs (not parents). For example, 100 ASPs have power of 80% to detect a locus with associated λ_s of 3.0 (Risch, 1990b, Figure 1) whereas detecting a locus with $\lambda_s = 2$ requires slightly more than 200 ASPs with the same power.

As suggested by Elston (1994), it may be more economical to carry out a two-stage search with an initial low density map and a low threshold, where results exceeding this threshold will later be followed up with more marker typing. For example, with power 80%, 100 ASPs will detect a locus of strength $\lambda_s = 3$ when the critical lod score level is 3.0, but they will detect a much weaker locus of $\lambda_s \approx 1.8$ with a critical lod score of 1.0 (Weeks and Lathrop, 1995, Figure 1).

To determine power in disequilibrium studies using the HHRR approach, Terwilliger and Ott (1992b) computed the probability that a chi-square test is significant at the 5% level for a marker with two equally frequent alleles and n families with one affected offspring and two parents. The disease locus was assumed to follow a recessive mode of inheritance, with marker and disease loci being separated by a recombination fraction θ. To detect a standardized disequilibrium of $D' = 0.20$, this furnishes a power of 0.95 with $\theta = 0$ and $n = 100$, a power of 0.63 with $\theta = 0.20$ and $n = 100$, power of 0.82 with $\theta = 0$ and $n = 50$, and power of 0.42 with $\theta = 0.20$ and $n = 50$.

More generally, one may assume, for example, a marker with four equally frequent alleles, where the *4* allele is in LD with the susceptibility allele, *d,* at a specific disease locus, which has two alleles. Let the disease and wild allele frequencies be $P(d) = 0.20$ and $P(+) = 0.80$, respectively. Table 15.2 shows the layout of the resulting haplotype frequencies, where the first four columns correspond to marker alleles and the first two rows

Table 15.2. Haplotype Frequencies between Assumed Marker and Disease Alleles

0.05 − *D/3*	0.05 − *D/3*	0.05 − *D/3*	0.05 + *D*	0.20
0.20 + *D/3*	0.20 + *D/3*	0.20 + *D/3*	0.20 − *D*	0.80
0.25	0.25	0.25	0.25	1

to alleles at the disease locus. Assume that a disequilibrium at 80% of its maximum value should be detected. In Table 15.2, the haplotype of interest (between marker allele *4* and disease allele *d*) has a maximum frequency of 0.20 (it cannot exceed the marginal frequency of 0.20). That is, $0.05 + D \leq 0.20$, so that the maximum disequilibrium is $D_{max} = 0.20 - 0.05 = 0.15$. For the standardized disequilibrium to be equal to $D' = D/D_{max} = 0.80$, the disequilibrium must be $D = 0.80 \times D_{max} = 0.80 \times 0.15 = 0.12$. With this, haplotype frequencies in Table 15.2 are obtained as $P(4d) = 0.05 + D = 0.17$, $P(4+) = 0.20 - D = 0.08$, $P(3d) = 0.05 - D/3 = 0.01$, $P(3+) = 0.20 + D/3 = 0.24$, and so on. Once this structure is in place, one can proceed to defining a suitable set of penetrances at the disease locus and carrying out a computer simulation. What constitutes a suitable disease model depends on the trait being studied. For schizophrenia, for example, based on Neuman and Rice's (1992) two-locus model discussed in Section 14.1, if the two disease loci have equal disease allele frequencies of 0.20 each, the corresponding single-locus marginal penetrances are given by 0, 0.014, and 0.126 for genotypes *++*, *+d*, and *dd,* respectively. As this is a model without phenocopies, one may want to assign some penetrance to the *++* geno-type. The simulation would involve writing a small computer program to generate a genotype (pair of haplotypes) for each of the parents and, based on parental genotypes, a genotype for the offspring. Those families with affected offspring would be ascertained for the analysis. For each affected offspring, the two transmitted and two nontransmitted alleles are recorded. For all offspring in the given sample size, a frequency table of transmitted versus nontransmitted marker alleles is set up and analyzed by chi-square, which constitutes the result for one replicate of the simulation. The proportion of replicates with chi-square exceeding a predefined significance level approximates the power.

For the TDT and other tests, based on computer simulation, Kaplan et al. (1997) published tables of power figures for various disease models and marker allele frequencies.

15.6. Problems

Problem 15.1. For rare, fully penetrant dominant and recessive traits with respective disease allele frequencies of p_d and p_r, derive the expressions of λ_o as a function of the allele frequencies. Assuming a trait prevalence of ½% for each trait, what are the numerical values for the λ risk ratios?

Problem 15.2. As mentioned in Section 15.2, the observed sib risk ratio for type 1 diabetes is 15. The two main contributing loci, IDDM1 and IDDM2, are associated with respective individual risk ratios of 3.1 and 1.3. Assume that all loci interact epistatically and the remaining diabetes loci are equally strong (same risk ratios) and have an associated risk ratio of 1.2 each. How many remaining loci are there?

Problem 15.3. Compute numerically the risk ratio, λ_s, for the following mendelian model: Dominant disease with full penetrance for genetic cases and penetrance $f = 0.02$ for non-genetic cases (phenocopies). The trait prevalence if $K = 0.10$. *Hint:* Use the MLINK program to carry out risk calculations.

Solutions to Study Problems

Solution 1.1. One proceeds as shown in Section 1.4 for the Haldane mapping function. From (1.3) one finds $x_{12} = \frac{1}{4} \ln[(1 + 2\theta_{12})/(1 - 2\theta_{12})]$ and the analogous expression for x_{23}. The sum, $x_{12} + x_{23}$, is obtained as $\frac{1}{4} \ln\{(1 + 2\theta_{12})(1 + 2\theta_{23})/[(1 - 2\theta_{12})(1 - 2\theta_{23})]\}$ and represents the map distance between loci *1* and *3*. The corresponding recombination fraction is obtained by substituting $x_{12} + x_{23}$ for x in the inverse of (1.3) so that, with $\exp[4(x_{12} + x_{23})] = (1 + 2\theta_{12})(1 + 2\theta_{23})/[(1 - 2\theta_{12})(1 - 2\theta_{23})]$, one obtains $\theta_{13} = (\theta_{12} + \theta_{23})/(1 + 4\theta_{12}\theta_{23})$.

Solution 1.2. In analogy to the previous problem, one finds $x_{12} + x_{23} = [\frac{1}{2}/(2 - k)] \ln\{[1 + 2\theta_{12}(2 - k)/(1 - 2\theta_{12})][1 + 2\theta_{23}(2 - k)/(1 - 2\theta_{23})]\}$ and $\exp[2(x_{12} + x_{23})(2 - k)] = [1 + 2\theta_{12}(2 - k)/(1 - 2\theta_{12})][1 + 2\theta_{23}(2 - k)/(1 - 2\theta_{23})]$. A somewhat lengthy calculation then leads to $\theta_{13} = (\theta_{12} + \theta_{23} - 2k\theta_{12}\theta_{23})/[1 + 4(1 - k)\theta_{12}\theta_{23}]$. Solving this expression for the interference parameter yields $k = [\theta_{12} + \theta_{23} - \theta_{13}(1 + 4\theta_{12}\theta_{23})]/[2\theta_{12}\theta_{23}(1 - 2\theta_{13})]$.

Solution 1.3. Under complete interference, there is at most one chiasma. But we also know that there is always at least one chiasma so that each chromosome shows exactly one chiasma. Then, half the strands (chromatids) are recombinant and half are nonrecombinant. According to the definition of map distance, therefore, the expected number of crossovers per strand is equal to $\frac{1}{2}$.

Solution 2.1. Subtracting equation (2.4) from (2.2) yields $(a - 1)/a^3$ as the difference between H and PIC. The inequality, $(a - 1)/a^3 < 0.01$ leads to a cubic equation which, after rearranging terms, may be solved iteratively as $a = [(a - 1)/0.01]^{1/3}$. The solution is 9.46, that is, with 10 or more equally frequent alleles, the difference between H and PIC is smaller than 0.01.

331

Solution 2.2. If markers were equally spaced, $m = 10$ markers would be sufficient because the distance between adjacent markers would be 10 cM; thus any new locus is never more than 5 cM away from the nearest marker. With random placement of markers, equation (2.9) with $L = 100$, $d = 5$, and $P = 0.95$ must be used. The result is $m \geq 29$ markers.

Solution 3.1. Based on the phenotype, the genotype must contain at least one A allele. If one of the parents has phenotype A- (genotype a/a), that tells us that a child with phenotype A+ must have genotype A/a.

Solution 3.2. Each parent has two possible genotypes, A/A with conditional probability $p^2/[p^2 + 2p(1 - p)] = p/(2 - p)$, and A/a with conditional probability $1 - p/(2 - p) = 2(1 - p)/(2 - p)$. For each of the $2 \times 2 = 4$ possible genotypic matings of mother and father, it is easy to determine the probability of their having an A+ child. All matings, except $A/a \times A/a$, produce only A+ children. For the $A/a \times A/a$ mating whose probability of occurrence is $[2(1 - p)/(2 - p)]^2$, the probability of an A- child (a/a genotype) is equal to ¼. Hence, the parents have an A+ child with probability $Q = 1 - (¼)[2(1 - p)/(2 - p)]^2 = (3 - 2p)/(2 - p)^2$. This probability tends to 1 as $p \to 1$ (the parents are both A/A) and tends to ¾ as $p \to 0$ (the parents are both A/a).

The answer to the second question is "No"; Q does not necessarily stay the same but may vary with the phenotypes of the children already born. Because the parental genotypes are unknown, offspring phenotypes may give clues as to what the parents' genotypes are. For example, if the first child has phenotype A-, this will identify both parental genotypes as A/a. Therefore, the second child (and each later child) has probability ¾ of being A+, which is different from Q unless $p = 0$.

Solution 3.3. Both L_1 and L_2 are correct likelihoods, but they refer to different sampling frames. L_1 is calculated for given birth order of the children, which is customary in human linkage analysis, as it is customary to calculate pedigree likelihoods for given sex of the pedigree members. L_2 refers to an event that comprises three different birth orders each of which has likelihood L_1. In calculations of likelihoods with respect to recombination fractions, one could use either L_1 or L_2. The constant factor between L_1 and L_2 cancels in the likelihood ratio usually formed.

Solution 3.4. Following formula $1 - \alpha^{1/n}$, with $n = 10$ and $\alpha = 0.10$, one finds a confidence interval of $(0, 0.206)$.

Solution 4.1. Yes, one should. However, in this case, the grandparental mating is a phase-unknown double backcross with only offspring. Hence, there is no information for linkage from that generation.

Solution 4.2. (1a) With $k = 1$ and $n = 5$, one has $\hat{\theta} = 1/5 = 0.20$. (1b) For unknown phase, the adjusted likelihood is $L^*(\theta) = 16[\theta(1 - \theta)^4 + \theta^4(1 - \theta)]$. Numerical evaluation of it with an accuracy to two decimal places in θ shows that its maximum, 1.3333, occurs at $\hat{\theta} = 0.21$. (2a) $\hat{\theta} = 1/4 = 0.25$. (2b) $L^*(\theta) = 8[\theta(1 - \theta)^3 + \theta^3(1 - \theta)]$ turns out to rise from 0 at $\theta = 0$ to a maximum at $\theta = 1/2$ so that the estimate of the recombination fraction is $\hat{\theta} = 1/2$.

Solution 4.3. The power of H_0 versus H_1 is given by $(1 - \theta)^{15}$. For $\theta = 0.01$, this yields a value of 0.86. For H_0 versus H_1, the power is given by $(1 - \theta_m)^7(1 - \theta_f)^6[1 + 7\theta_m(1 - 2\theta_f) + 6\theta_f]$. For $\theta = \theta_m = \theta_f$, this reduces to $(1 - \theta)^{14}(1 + 14\theta)$ and, for $\theta = 0.01$, results in 0.99.

Solution 4.4. For k recombinants in $n = 20$ meioses, Z_{max} is given by equation (4.11), and the upper bound to the significance level is given by $p_u = 10^{-Z_{max}}$ (4.10). The actual significance level p may be obtained using the BINOM program. This furnishes the following results:

k	Z_{max}	p_u	p
1	4.30	0.00005	0.00002
2	3.20	0.0006	0.0002
3	2.35	0.0045	0.0013
4	1.67	0.0212	0.0059
5	1.14	0.0731	0.0207

Solution 4.5. Sometimes, people are impressed by a strongly negative lod score. However, because it occurs at $\theta = 0$, the simple interpretation of this finding proceeds as follows. One or more known recombinants lead to a lod score of $-\infty$ at $\theta = 0$. A strongly negative lod score at $\theta = 0$ implies that almost certainly there was at least one recombinant in the data but, perhaps as a consequence of incomplete penetrance, one cannot tell for certain.

Solution 5.1. Parent 1 can produce only two types of gametes, *A1* and *B1,* with probability 1/2 each, because of the four possible gametes two each are undistinguishable. Analogously, parent 2 potentially produces gametes *C1* and *C2* with probability 1/2 each, because the two *C* cannot be distinguished. There are then four offspring genotypes, *A1/C1*, *A1/C2*, *B1/C1*, and *B1/C2*, with probabilities of occurrence of ¼ each. These probabilities do not contain θ (or r) so that no information on the recombination fraction is available.

Solution 5.2. The crucial fact in such ascertainment problems is that the lod scores $Z(\theta)$ used after selection are the same as the ones without selection, but the class probabilities change owing to selection (in other words, the lod scores used are no longer appropriate for the data conditional on ascertainment). When class 4 individuals are discarded, only individuals in classes 1 through 3 occur, the corresponding class probabilities being given by $f_i = p_i/(p_1 + p_2 + p_3)$, for example, $f_1 = (1 - r)^2/[1 + 2r(1 - r)]$. The expected lod score is then given by $\Sigma f_i Z_i(\theta)$. Work is simplified by omitting the "4" in each of the three lod scores—this will add a constant to the expected lod score but will not change the estimate of θ because the derivative of a constant is zero. Also, natural logs instead of decimal logs are preferable—this multiplies the equation by a constant factor that drops out when the derivative is set equal to zero. Once this is done, one may collect terms of θ so that the expected log likelihood is given by

$$\ln[L(\theta)] = (2f_1 + f_2)\ln(1 - \theta) + (f_2 + 2f_3)\ln(\theta).$$

The first derivative is obtained as

$$d\ln(L)/d\theta = (f_2 + 2f_3)/\theta - (2f_1 + f_2)/(1 - \theta).$$

Setting this equal to zero and solving the resulting equation for θ leads to $\tilde{\theta} = \frac{1}{2}f_2 + f_3$, which is the point of θ at which the expected log likelihood, or expected lod score, has its maximum. That it is a maximum rather than a minimum may be verified by showing that the second derivative with respect to θ is negative at $\theta = \tilde{\theta}$. Substituting the f_i by the corresponding expressions in r (true recombination fraction), one finds that $\tilde{\theta} = r(2 - r)/[1 + 2r(1 - r)]$, and this is larger than r except at $r = 0$ and $r = \frac{1}{2}$. Section 11.2 provides additional material on this case.

Solution 5.3. Proceeding as outlined in Section 5.5, you will find that for the offspring genotypes only two distinct probabilities occur. Using the numbering scheme of Table 5.3, combining phenotypes 1 + 3 + 5 + 7 + 9 leads to a class with associated probability of $2r(1 - r)$, which is the same as the probability for one of the two classes in the phase unknown double backcross with two offspring.

Solution 5.4. One finds the following three phenotype classes among the offspring where, for example, genotypes T/t or T/T lead to the dominant phenotype T, and q is the first derivative of p with respect to r:

Phenotype	p	q^2/p	$Z(\theta)$
T-D	$\frac{1}{4}(2 + r^2)$	$r^2/(2 + r^2)$	$\log[(4/9)(2 + \theta^2)]$
T-d, t-D	$\frac{1}{2}(1 - r^2)$	$2r^2/(1 - r^2)$	$\log[(4/3)(1 - \theta^2)]$
t-d	$\frac{1}{4}r^2$	1	$2\log(2\theta)$

	$r = 0$	0.1	0.2	0.3	0.4	0.5
$i(r)$	1	1.025	1.103	1.241	1.455	1.778
$E[Z(r)]$	0.037	0.032	0.022	0.011	0.003	0

The results presented in the preceding table show the unusual phenomenon that, for r approaching $\frac{1}{2}$, the expected lod score decreases (which is normal) while the expected information increases. Therefore, with data from this mating type, the recombination fraction estimate has smallest variance at $\theta = \frac{1}{2}$.

Solution 5.5. The second parent is $A1/A1$ or $A1/A2$ or $A2/A2$ with the respective unconditional frequencies p^2, $2p(1 - p)$, and $(1 - p)^2$. Given the first or third genotype of this parent, the ELOD is $E_1 = r\log(2r) + (1 - r)\log(2 - 2r)$. With genotype $A1/A2$, three offspring genotype classes exist, whose frequencies are $\frac{3}{4}(1 - r)$, $\frac{3}{4}r$, and $\frac{1}{4}$. The corresponding ELOD is $E_2 = \frac{3}{4}(1 - r)\log(2 - 2r) + \frac{3}{4}r\log(2r)$. The unconditional ELOD is thus obtained as $E(Z) = 2p(1 - p)E_2 + [1 - 2p(1 - p)]E_1$. This example shows a case in which gene frequencies enter the calculation of lod scores. Obviously, E_2 is smaller than E_1. The overall ELOD will be highest when the genotype $A1/A2$ of the second parent has low probability, and this is the case for small or high values of p.

Solution 5.6. Because each parent is doubly heterozygous (*1/2, 1/2*) with unknown phase, there are four possible phase combinations, each occurring with equal probability. For each phase combination, one computes the probability of the n offspring phenotypes (*1/2, 1/2*). For example, assuming genotypes *11/22* for both parents, one prepares a table whose marginals are given by the probabilities of the gametes (haplotypes) that each parent can produce. In the body of the table are the phenotype probabilities for one offspring.

	$P(11) = \frac{1}{2}(1 - \theta)$	$P(22) = \frac{1}{2}(1 - \theta)$	$P(12) = \frac{1}{2}\theta$	$P(21) = \frac{1}{2}\theta$
$P(11) = \frac{1}{2}(1 - \theta)$	0	$\frac{1}{4}(1 - \theta)^2$	0	0
$P(22) = \frac{1}{2}(1 - \theta)$	$\frac{1}{4}(1 - \theta)^2$	0	0	0
$P(12) = \frac{1}{2}\theta$	0	0	0	$\frac{1}{4}\theta^2$
$P(21) = \frac{1}{2}\theta$	0	0	$\frac{1}{4}\theta^2$	0

For this phase combination, the probability of a *1/2* offspring is thus $\frac{1}{2}(1 - \theta)^2 + \frac{1}{2}\theta^2$, and for *n* offspring it is this quantity raised to the *n*th power. It turns out that phase combination *12/12* × *12/12* yields the same offspring probabilities. For phase combinations *11/22* × *12/21* and *12/21* × *11/22*, one finds an offspring probability of $[\theta(1 - \theta)]^n$ each. After some manipulations the likelihood ratio is obtained as $L(\theta)/L(\frac{1}{2}) = 2^{n-1}\{[(1 - \theta)^2 + \theta^2]^n + [2\theta(1 - \theta)]^n\}$. At $\theta = 0$, this is equal to 2^{n-1}, which is equal to 1 for $n = 1$ and is larger than 1 for n > 1. Hence, the mating is uninformative for linkage with only one offspring but informative for linkage with more than one offspring.

Solution 5.7. For a phase-known double backcross family of size 6, with $r = 0.10$, the calculation of $E[Z(r)] = \Sigma_k Z(k; r)P(k)$ and $E(Z_{max}) = \Sigma_k Z_{max}(k)P(k)$ proceeds as shown in the following table:

k	$Z(0.10)$	Z_{max}	$P(k)$	$Z(0.1) \times P(k)$	$Z_{max} \times P(k)$
0	1.532	1.806	0.531441	0.814	0.960
1	0.577	0.632	0.354294	0.204	0.224
2	−0.377	0.148	0.098415	−0.037	0.014
3	−1.331	0	0.014580	−0.019	0
4	−2.285	0	0.001215	−0.003	0
5	−3.240	0	0.000054	−0.000	0
6	−4.194	0	0.000001	−0.000	0
			Weighted average	0.959	1.198

For a single family of size 3 (Table 5.1), one has ELOD = 0.480 and $E(Z_{max}) = 0.676$. Doubling these values for two families of size 3 each (one family of size 6) yields 2 × 0.480 = 0.960 for the ELOD, which is what the table above furnishes (the difference of 0.001 must be due to rounding errors), and 2 × 0.676 = 1.352 for $E(Z_{max})$, which is much larger than the correct value of 1.198.

Solution 6.1. Starting with $d\theta/dx = 1 - 4\theta^2$, one computes the second derivative (notice that θ is the function, not the variable with respect to which one differentiates), $d^2\theta/dx^2 = -8\theta(d\theta/dx) = -8\theta(1 - 4\theta^2) =$

$-8\theta + 32\theta^3$. From this, the third derivative is obtained as $d^3\theta/dx^3 = -8(dr/dx) + 96\theta^2(d\theta/dx) = (96\theta^2 - 8)(1 - 4\theta^2)$, which is equal to -8 for $\theta = 0$, violating condition (6.20) for multilocus feasibility.

Solution 6.2. A set of closely linked markers is required, with a marker being located at each chromosome end. No two adjacent loci must have a recombination fraction larger than, say, 10%. Then, the recombination fraction is essentially equal to the map distance, and the sum of all recombination fractions in the different intervals is equal to the total map length.

Solution 6.3. For the Haldane map function (use equation [6.11] with $\gamma = 1$), one finds $\theta_{AC} = 0.122$, and the Kosambi map function predicts (equation [6.16]) $\theta_{AC} = 0.128$. The difference between the two values is 0.006, corresponding to a relative difference of approximately 5%.

Solution 6.4. Using equation (1.9) or the MAPFUN program, one translates $\theta_{AB} = 0.05$ and $\theta_{BC} = 0.08$ into map distances, $x_{AB} = 0.0513$ and $x_{BC} = 0.0835$. The map distance over the two intervals is then $x_{AC} = x_{AB} + x_{BC} = 0.1348$, which is retransformed using equation (1.8) into $\theta_{AC} = 0.1257$. With this, equation (6.10) furnishes $\gamma = \frac{1}{2}(0.05 + 0.08 - 0.1257)/(0.05 \times 0.08) = 0.54$.

Solution 6.5. (1) This chromosome shows an average of 1.5 chiasmata. Because each chiasma leads to a crossover with probability $\frac{1}{2}$, the average number of crossovers is given by $1.5/2 = 0.75$. (2) Either by hand calculation or using the CROSSOVR program, one finds that 0, 1, and 2 crossovers occur with the respective probabilities 0.375, 0.500, and 0.125.

Solution 7.1. One needs to find that age, x, for which $F(x) = 0.80$. Through linear interpolation between $x_1 = 5$ and $x_2 = 40$, the 80% value of F is found at age $x = 5 + 0.80 \times (40 - 5) = 33$ years.

Solution 7.2. An easy way to solve problems such as this is by way of a "flow diagram" in which a succession of conditions and outcomes are listed. For each condition, all possible outcomes with their conditional probabilities are given. The relevant diagram for this and the next problem is shown in Figure 7.4. For part (a) of this problem, one focuses on the left side of the diagram, where y_1 is the desired probability that the woman is unaffected at age 80 given she is unaffected at age 60 and is susceptible.

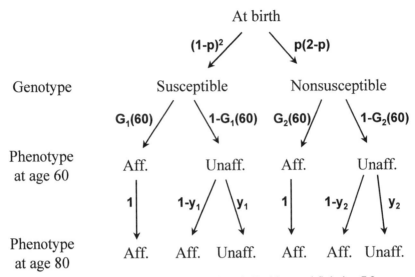

Figure 7.4. Diagram for risk calcuations in Problem and Solution 7.2.

Given susceptibility, her probability of being affected at age 80 is read off Figure 7.2 (Chapter 7) as 0.8 so that her probability of being unaffected at age 80 is 0.2. According to the left side of Figure 7.4, this is equal to $0.2 = [1 - G_1(60)]y_1$, which is solved for $y_1 = 0.2/[1 - G_1(60)]$. With $G_1(60) \approx 0.55$ from Figure 7.2, we find $y_1 = 0.2/0.45 = 0.44$. Analogously, if she is unsusceptible, we read off Figure 7.2, $G_2(60) \approx 0.04$ and know that she is affected at age 80 with probability ≈ 0.08. Thus, $1 - 0.08 = [1 - G_2(60)]y_2$ is solved for $y_2 = 0.92/0.96 = 0.96$.

Solution 7.3. If susceptibility status is not known (it usually is not), the desired probability cannot directly be obtained as above but only after the following first step: Let $U60$ and $U80$ denote the respective events that a woman is unaffected at ages 60 and 80. Following rules of conditional probability calculus, we write $P(U80|U60) = P(U80,U60)/P(U60)$. Note that $U80$ *and* $U60$ is the same thing as $U80$ so that $P(U80|U60) = P(U80)/P(U60)$. Numerator and denominator of this expression are now expanded as follows: $P(U80) = P(U80|\text{susceptible})P(\text{susceptible}) + P(U80|\text{nonsusceptible})P(\text{nonsusceptible})$. We know from Solution 7.2 that $P(U80|\text{susceptible}) = 0.20$. Also, with $p = 0.0033$ being the disease allele frequency, $P(\text{susceptible}) = 1 - (1 - p)^2 = p(2 - p) = 0.0066$. Thus, $P(U80) = 0.20 \times 0.0066 + 0.92 \times 0.9934 = 0.92$. Analogously, $P(U60) = (PU60|\text{susceptible})P(\text{susceptible}) + P(U60|\text{nonsusceptible})$

$P(\text{nonsusceptible}) = (1 - 0.55) \times 0.0066 + (1 - 0.04) \times 0.9934 = 0.9566$. Therefore, the desired probability is obtained as $P(U80)/P(U60) = 0.96$.

Solution 8.1. For these calculations, constant terms in $f(x)$ may be omitted so that one can write $f(x) = \exp(-\tfrac{1}{2}x^2) + \exp[-\tfrac{1}{2}(x - m)^2]$. The first derivative is calculated as $f'(x) = -x \exp(-\tfrac{1}{2}x^2) - (x - m) \exp[-\tfrac{1}{2}(x - m)^2]$. For the second derivative, evaluated at $x = \tfrac{1}{2}m$, one obtains the condition $f''(\tfrac{1}{2}m) = [-2 + 2(\tfrac{1}{2}m)^2] \exp[-\tfrac{1}{2}(\tfrac{1}{2}m)^2] > 0$. For finite m, the exponential term on the left of this inequality is nonzero so that one divides left and right sides by this term and finds $(\tfrac{1}{2}m)^2 > 1$ or $m > 2$ (or $m < -2$) as stated.

Solution 9.1. The lod score is $Z(\theta) = \log[2\theta^2 + 2(1 - \theta)^2]$.

Solution 9.2. With $p = 0$, one obtains $Z = \log[4\theta(1 - \theta)]$, and with $p = 1$, the lod score is $Z = 0$. In the latter case, none of the parents is doubly heterozygous; therefore, the mating is uninformative for linkage.

Solution 9.3. As usual, one makes a table of haplotypes produced by each parent. In case of mating type I, this yields a 4×4 table. Each cell contains an offspring genotype with associated probability of occurrence, which is the product of the frequencies of the haplotypes making up this genotype. Then one collects cells leading to the same phenotype. For type I, this results in eight offspring classes, four for affected and four for unaffected offspring. Combining offspring classes with equal frequencies into one class each reduces this list to six classes as follows:

Phenotype	Probability	Lod Score at $\theta = r$
Affected		
1/3	$(1 - r)^2/4$	$\log[4(1 - r)^2]$
2/3, 1/4	$r(1 - r)/2$	$\log[4r(1 - r)]$
2/4	$r^2/4$	$\log(4r^2)$
Unaffected		
1/3	$r(1 - r)/2 + r^2/4$	$\log[(8/3)r(1 - r) + (4/3)r^2]$
2/3, 1/4	$[r^2 + r(1 - r) + (1 - r)^2]/2$	$\log[(4/3)\{r^2 + r(1 - r) + (1 - r)^2\}]$
2/4	$r(1 - r)/2 + (1 - r)^2/4$	$\log[(8/3)r(1 - r) + (4/3)(1 - r)^2]$

For mating type II, only the haplotypes of the doubly heterozygous parent are relevant and lead to a table of four entries. Two each of these are equal so that only two probabilities need to be considered. Expected lod scores, E_I and E_{II}, are obtained as weighted averages of the lod scores, weighted by their probabilities occurrence. These ELODs represent linkage information per offspring. For n offspring, ELODs must be multiplied by n. For $n = 1$, at $r \approx 0$, one obtains $E_I = 0.2442$, $E_{II} = 0.3010$, and $E_I/E_{II} = 0.8112$ or $E_{II}/E_I = 1.23$. Thus, mating type II provides 23% more linkage information than mating type I even though only one parent is informative for linkage. At $r = 0.05$, the corresponding ratio increases to $E_{II}/E_I = 1.29$, and in the limit, $r \to 0.50$, $E_{II}/E_I \to 1.50$. So, mating type II is clearly better than I.

Solution 10.1. For each of the bolded likelihood values in Table 10.5, the value of α_3 is calculated from the values of α_1 and α_2. One finds that only the values 0, 0.05, and 0.10 occur. Hence, the 3.9-unit support interval for α_3 is given by (0, 0.10). With a 3-unit support interval, the following support intervals are found: (0.35, 0.70) for α_1, (0.30, 0.65) for α_2, and (0, 0.05) for α_3.

Solution 10.2. The standard errors of $\hat{\theta}$ at $\alpha = 0.9$ and 0.5 are equal to 0.060 and 0.151, respectively (Table 10.6). The increase in the number of observations required is given by the inverse of the ratio of the variances (Section 5.10), that is, by $(0.151/0.060)^2 = 6.3$. Hence, when $\alpha = 0.5$, 63 families furnish a θ estimate as precise as the one obtained from 10 families when $\alpha = 0.9$.

Solution 11.1. Because class 4 offspring (Table 5.4) are now taken to be double nonrecombinants each, their lod score is the same as that for class 1 individuals. Hence, one has the following three classes with their probabilities p of occurrence and associated lod scores Z:

Class	p	Z
1 + 4	$\frac{1}{2}r^2 + (1 - r)^2$	$\log(4) + 2 \times \log(1 - \theta)$
2	$2r(1 - r)$	$\log(4) + \log(\theta) + \log(1 - \theta)$
3	$\frac{1}{2}r^2$	$\log(4) + 2 \times \log(\theta)$

Computing the weighted average of Z over the three classes leads to $E_3 = \Sigma pZ = \log(4) + p_1\log(1 - \theta) + p_2\log(\theta)$ given in equation (11.3), where $p_1 = 1 + (1 - r)^2$ and $p_2 = r(2 - r)$. The derivative of E_3 with respect to θ is proportional to $(p_2/\theta) - p_1/(1 - \theta)$. Setting this equal to zero and solving for θ leads to $\tilde{\theta} = r(1 - \frac{1}{2}r)$. The asymptotic bias is equal to $b = \tilde{\theta} - r = -\frac{1}{2}r^2$.

Solution 11.2. From Table 11.3, a relative ELOD of 0.92 is read off. To obtain the same ELOD as if no misclassification were present, the number of offspring must be increased by a factor of $1/0.92 = 1.087$ or by close to 10%.

Solution 12.1. The penetrances, P(phenotype|genotype), are given in the table below (d = disease allele, n = normal allele):

Genotype		Female Phenotype			Male Phenotype	
Female	Male	CK High	CK Low	Unaffected[a]	Affected	Unaffected
n/n	n	0.05	0.95	1	0	1
n/d	d	0.70	0.30	1	1	0

[a]CK value unknown.

Solution 13.1. Consider disease alleles + (normal) and d (disease, dominant), and a marker with alleles *1, 2, 3, 4*. The two parents are assumed to have phase-known genotypes $d1/+2$ and $+3/+4$. Each parent passes one of the two haplotypes with probability ½ to each offspring. Thus, each sib has four equally likely genotypes: $d1/+3$, $d1/+4$, $+2/+3$, $+2/+4$. To inspect the genotypes of an ASP, form a 4 × 4 table with rows corresponding to genotypes of sib 1 and columns to genotypes of sib 2. Then only one quadrant (4 out of the 16 cells) corresponds to the situation that both offspring are affected. Two of these cells show one allele shared IBD and the other two cells show two alleles IBD. For example, with $d1/+3$ for sib 1 and $d1/+4$ for sib 2, only the *1* allele is shared.

Solution 13.2. The test statistic turns out to be $X = 2.4964$ so that $p = 0.0063$ (one-sided). For the marker tested (FGF3), some parents were evidently unavailable as the total number of parents scored was 301 versus $n = 119$ ASPs. For the mean test (parents scored), the p-value is obtained as 0.0046 which is better than the result for the minmax test. Presumably, this is largely due to the increased number of observations available to the mean test.

Solution 13.3. The sole effect of knowing the affection status of the first (untested) child is to make the parents unequivocally known to be heterozygous carriers of the CF gene. (1) Without marker typing, the unborn child has probability 1/4 of being homozygous for the CF gene. (2) With the marker types, each parent is a double heterozygote, phase unknown. The father has genotypes *CF B/+ C* or *CF C/+ B* (+ = normal allele), the mother is *CF A/+ B* or *CF B/+ A*. Based on Table 13.1, the first phase in the father has probability $2 \times 0.0173 \times 0.431 = 0.014913$, and the second phase has probability $2 \times 0.00056 \times 0.137 = 0.000153$. Because these are only two possibilities, their conditional probabilities of occurrence are obtained by scaling them so that they sum to 1, which yields 0.99 and 0.01. Analogously, the two phases of the mother have conditional probabilities of occurrence of 0.04 and 0.96. This result nicely demonstrates how different the phase probabilities can be under linkage disequilibrium (under linkage equilibrium they are ½ each). Without recombination, the parents have a child with *CF/CF* genotype only for phase I in the father and phase II in the mother. The probability that a child with marker typing *B/B* has cystic fibrosis is thus approximately obtained as $0.99 \times 0.96 = 0.95$.

Solution 13.4. (1) Each of the parents must have genotype *CF/N*, where *CF* stands for a disease allele and *N* denotes the normal allele. Their offspring is expected to have genotypes *CF/CF* (affected), *CF/N*, and *N/N* in the proportions ¼, ½, and ¼, respectively. The proband is known to be unaffected, so he can have only one of the latter genotypes. Hence, the conditional probability of being *CF/N* is obtained as ½/(½ + ¼) = ⅔. (2) This situation is easy to handle when one distinguishes two different *CF* (disease) alleles, *CFΔ* being the disease allele with the ΔF_{508} mutation and *CFm* being a disease allele other than *CFΔ*, where *CF* (=*CFΔ* or *CFm*) without an additional symbol represents any *CF* allele. One now writes down the possible genotypes for the proband, given that he is unaffected, as shown in Figure 13.4. Each arrow reflects a conditional probability given the situation indicated at the origin of the arrow.

As calculated under (1), the proband is *CF/N* with probability ⅔, and this *CF* allele is randomly picked from the population. Hence, with probability ¼ it is not equal to the ΔF_{508} mutation. The total probability of a *CFm/N* genotype is given by ⅔ × ¼ = ⅙. Also, the *N/N* genotype has probability of occurrence ⅓. Because these are the only two possible genotypes, normalizing their probabilities to sum to 1 yields a conditional probability of ⅓ of being a *CF* carrier, down from ⅔ without test for the ΔF_{508} mutation.

Solution 13.5. Following equation (13.9), the highest disequilibrium, $D = ¼$, is obtained for allele frequencies of ½ at each locus.

Solution 13.6. Haplotype frequencies in each population are as follows. *Population 1*: $P(AB) = 0.18$, $P(Ab) = 0.42$, $P(aB) = 0.12$,

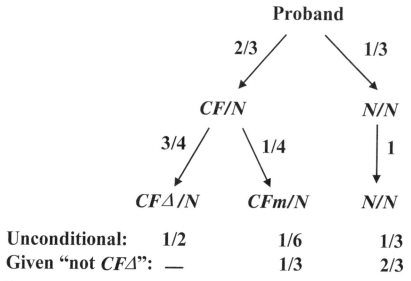

Figure 13.4. Scheme for calculating risk in Problem 13.4.

$P(ab) = 0.28$. *Population 2*: $P(AB) = 0.18$, $P(Ab) = 0.02$, $P(aB) = 0.72$, $P(ab) = 0.08$. Averaging haplotype frequencies leads to the following haplotype frequencies in the mixed population: $P(AB) = 0.18$, $P(Ab) = 0.22$, $P(aB) = 0.42$, $P(ab) = 0.18$. The resulting disequilibrium parameters are $D = -0.06$, $D_{min} = -0.24$, $D' = 0.25$. Thus, alleles A and B will be negatively associated.

Solution 14.1. At each locus, genotype probabilities are, for example, $P(dd) = p^2$, $P(nn) = (1 - p)^2$, $P(nd$ or $dd) = 1 - (1 - p)^2$. *Epistasis*: $K = f[1 - (1 - p)^2]^2 = f p^2(2 - p)^2$. *Heterogeneity*: $K = f p^2 + f p^2 - f p^4 = f p^2(2 - p^2)$. *Threshold*: $K = f[2 \times 2p(1 - p)p^2 + p^4] = f p^3(4 - 3p)$.

Solution 14.2. Genotype nd at locus 1: given dd at locus 2, the probability of being affected is 0.35. As dd at locus 2 occurs with probability $0.101^2 = 0.010$, the total probability of being affected is given by $0.35 \times 0.010 = 0.004$, which is the penetrance for the nd genotype at locus 1. For the dd genotype at locus 1, one obtains 0.067 as the penetrance. For genotypes nn, nd, and dd at locus 2, the respective penetrances are obtained as 0, 0.044, and 0.204. It is interesting that at both loci, the nd penetrance is approximately equal to the square of the dd penetrance. At each locus, the predicted trait prevalence (weighted sum of penetrances with genotype probabilities as weights) is equal to 0.01 as it should (this is what it is for the two-locus model). Both loci are intermediate between recessive and dominant.

Solution 15.1. Dominant trait: Assuming that the affected parent's mate is unaffected, the recurrence risk to an offspring is ½. Population prevalence is $K = 1 - (1 - p_d)^2 \approx 2p_d$ so that $\lambda = 1/(4p_d)$. With $K = 0.005$, one has $p_d = 0.0025$ and $\lambda = 100$. *Recessive trait*: Again, it is safe to assume that the affected parent's mate is unaffected. An unaffected individual has probability $2p_r/(1 + p_r)$ of being a heterozygous carrier and probability $(1 - p_r)/(1 + p_r)$ of not being a carrier. In the first case, the recurrence risk to the offspring is ½ (this is the probability with which the unaffected mate passes a disease allele), and in the second case it is 0. The weighted average of the recurrence risk turns out to be $p_r/(1 + p_r)$. With the population prevalence given by $K = p^2$, one obtains $\lambda = 1/[p_r(1 + p_r)] \approx 1/p_r$. For $K = 0.005$, one finds $p_r = 0.07$ and $\lambda = 14$.

Solution 15.2. The (remaining) risk ratio not accounted for by the two known IDDM loci is given by $15/(3.1 \times 1.3) = 3.722$. One needs the solution of $3.722 = (1.2)^n$, where n is the number of the remaining loci with a risk ratio of 1.2 each. One finds $n = \log(3.722)/\log(1.2) \approx 7$.

Solution 15.3. Consider genotypes *nn, nd, dd* with respective penetrances $f, f,$ and 1, and genotype probabilities $(1 - p)^2$, $2p(1 - p)$, and p^2. The population prevalence is given by $K = f(1 - p^2) + p^2$ so that $p = \sqrt{(K - f)/(1 - f)} = 0.2857$. With these values for penetrances $(f = 0.02)$ and allele frequencies, a pedigree file is created consisting of two parents and two offspring (sib 1 and sib 2). One may also define a marker locus with two alleles with everybody having the same homozygous marker genotype as some linkage programs do not run with just one locus, but the locus is not used here in any way. At the disease locus, all individuals are coded as having "unknown" phenotype except sib 1 who is affected. Make certain that sib 2 (possibly the last person in the pedigree list) is flagged as being the "proband" (the LINKAGE programs designate that person as the proband for whom risk calculations are done). For genotypes *nn, nd,* and *dd* of sib 2, the MLINK program will calculate the respective risks (genotype risks!) 0.2041, 0.4490, and 0.3469. Now, these numbers are used to compute the probability that sib 2 is affected, that is, a weighted average of the penetrances with weights being given by the genotype probabilities (risks). One obtains $(0.2041 + 0.4490) \times 0.02 + 0.3469 = 0.3600$, which is the recurrence risk to sib 2. Division by the population trait prevalence of 0.10 leads to the result, $\lambda_s = 3.60$. With $f = 0$ (no phenocopies), one obtains $\lambda_s = 4.27$.

References

Akaike H. 1985. Prediction and entropy. In *A Celebration of Statistics. The ISI Centenary Volume,* edited by AC Atkinson, SE Fienberg. New York: Springer, pp 1–24

Ala-Kokko L, Baldwin CT, Moskowitz RW, Prockop DJ. 1990. Single base mutation in the type II procollagen gene (COL2A1) as a cause of primary osteoarthritis associated with a mild chondrodysplasia. *Proc Natl Acad Sci USA* 87:6565–6568

Allison DB. 1997. Transmision–disequilibrium tests for quantitative traits. *Am J Hum Genet* 60:676–690

Allison DB, Heo M, Schork NJ, Wong S-L, Elston RC. 1998. Extreme selection strategies in gene mapping studies of oligogenic quantitative traits do not always increase power. *Hum Hered* 48:97–107

Almasy L, Blangero J. 1998. Multipoint quantitative-trait linkage analysis in general pedigrees. *Am J Hum Genet* 62:1198–1211

Amos CI. 1994. Robust variance-components approach for assessing genetic linkage in pedigrees. *Am J Hum Genet* 54:535–543

Amos CI, Elston RC, Bonney GE, Keats BJB, Berenson GS. 1990. A multivariate method for detecting genetic linkage, with application to a pedigree with an adverse lipoprotein phenotype. *Am J Hum Genet* 47:247–254

Anderson S, Bankier AT, Barrell BG, de Bruijin MHL, Coulson AR, Drouin J, Eperon IC, Nierlich DP, Rose BA, Sanger F, Schreier PH, Smith AJH, Staden R, Young IG. 1981. Sequence and organization for the human mitochondrial genome. *Nature* 290:457–465

Angrist M, Jing S, Bolk S, Bentley K, Nallasamy S, Halushka M, Fox GM, Chakravarti A. 1998. Human GFRA1: Cloning, mapping, genomic structure, and evaluation as a candidate gene for Hirschsprung disease susceptibility. *Genomics* 48:354–362

Armitage P, Berry G. 1987. *Statistical Methods in Medical Research.* Oxford: Blackwell

Arnheim N, Li H, Cui X. 1990. Review: PCR analysis of DNA sequences in single cells: Single sperm gene mapping and genetic disease diagnosis. *Genomics* 8:415–419

Arveiler B, de Saint-Basile G, Fischer A, Griscelli C, Mandel JL. 1990. Germ-line mosaicism simulates genetic heterogeneity in Wiscott–Aldrich syndrome. *Genomics* 46:906–911

Ayala FJ. 1997. Vagaries of the evolutionary clock. *Proc Natl Acad Sci USA* 94:7776–7783

Bailey NTJ. 1961. *Introduction to the Mathematical Theory of Genetic Linkage.* Oxford: Clarendon Press

Barcellos LF, Klitz W, Field LL, Tobias R, Bowcock AM, Wilson T, Nelson MP, Nagatomi J, Thomson G. 1997. Association mapping of disease loci, by use of a pooled DNA genomic screen. *Am J Hum Genet* 61:734–747

Barnard GA. 1949. Statistical inference. *J Roy Statist Soc* B11:115–139

Barr CL, Sandor P. 1998. Current status of genetic studies of Gilles de la Tourette syndrome. *Can J Psychiatry* 43:351–357

Barratt RW, Newmeyer D, Perkins DD, Garnjobst L. 1954. Map construction in *Neurospora*. *Adv Genet* 6:1–93

Bateson W. 1913. *Mendel's Principles of Heredity*. Cambridge: Cambridge University Press

Baur MP, Elston RC, Gurtler H, Henningsen K, Hummel K, Matsumoto H, Mayr W, Morris JW, Niejenhuis L, Polesky H, Salmon D, Valentin J, Walkers R. 1986. No fallacies in the formulation of the paternity index. *Am J Hum Genet* 39:528–536

Beaudet AL, Feldman GL, Fernbach SD, Buffone GH, O'Brien WE. 1989. Linkage disequilibrium, cystic fibrosis, and genetic counseling. *Am J Hum Genet* 44:319–326

Bell J, Haldane JBS. 1937. The linkage between the genes for colour-blindness and haemophilia in man. *Proc Roy Soc Ser B* 123:119–150

Bennett JH, Rhodes RA, Robson HN. 1959. A possible genetic basis for kuru. *Am J Hum Genet* 11:169–187

Berg K, Heiberg A. 1976. Linkage studies on familial hyperlipoproteinemia with xanthomatosis: Normal lipoprotein markers and the C3 polymorphism. *Cytogenet Cell Genet* 16:266–270

——. 1978. Linkage between familial hypercholesterolemia with xanthomatosis and the C3 polymorphism confirmed. *Cytogenet Cell Genet* 22:621–623

Bernstein F. 1931. Zur Grundlegung der Chromosomentheorie der Vererbung beim Menschen. *Z Abst Vererb* 57:113–138

Bhat A, Heath SC, and Ott J. 1999. Heterogeneity for multiple disease loci in linkage analysis. *Hum Hered* (in press)

Bickeböller H, Clerget-Darpoux F. 1995. Statistical properties of the allelic and genotypic transmission/disequilibrium test for multiallelic markers. *Genet Epidemiol* 12:865–870

Bird TD, Kraft GH. 1978. Charcot–Marie–Tooth disease: Data for genetic counseling relating age to risk. *Clin Genet* 14:43–49

Bishop DT. 1985. The information content of phase-known matings for ordering genetic loci. *Genet Epidemiol* 2:349–361

Bishop DT, Williamson JA. 1990. The power of identity-by-state methods for linkage analysis. *Am J Hum Genet* 46:254–265

Blackwelder WC, Elston RC. 1985. A comparison of sib-pair linkage tests for disease susceptibility loci. *Genet Epidemiol* 2:85–97

Bodmer WF. 1986. Human genetics: The molecular challenge. *Cold Spring Harb Symp Quant Biol* 51:1–13

Bodmer WF, Bailey CJ, Bodmer J, Bussey HJR, Ellis A, Gorman P, Lucibello FC, Murday VA, Rider SH, Scambler P, Sheer D, Solomon E, and Spurr NK. 1987. Localization of the gene for familial adenomatous polyposis on chromosome 5. *Nature* 328:614–616

Boehnke M. 1986. Estimating the power of a proposed linkage study: A practical computer simulation approach. *Am J Hum Genet* 39:513–527

———. 1991. Allele frequency estimation from data on relatives. *Am J Hum Genet* 48:22–25

Boehnke M, Arnheim N, Li H, Collins FS. 1989. Fine structure genetic mapping of human chromosomes using the polymerase chain reaction on single sperm: Experimental design considerations. *Am J Hum Genet* 45:21–32

Boehnke M, Cox NJ. 1997. Accurate inference of relationships in sib-pair linkage studies. *Am J Hum Genet* 61:423–429

Bolling DR, Murphy EA. 1979. Finite sample properties of maximum likelihood estimates of the recombination fraction in double backcross matings in man. *Am J Med Genet* 3:81–95

Bonney GE. 1984. On the statistical determination of major gene mechanisms in continuous human traits: Regressive models. *Am J Med Genet* 18:731–749

———. 1992. Compound regressive models for family data. *Hum Hered* 42:28–41

Botstein D, White RL, Skolnick MH, Davies RW. 1980. Construction of a genetic linkage map in man using restriction fragment length polymorphisms. *Am J Hum Genet* 32:314–331

Box GEP, Cox DR. 1964. An analysis of transformation. *J Roy Statist Soc* 26B: 211–252

Brenner S. 1990. The human genome: The nature of the enterprise. *Ciba Found Symp* 149:6–12

Brookfield JFY. 1989. Analysis of DNA fingerprinting data in cases of disputed paternity. *IMA J Math Appl Med & Biol* 6:111–131

Brzustowicz LM, Honer WG, Chow EW, Hogan J, Hodgkinson K, Bassett AS. 1997. Use of a quantitative trait to map a locus associated with severity of positive symptoms in familial schizophrenia to chromosome 6p. *Am J Hum Genet* 61:1388–1396

Brzustowicz LM, Lehner T, Castilla LH, Penchaszadeh GK, Wilhelmsen KC, Daniels R, Davies KE, Leppert M, Ziter F, Wood D, Dubowitz V, Zerres K, Hausmanowa-Petrusewicz I, Ott J, Munsat TL, Gilliam TC. 1990. Genetic mapping of chronic childhood-onset spinal muscular atrophy to chromosome 5q11.2-12.3. *Nature* 344:540–541

Brzustowicz LM, Mérette C, Xie X, Townsend L, Gilliam TC, Ott J. 1993. Molecular and statistical approaches to the detection and correction of errors in genotype databases. *Am J Hum Genet* 53:1137–1145

Buetow KH. 1991. Influence of aberrant observations on high-resolution linkage analysis outcomes. *Am J Hum Genet* 49:985–994

Bulle F, Chiannilkulchai N, Pawlak A, Weissenbach J, Gyapay G, Guellaën G. 1997. Identification and chromosomal localization of human genes containing CAG/CTG repeats expressed in testis and brain. *Genome Res* 7:705–715

Cann RL, Stoneking M, Wilson AC. 1987. Mitochondrial DNA and human evolution. *Nature* 325:31–36

Cannings C, Thompson EA. 1977. Ascertainment in the sequential sampling of pedigrees. *Clin Genet* 12:208–212

Cannings C, Thompson EA, Skolnick MH. 1978. Probability functions on complex pedigrees. *Adv Appl Prob* 10:26–61

Cannon-Albright LA, Skolnick MH. 1996. The genetics of familial breast cancer. *Semin Oncol* 23(suppl 2):1–5

Cantor RM, Rotter JI. 1986. Sample-size considerations and strategies for linkage analysis in autosomal recessive disorders. *Am J Hum Genet* 39:25–37

Carter TC, Falconer DS. 1951. Stocks for detecting linkage in the mouse and the theory of their design. *J Genet* 50:307–323

Cassidy SB, Schwartz S. 1998. Prader–Willi and Angelman syndromes. Disorders of genomic imprinting. *Medicine (Baltimore)* 77:140–151

Cavalli-Sforza LL. 1990. Cultural transmission and nutrition. In *Genetic Variation and Nutrition,* edited by AP Simopoulos, B Childs. Basel: Karger, pp 35–48

Cavalli-Sforza LL, Bodmer WF. [1971] 1977. *The Genetics of Human Populations.* Paperback reprint. San Francisco: Freeman

Cavalli-Sforza LL, King MC. 1986. Detecting linkage for genetically heterogeneous diseases and detecting heterogeneity with linkage data. *Am J Hum Genet* 38:599–616

Ceppellini R, Siniscalco M, Smith CAB. 1955. The estimation of gene frequencies in a random-mating population. *Ann Hum Genet* 20:97–115

Chakraborty R. 1987. Further consideration of difficulties of estimating familial risks from pedigree data. *Hum Hered* 37:222–228

Chakraborty R, Kimmel M, Stivers DN, Davison LJ, Deka R. 1997. Relative mutation rates at di-, tri-, and tetranucleotide microsatellite loci. *Proc Natl Acad Sci USA* 94:1041–1046

Chakravarti A, Badner JA, Li CC. 1987. Tests of linkage and heterogeneity in Mendelian diseases using identity by descent scores. *Genet Epidemiol* 4:255–266

Chakravarti A, Li CC, Buetow KH. 1984. Estimation of the marker gene frequency and linkage disequilibrium from conditional marker data. *Am J Hum Genet* 36:177–186

Chakravarti A, Slaugenhaupt SA. 1987. Methods for studying recombination on chromosomes that undergo nondisjunction. *Genomics* 1:35–42

Chen WJ, Faraone SV, Orav EJ, Tsuang MT. 1993. Estimating age at onset distributions: The bias from prevalent cases and its impact on risk estimation. *Genet Epidemiol* 10:43–59

Cheung VG, Gregg JP, Gogolin-Ewens KJ, Bandong J, Stanley CA, Baker L, Higgins MJ, Nowak NJ, Shows TB, Ewens WJ, Nelson SF, Spielman RS. 1998. Linkage-disequilibrium mapping without genotyping. *Nat Genet* 18:255–230

Cheung VG, Nelson SF. 1998. Genomic mismatch scanning identifies human genomic DNA shared identical by descent. *Genomics* 47:1–6

Chiano MN, Yates JRW. 1995. Linkage detection under heterogeneity and the mixture problem. *Ann Hum Genet* 59:83–95

Chotai J. 1984. On the lod score method in linkage analysis. *Ann Hum Genet* 48:359–378

Claus EB, Risch N, Thompson WD. 1991. Genetic analysis of breast cancer in the cancer and steroid hormone study. *Am J Hum Genet* 48:232–242

Claverie J-M. 1997. Computational methods for the identification of genes in vertebrate genomic sequences. *Hum Mol Genet* 6:1735–1744

Clerget-Darpoux FM. 1982. Bias of the estimated recombination fraction and lod score due to an association between a disease gene and a marker. *Ann Hum Genet* 46:363–372

Clerget-Darpoux F, Babron M-C, Bonaïti-Pellié C. 1987. Power and robustness of the linkage homogeneity test in genetic analysis of common disorders. *J Psychiatr Res* 21:625–630

———. 1990. Assessing the effect of multiple linkage tests in complex diseases. *Genet Epidemiol* 7:245–253

Clerget-Darpoux F, Babron MC, Prum B, Lathrop GM, Deschamps I, Hors J. 1988. A new method to test genetic models in HLA associated diseases: The MASC method. *Ann Hum Genet* 52:247–258

Clerget-Darpoux F, Bonaïti-Pellié C, Hochez J. 1986. Effects of misspecifying genetic parameters in lod score analysis. *Biometrics* 42:393–399

Cleves MA, Elston RC. 1997. Alternative test for linkage between two loci. *Genet Epidemiol* 14:117–131

Cockerham CC, Weir BS. 1983. Linkage between a marker locus and a quantitative trait of sibs. *Am J Hum Genet* 35:263–273

Cohen J. 1990. Things I have learned (so far). *Amer Psychol* 45:1304–1312

Cohen JE. 1976. The distribution of the chi-squared statistic under clustered sampling from contingency tables. *J Am Statist Assoc* 71:665–670

Collins A, Frézal J, Teague J, Morton NE. 1996a. A metric map of humans: 23,500 loci in 850 bands. *Proc Natl Acad Sci USA* 93:14771–14775

Collins A, Morton NE. 1995. Nonparametric tests for linkage with dependent sib pairs. *Hum Hered* 45:311–318

Collins A, Teague J, Keats BJ, Morton NE. 1996b. Linkage map integration. *Genomics* 36:157–162

Collins FS. 1995. Positional cloning moves from perditional to traditional. *Nat Genet* 9:347–350

Collins FS, Guyer MS, Chakravarti A. 1997. Variations on a theme: Cataloging human DNA sequence variation. *Science* 278:1580–1581

Comuzzie AG, Allison DB. 1998. The search for human obesity genes. *Science* 280:1374–1377

Comuzzie AG, Mahaney MC, Almasy L, Dyer TD, Blangero J. 1997. Exploiting pleiotropy to map genes for oligogenic phenotypes using extended pedigree data. *Genet Epidemiol* 14:975–980

Conneally PM, Edwards JH, Kidd KK, Lalouel J-M, Morton NE, Ott J, White R. 1985. Report of the committee on methods of linkage analysis and reporting. *Cytogenet Cell Genet* 40:356–359

Cook PJL, Robson EB, Buckton KE, Jacobs PA, Polani PE. 1974. Segregation of genetic markers in families with chromosome polymorphisms and structural rearrangements involving chromosome 1. *Ann Hum Genet* 37:261–274

Cooper HL, Hernits R. 1963. A familial chromosome variant in a subject with anomalous sex differentiation. *Am J Hum Genet* 15:465–475

Cotterman CW. 1969. Factor-union phenotype systems. In *Computer Applications in Genetics,* edited by NE Morton. Honolulu: University of Hawaii Press, pp 1–19

Crow JF. 1966. The quality of people: Human evolutionary changes. *Bioscience* 16:863–867

Curtis D, Sham PC. 1995a. Model-free linkage analysis using likelihoods. *Am J Hum Genet* 57:703–716

———. 1995b. A note on the application of the transmission disequilibrium test when a parent is missing. *Am J Hum Genet* 56:811–812

Dao D, Frank D, Qian N, O'Keefe D, Vosatka RJ, Walsh CP, Tycko B. 1998. IMPT1, an imprinted gene similar to polyspecific transporter and multi-drug resistance genes. *Hum Mol Genet* 7:597–608

Dausset J, Cann H, Cohen D, Lathrop M, Lalouel J-M, White R. 1990. Centre d'Etude du Polymorphisme Humain (CEPH): Collaborative genetic mapping of the human genome. *Genomics* 6:575–577

Davies JL, Kawaguchi Y, Bennett ST, Copeman JB, Cordell HJ, Pritchard LE, Reed PW, Gough SC, Jenkins SC, Palmer SM, Balfour KM, Rowe BR, Farrall M, Barnett AH, Bain SC, Todd JA. 1994. A genome-wide search for human type 1 diabetes susceptibility genes. *Nature* 371:130–136

Davies K. 1990. Complimentary endeavours. *Nature* 348:110–111

Davis S, Schroeder M, Goldin LR, Weeks DE. 1996. Nonparametric simulation-based statistics for detecting linkage in general pedigrees. *Am J Hum Genet* 58:867–880

Davis S, Weeks DE. 1997. Comparison of nonparametric statistics for the detection of linkage in nuclear families: Single-marker evaluation. *Am J Hum Genet* 61:1431–1444

Defrise-Gussenhoven E. 1962. Hypothèses de dimérie et de non-pénétrance. *Acta Genet (Basel)* 12:65–96

Deka R, Chakravarti A, Surti U, Hauselman E, Reefer J, Majumder PP, Ferrell RE. 1990. Genetics and biology of human ovarian teratomas. II. Molecular analysis of origin of nondisjunction and gene-centromere mapping of chromosome I markers. *Am J Hum Genet* 47:644–655

Dempster AP, Laird NM, Rubin DB. 1977. Maximum likelihood from incomplete data via the EM algorithm. *J Roy Statist Soc* 39B:1–38

Dib C, Faure S, Fizames C, Samson D, Drouot N, Vignal A, Millasseau P, Marc S, Hazan J, Seboun E, Lathrop M, Gyapay G, Morissette J, Weissenbach J. 1996. A comprehensive genetic map of the human genome based on 5,264 microsatellites. *Nature* 380:152–154

Dizier M-H, Babron M-C, Clerget-Darpoux F. 1996. Conclusions of LOD-score analysis for family data generated under two-locus models. *Am J Hum Genet* 58:1338–1346

Dobbie Z, Heinimann K, Bishop DT, Müller H, Scott RJ. 1997. Identification of a modifier gene locus on chromosome 1p35-36 in familial adenomatous polyposis. *Hum Genet* 99:653–657

Donahue RP, Bias WB, Renwick JH, McKusick VA. 1968. Probable assignment of the Duffy blood group locus to chromosome 1 in man. *Proc Natl Acad Sci USA* 61:949–955

Donis-Keller H, Green P, Helms C, Cartinhour S, Weiffenbach B, Stephens K, Keith TP, Bowden DW, Smith DR, Lander ES, Botstein D, Akots G, Rediker KS, Gravius T, Brown VA, Rising MB, Parker C, Powers JA, Watt DE, Kauffman ER, Bricker A, Phipps P, Muller-Kahle H, Fulton TR, Ng S, Schumm JW, Braman JC, Knowlton RG, Barker DF, Crooks SM, Lincoln SE, Daly MJ, Abrahamson J. 1987. A genetic linkage map of the human genome. *Cell* 51:319–337

Dorn CR, Schneider R. 1976. Inbreeding and canine mammary cancer: A retrospective study. *J Natl Cancer Inst* 57:545–548

Dubay C, Vincent M, Samani NJ, Hilbert P, Kaiser MA, Beressi JP, Kotelevtsev Y, Beckmann JS, Soubrier F, Sassard J, Lathrop GM. 1993. Genetic determinants of diastolic and pulse pressure map to different loci in Lyon hypertensive rats. *Nat Genet* 3:354–357

Dupuis J, Brown PO. Siegmund D. 1995. Statistical methods for linkage analysis of complex traits from high-resolution maps of identity by descent. *Genetics* 140: 843–856

Durham LK, Feingold E. 1997. Genome scanning for segments shared identical by descent among distant relatives in isolated populations. *Am J Hum Genet* 61:830–842

Durner M, Greenberg DA, Hodge SE. 1992. Inter- and intrafamilial heterogeneity: Effective sampling strategies and comparison of analysis methods. *Am J Hum Genet* 51:859–870

———. 1996. Phenocopies versus genetic heterogeneity: Can we use phenocopy frequencies in linkage analysis to compensate for heterogeneity? *Hum Hered* 46:265–273

Dyck PJ, Ott J, Moore SB, Swanson CJ, Lambert EH. 1983. Linkage evidence for genetic heterogeneity among kinships with hereditary motor and sensory neuropathy type 1. *Mayo Clin Proc* 58:430–435

Easton DF, Bishop DT, Ford D, Crockford GP. 1993. Genetic linkage analysis in familial breast and ovarian cancer: Results from 214 families. The Breast Cancer Linkage Consortium. *Am J Hum Genet* 52:678–701

Edwards AWF. 1989. Probability and likelihood in genetic counselling. *Clin Genet* 36:209–216

———. 1992. *Likelihood,* expanded edition. Baltimore, Maryland: Johns Hopkins University Press

———. 1996. The early history of the statistical estimation of linkage. *Ann Hum Genet* 60:237–249

Edwards JH. 1960. The simulation of Mendelism. *Acta Genet* 10:63–70

———. 1971. The analysis of X-linkage. *Ann Hum Genet* 34:229–259

———. 1972. Linkage studies. In *Perspectives of Cytogenetics: The Next Decade,* edited by SW Wright, BF Crandall, L Boyer. Springfield, Illinois: Charles C Thomas, pp 97–114

———. 1976. The interpretation of lod scores in linkage analysis. *Cytogenet Cell Genet* 16:289–293

———. 1980. Allelic association in man. In *Population Structure and Genetic Disorders,* edited by AW Ericksson, HR Forsius, HR Nevanlinna, PL Workman, RK Norio. New York: Academic Press, pp 239–255

———. 1987. Exclusion mapping. *J Med Genet* 24:539–543

———. 1989a. The locus positioning problem. *Ann Hum Genet* 53:271–275

———. 1989b. Familiarity, recessivity and germline association. *Ann Hum Genet* 53:33–47

Efron B. 1982. *The Jacknife, the Bootstrap and Other Resampling Plans.* CBMS-NSF Regional Conference Series in Applied Mathematics, Monograph 38. Philadelphia: SIAM

Elandt-Johnson RC. 1971. *Probability Models and Statistical Methods in Genetics.* New York: Wiley

Elmslie FV, Rees M, Williamson MP, Kerr M, Kjeldsen MJ, Pang KA, Sundqvist A, Friis ML, Chadwick D, Richens A, Covanis A, Santos M, Arzimanoglou A,

Panayiotopoulos CP, Curtis D, Whitehouse WP, Gardiner RM. 1997. Genetic mapping of a major susceptibility locus for juvenile myoclonic epilepsy on chromosome 15q. *Hum Mol Genet* 6:1329–1334

Elston RC. 1973. Ascertainment and age of onset in pedigree analysis. *Hum Hered* 23:105–112

———. 1994. *P* values, power, and pitfalls in the linkage analysis of psychiatric disorders. In *Genetic Approaches to Mental Disorders,* edited by ES Gershon and CR Cloninger. Washington, DC: American Psychiatric Press, pp 3–21

Elston RC, George VT, Severtson F. 1992. The Elston–Stewart algorithm for continuous genotypes and environmental factors. *Hum Hered* 42:16–27

Elston RC, Johnson WD. 1994. *Essentials of Biostatistics,* 2nd edition. Philadelphia: Davis

Elston RC, Lange K. 1975. The prior probability of autosomal linkage. *Ann Hum Genet* 38:341–350

Elston RC, Lange K, Namboodiri KK. 1976. Age trends in human chiasma frequencies and recombination fractions. II. Method for analyzing recombination fractions and applications to the ABO:Nail–Patella linkage. *Am J Hum Genet* 28:69–76

Elston RC, Namboodiri KK, Go RCP, Siervogel RM, Glueck CJ. 1976. Probable linkage between essential familial hypercholesterolemia and third complement (C3). *Cytogenet Cell Genet* 16:294–297

Elston RC, Stewart J. 1971. A general model for the analysis of pedigree data. *Hum Hered* 21:523–542

Engel E. 1980. A new concept: Uniparental disomy and its potential effect, isodisomy. *Am J Med Genet* 6:137–143

Evans SN, McPeek MS, Speed TP. 1993. A characterisation of crossover models that possess map functions. *Theoret Popul Biol* 43:80–90

Ewens WJ. 1991. Ascertainment biases and their resolution in biological surveys. In *Handbood of Statistics, Volume 8,* edited by CR Rao and R Chakraborty. New York: Elsevier, pp 29–61

Fain PR, Wright E, Willard HF, Stephens K, Barker DF. 1989. The order of loci in the pericentric region of chromosome 17, based on evidence from physical and genetic breakpoints. *Am J Hum Genet* 44:68–72

Falk CT, Edwards JH. 1970. A computer approach to the analysis of family genetic data for detection of linkage. *Genetics* 64:s18

Falk CT, Rubinstein P. 1987. Haplotype relative risks: An easy reliable way to construct a proper control sample for risk calculations. *Ann Hum Genet* 51:227–233

Fann CSJ, Ott J. 1995. Parsimonious estimation of sex-specific map distances by stepwise maximum likelihood regression. *Genomics* 29:571–575

Faraway JJ. 1993. Distribution of the admixture test for the detection of linkage under heterogeneity. *Genet Epidemiol* 10:75–83

Feingold E, Siegmund DO. 1997. Strategies for mapping heterogeneous recessive traits by allele-sharing methods. *Am J Hum Genet* 60:965–978

Feller WF. 1968. *An Introduction to Probability Theory and Its Applications, Vol I,* 3rd edition. New York: Wiley

Felsenstein J. 1979. A mathematically tractable family of genetic mapping functions with different amounts of interference. *Genetics* 91:769–775

Ferguson-Smith MA, Ellis PM, Mutchinick O, Glen KP, Côté GB, Edwards JH. 1975. Centromeric linkage. *Cytogenet Cell Genet* 14:300–307

Fijneman RJ, de Vries SS, Jansen RC, Demant P. 1996. Complex interactions of new quantitative trait loci, Sluc1, Sluc2, Sluc3, and Sluc4, that influence the susceptibility to lung cancer in the mouse. *Nat Genet* 14:465–467

Fisher E, Scambler P. 1994. Human haploinsufficiency—One for sorrow, two for joy. *Nat Genet* 7:5–7

Fisher RA, 1922a. On the mathematical foundations of theoretical statistics. *Phil Trans Roy Soc* A202:309–368

———. 1922b. The systematic location of genes by means of crossover observations. *Amer Naturalist* 56:406–411

———. 1925. Theory of statistical estimation. *Proc Camb Phil Soc* 22:700–725

———. 1935a. The detection of linkage with dominant abnormalities. *Ann Eugen* 6:187–201

———. 1935b. The detection of linkage with recessive abnormalities. *Ann Eugen* 6:339–351

———. 1954. The experimental study of multiple crossing-over. *Caryologia* 6(suppl):227–231

———. 1960. *The Design of Experiments.* Edinburgh: Oliver & Boyd

———. 1970. *Statistical Methods for Research Workers,* 14th edition. New York: Hafner Press

Fishman PM, Suarez B, Hodge SE, Reich T. 1978. A robust method for the detection of linkage in familial diseases. *Am J Hum Genet* 30:308–321

Folstein SE. 1989. *Huntington's Disease.* Baltimore: Johns Hopkins University Press

Frankel WN, Schork NJ. 1996. Who's afraid of epistasis? *Nat Genet* 14:371–373

Freimer NB, Sandkuijl LA, Blower SM. 1993. Incorrect specification of marker allele frequencies: Effects of linkage analysis. *Am J Hum Genet* 52:1102–1110

Fulker DW, Cardon LR. 1994. A sib-pair approach to interval mapping of quantitative trait loci. *Am J Hum Genet* 54:1092–1103

Gajdusek DC, Gibbs CJ, Alpers M. 1966. Experimental transmission of a kuru-like syndrome to chimpanzees. *Nature* 209:794–796

Gangloff S, Lieber MR, Rothstein R. 1994. Transcription, topoisomerases and recombination. *Experientia* 50:261–269

Gedde-Dahl T Jr, Fagerhol MK, Cook PJL, Noades J. 1972. Autosomal linkage between the Gm and Pi loci in man. *Ann Hum Genet* 35:393–399

Gelb BD, Willner JP, Dunn TM, Kardon NB, Verloes A, Poncin J, Desnick RJ. 1998. Paternal uniparental disomy for chromosome 1 revealed by molecular analysis of a patient with pycnodysostosis. *Am J Hum Genet* 62:848–854

Génin E, Clerget-Darpoux F. 1996. Association studies in consanguineous populations. *Am J Hum Genet* 58:861–866

Gilliam TC, Brzustowicz LM, Castilla LH, Lehner T, Penchaszadeh GK, Daniels RJ, Byth BC, Knowles J, Hislop JE, Shapira Y, Dubowitz V, Munsat TL, Ott J, Davies KE. 1990. Genetic homogeneity between acute and chronic forms of spinal muscular atrophy. *Nature* 345:823–825

Giver CR, Grosovsky AJ. 1997. Single and coincident intragenic mutations attributable to gene conversion in a human cell line. *Genetics* 146:1429–1439

Goldgar DR, Fain PR. 1988. Models of multilocus recombination: Nonrandomness in chiasma number and crossover positions. *Am J Hum Genet* 43:38–45

Goldgar DR, Fain PR, Kimberling WJ. 1989. Chiasma-based models of multilocus recombination: Increased power for exclusion mapping and gene ordering. *Genomics* 5:283–290

Goldgar DR, Green P, Parry DM, Mulvihill JJ. 1989. Multipoint linkage analysis in Neurofibromatosis type I: An international collaboration. *Am J Hum Genet* 44:6–12

Goldstein M, Dillon WR. 1978. *Discrete Discriminant Analysis.* New York: Wiley

Goldstein DR, Zhao H, Speed TP. 1997. The effects of genotyping errors and interference on estimation of genetic distance. *Hum Hered* 47:86–100

González-Pastor JR, San Millán JL, Moreno F. 1994. The smallest gene known. *Nature* 369:281

Goodfellow P. 1995. Complementary endeavours. *Nature* 377:285–286

Gordon D, Heath S, Ott J. 1999. True pedigree errors more frequent than apparent errors for single nucleotide polymorphisms. *Hum Hered* (in press)

Göring HH, Ott J. 1997. Relationship estimation in affected sib pair analysis of late-onset diseases. *Eur J Hum Genet* 5:69–77

Goss SJ, Harris H. 1975. New method for mapping genes in human chromosomes. *Nature* 255:680–684

Gottesman II, Shields J. 1982. *Schizophrenia: The Epigenetic Puzzle.* New York: Cambridge University Press

Gough NM, Gearing DP, Nicola NA, Baker E, Pritchard M, Callen DF, Sutherland GF. 1990. Localization of the human GM-CSF receptor gene to the X-Y pseudoautosomal region. *Nature* 345:734–736

Greenberg DA. 1986. The effect of proband designation on segregation analysis. *Am J Hum Genet* 39:329–339

———. 1989. Inferring mode of inheritance by comparison of lod scores. *Am J Med Gen* 34:480–486

Greenberg DA, Hodge SE. 1989. Linkage analysis under ''random'' and ''genetic'' reduced penetrance. *Genet Epidemiol* 6:259–264

Grigorenko EL, Wood FB, Meyer MS, Hart LA, Speed WC, Shuster A, Pauls DL. 1997. Susceptibility loci for distinct components of developmental dyslexia on chromosomes 6 and 15. *Am J Hum Genet* 60:27–39

Grimm T, Müller B, Dreier M, Kind E, Bettecken T, Meng G, Müller CR. 1989. Hot spot of recombination within DXS164 in the Duchenne muscular dystrophy gene. *Am J Hum Genet* 45:368–372

Grön K, Aula P, Peltonen L. 1990. Linkage of aspartylglucosaminuria (AGU) to marker loci on the long arm of chromosome 4. *Hum Genet* 85:233–236

Guigó R. 1997. Computational gene identification. *J Mol Med* 75:389–393

Gulcher JR, Jonsson P, Kong A, Kristjansson K, Frigge ML, Karason A, Einarsdottir IE, Stefansson H, Einarsdottir AS, Sigurthoardottir S, Baldursson S, Bjornsdottir S, Hrafnkelsdottir SM, Jakobsson F, Benedickz J, Stefansson K. 1997. Mapping of a familial essential tremor gene, FET1, to chromosome 3q13. *Nat Genet* 17:84–87

Guo S-W. 1997. Linkage disequilibrium measures for fine-scale mapping: A comparison. *Hum Hered* 47:301–314

Guo S-W, Xiong M. 1997. Estimating the age of mutant disease alleles based on linkage disequilibrium. *Hum Hered* 47:315–337

Gusella J, Wexler NS, Conneally PM, Naylor SL, Anderson MA, Tanzi RE, Watkins PC, Ottina K, Wallace MR, Sakaguchi AY, Young AB, Shoulson I, Bonilla E, Martin JB. 1983. A polymorphic DNA marker genetically linked to Huntington's disease. *Nature* 306:234–238

Hadlow WJ. 1959. Scrapie and kuru. *Lancet* 2:289–290

Haines JL, Pericak-Vance MA (editors). 1998. *Approaches to Gene Mapping in Complex Human Diseases.* New York: Wiley-Liss

Haldane JBS. 1919. The combination of linkage values and the calculation of distances between the loci of linked factors. *J Genet* 8:299–309

———. 1922. Sex ratio and unisexual sterility in hybrid animals. *J Genet* 12:101–109

———. 1935. The rate of spontaneous mutation of a human gene. *J Genet* 31:317–326

———. 1985.The future of biology. In *On Being the Right Size and Other Essays—J.B.S. Haldane,* edited by JM Smith. Oxford, New York: Oxford University Press

Haldane JBS, Crew FAE. 1925. Change of linkage in poultry with age. *Nature* 115:641

Haldane JBS, Smith CAB. 1947. A new estimate of the linkage between the genes for colour-blindness and haemophilia in man. *Ann Eugen* 14:10–31

Hall JM, Lee MK, Newman B, Morrow JE, Anserson LA, Huey B, King M-C. 1990. Linkage of early-onset familial breast cancer to chromosome 17q21. *Science* 250:1684–1689

Hammersley JM, Handscomb DC. 1983. *Monte Carlo Methods.* New York: Chapman & Hall

Hampe J, Mrowka R, Marczinek K, Nurnberg P. 1997. A novel standardization method for two-dimensional DNA fingerprints. *Electrophoresis* 18:2874–2879

Harris H, Hopkinson DA, Edwards YH. 1977. Polymorphism and the subunit structure of enzymes. A contribution to the neutralist–selectionist controversy. *Proc Natl Acad Sci USA* 74:698–701

Hartl DL. 1988. *A Primer of Population Genetics.* Sunderland, Massachusetts: Sinauer Associates

Hartl DL, Clark AG. 1989. *Principles of Population Genetics.* Sunderland, Massachusetts: Sinauer Associates

Haseman JK, Elston RC. 1972. The investigation of linkage between a quantitative trait and a marker locus. *Behav Genet* 2:3–19

Hashimoto L, Habita C, Beressi JP, Delepine M, Besse C, Cambon-Thomsen A, Deschamps I, Rotter JI, Djoulah S, James MR, Froguel P, Weissenbach J, Lathrop GM, Julier C. 1994. Genetic mapping of a susceptibility locus for insulin-dependent diabetes mellitus on chromosome 11q. *Nature* 371:161–164

Hasstedt SJ. 1982. A mixed model likelihood approximation for large pedigrees. *Comp Biomed Res* 15:295–307

Hasstedt SJ, Cartwright PE. 1981. *PAP—Pedigree Analysis Package.* University of Utah, Department of Medical Biophysics and Computing, Technical Report No. 13. Salt Lake City, Utah

Hauser ER, Boehnke M, Guo SW, Risch N. 1996. Affected-sib-pair interval mapping and exclusion for complex genetic traits: Sampling considerations. *Genet Epidemiol* 13:117–137

Heath SC. 1997. Markov chain Monte Carlo segregation and linkage analysis for oligogenic models. *Am J Hum Genet* 16:748–760

———. 1998. Generating consistent genotypic configurations for multi-allelic loci and large complex pedigrees. *Hum Hered* 48:1–11

Heimbuch RC, Matthysse S, Kidd KK. 1980. Estimating age-of-onset distributions for disorders with variable onset. *Am J Hum Genet* 32:564–574

Hendricks RW, Mensink EJBM, Kraakman MEM, Thompson A, Schuurman RKB. 1989. Evidence for male X chromosomal mosaicism in X-linked agammaglobulinemia. *Hum Genet* 83:267–270

Herskind AM, McGue M, Holm NV, Sørensen TIA, Harvald B, Vaupel JW. 1996. The heritability of human longevity: A population-based study of 2872 Danish twin pairs born 1870–1900. *Hum Genet* 97:319–323

Heuch I, Li FHF. 1972. PEDIG—A computer program for calculation of genotype probabilities using phenotype information. *Clin Genet* 3:501–504

Hill AP. 1975. Quantitative linkage: A statistical procedure for its detection and estimation. *Ann Hum Genet* 38:439–449

Hill WG. 1974. Estimation of linkage disequilibrium in randomly mating populations. *Heredity* 33:229–239

Hodge SE. 1984. The information contained in multiple sibling pairs. *Genet Epidemiol* 1:109–122

Hodge SE, Anderson CE, Neiswanger K, Sparkes RS, Rimoin DL. 1983. The search for heterogeneity in insulin-dependent diabetes mellitus (IDDM): Linkage studies, two-locus models, and genetic heterogeneity. *Am J Hum Genet* 35:1139–1155

Hodge SE, Elston RC. 1994. Lods, wrods, and mods: The interpretation of lod scores calculated under different models. *Genet Epidemiol* 11:329–342

Hodge SE, Flodman PL, Duryea MF, Spence MA. 1998. Estimating recombination fraction separately for males and females: A counterintuitive result. *Hum Hered* 48:42–48

Hogben L. 1932. The genetic analysis of familial traits. II. Double gene substitutions, with special reference to hereditary dwarfism. *J Genet* 25:211–240

Holliday R. 1964. A mechanism for gene conversion in fungi. *Genet Res* 5:282–304

Holmans P. 1993. Asymptotic properties of affected-sib-pair linkage analysis. *Am J Hum Genet* 52:362–374

Holmgren G, Haettner E, Nordenson I, Sandgren O, Steen L, Lundgren E. 1988. Homozygosity for the transthyretin-met^{30}-gene in two Swedish sibs with familial amyloidotic polyneuropathy. *Clin Genet* 34:333–338

Hopfield JJ. 1982. Neural networks and physical systems with emergent collective computational abilities. *Proc Natl Acad Sci USA* 79:2554–2558

Houwen RH, Baharloo S, Blankenship K, Raeymaekers P, Juyn J, Sandkuijl LA, Freimer NB. 1994. Genome screening by searching for shared segments: Mapping a gene for benign recurrent intrahepatic cholestasis. *Nat Genet* 8:380–386

Hsiao K, Baker HF, Crow TJ, Poulter M, Owen F, Terwilliger JD, Westaway D, Ott J, Prusiner SB. 1989. Linkage of a prion protein missense variant to Gerstmann–Sträussler syndrome. *Nature* 338:342–345

Huether CA, Murphy EA. 1980. Reduction of bias in estimating the frequency of recessive genes. *Am J Hum Genet* 32:212–222

Hurst LD, McVean G, Moore T. 1996. Imprinted genes have few and small introns. *Nat Genet* 12:234–237

Hyer RN, Julier C, Buckley JD, Trucco M, Rotter J, Spielman R, Barnett A, Bain S, Boitard C, Deschamps I, Todd JA, Bell JI, Lathrop GM. 1991. High-resolution linkage mapping for susceptibility genes in human polygenic disease: Insulin-dependent diabetes mellitus and chromosome 11q. *Am J Hum Genet* 48:243–257

Idury RM, Elston RC. 1997. A faster and more general hidden Markov model algorithm for multipoint likelihood calculations. *Hum Hered* 47:197–202

Irwin M, Cox N, Kong A. 1994. Sequential imputation for multilocus linkage analysis. *Proc Natl Acad Sci USA* 91:11684–11688

Janssen B, Halley D, Sandkuijl L. 1997. Linkage analysis under locus heterogeneity: Behaviour of the A-test in complex analyses. *Hum Hered* 47:223–233

Järvelä I, Schleutker J, Haataja L, Santavuori P, Puhakka L, Manninen T, Palotie A, Sandkuijl LA, Renlund M, White R, Aula P, Peltonen L. 1991. Infantile form of neuronal ceroid lipofuscinoses (CLN1) maps to the short arm of chromosome 1. *Genomics* 9:170–173

Jeffreys AJ, Wilson V, Thein SL. 1985. Individual-specific 'fingerprints' of human DNA. *Nature* 316:76–79

Johnson NL, Kotz S, 1970. *Continuous Univariate Distributions—2.* Boston: Houghton Mifflin

———. 1972. *Distributions in Statistics: Continuous Multivariate Distributions.* New York: Wiley

Johnson SM. 1963. Generation of permutations by adjacent transposition. *Math Comp* 17:282–285

Judge SJ. 1990. Does the eye grow into focus? *Nature* 345:477–478

Juneja RK, Weitkamp LR, Stratil A, Gahne B, Guttormsen SA. 1988. Further studies of the plasma α_1B-glycoprotein polymorphism: Two new alleles and allele frequencies in Caucasians and in American Blacks. *Hum Hered* 38:267–272

Kainulainen K, Pulkkinen L, Savolainen A, Kaitila I, Peltonen L. 1990. Location on chromosome 15 of the gene defect causing Marfan syndrome. *New Engl J Med* 323:935–939

Kanaar R, Hoeijmakers JHJ. 1998. Genetic recombination: From competition to collaboration. *Nature* 391:335–338

Kanno H, Huang IY, Kan YW, Yoshida A. 1989. Two structural genes on different chromosomes are required for encoding the major subunit of human red cell glucose-6-phosphate dehydrogenase. *Cell* 58:595–606

Kaplan NL, Martin ER, Weir BS. 1997. Power studies for the transmission/disequilibrium tests with multiple alleles. *Am J Hum Genet* 60:691–702

Karlin S. 1984. Theoretical aspects of genetic map functions in recombination processes. In *Human Population Genetics. The Pittsburgh Symposium,* edited by A Chakravarti. New York: Van Nostrand Reinhold Company, pp 209–228

Karlin S, Liberman U. 1978. Classifications and comparisons of multilocus recombination distributions. *Proc Natl Acad Sci USA* 75:6332–6336

Karlin S, Taylor HM. 1975. *A First Course in Stochastic Processes.* New York: Academic Press

Keats B, Ott J, Conneally M. 1989. Report of the committee on linkage and gene order. *Cytogenet Cell Genet* 51:459–502

Keats BJB, Sherman SL, Morton NE, Robson EB, Buetow KH, Cann HM, Cartwright PE, Chakravarti A, Francke U, Green PP, Ott J. 1991. Guidelines for human linkage maps. An international system for human linkage maps (ISLM, 1990). *Genomics* 9:557–560

Keats BJB, Sherman SL, Ott J. 1990. Report of the committee on linkage and gene order. *Cytogenet Cell Genet* 55:387–394

Keith TP, Green P, Reeders ST, Brown VA, Phipps P, Bricker A, Falls K, Rediker KS, Powers JA, Hogan C, Nelson C, Knowlton R, Donis-Keller H. 1990. Genetic linkage map of 46 DNA markers on human chromosome 16. *Proc Natl Acad Sci USA* 87:5754–5758

Kendler KS. 1983. Overview: A current perspective on twin studies of schizophrenia. *Am J Psychiatry* 140:1413–1425

Kendler KS, Pedersen NL, Neale MC, Mathe AA. 1995. A pilot Swedish twin study of affective illness including hospital- and population-ascertained subsamples: Results of model fitting. *Behav Genet* 25:217–232

Kerem E, Corey M, Kerem B, Rommens J, Markiewicz D, Levison H, Tsui L-C, Durie P. 1990. The relation between genotype and phenotype in cystic fibrosis—Analysis of the most common mutation (DF_{508}). *New Engl J Med* 323:1517–1522

Kerem B, Rommens JM, Buchana JA, Markiewicz D, Cox TK, Chakravarti A, Buchwald M, Tsui L-C. 1989. Identification of the cystic fibrosis gene: Genetic analysis. *Science* 245:1073–1080

Khoury MJ, Beaty TH, Cohen BH. 1993. *Fundamentals of Genetic Epidemiology.* New York: Oxford University Press

Kidd KK, Ott J. 1984. Power and sample size in linkage studies. *Cytogenet Cell Genet* 37:510–511

Kidwell MG, Lisch DR. 1998. Transposons unbound. *Nature* 393:22–23

Kimberling WJ, Weston MD, Möller C, Davenport SLH, Shugart YY, Priluck IA, Martini A, Milani M, Smith RJ. 1990. Localization of Usher syndrome type II to chromosome 1q. *Genomics* 7:245–249

Kloepfer HW. 1946. An investigation of 171 possible linkage relationships in man. *Ann Eugen* 13:35–71

Knapp M. 1997. The affected sib pair method for linkage analysis. In *Genetic Mapping of Disease Genes,* edited by I-H Pawlowitzki, JH Edwards, EA Thompson. New York: Academic Press, pp 147–157

Knapp M, Seuchter SA, Baur MP. 1994a. Linkage analysis in nuclear families. 2: Relationship between affected sib-pair tests and lod score analysis. *Hum Hered* 44:44–51

———. 1994b. Two-locus disease models with two marker loci: The power of affected-sib-pair tests. *Am J Hum Genet* 55:1030–1041

Knowles JA, Shugart Y, Banerjee P, Gilliam TC, Lewis CA, Jacobson SG, Ott J. 1994. Identification of a locus, distinct from RDS-peripherin, for autosomal recessive retinitis pigmentosa on chromosome 6p. *Hum Molec Genet* 3:1401–1403

Koeleman BPC, Reitsma PH, Allaart CF, Bertina RM. 1994. Activated protein C resistance as an additional risk factor for thrombosis in protein C deficient families. *Blood* 84:1031–1035

Kong A. 1991. Efficient methods for computing linkage likelihoods of recessive diseases in inbred pedigrees. *Genet Epidemiol* 8:81–103

Kong A, Cox NJ. 1997. Allele-sharing models: Lod scores and accurate linkage tests. *Am J Hum Genet* 61:1179–1188

Kong A, Frigge M, Irwin M, Cox N. 1992. Importance sampling. I. Computing multimodel *p* values in linkage analysis. *Am J Hum Genet* 51:1413–1429

Koob MD, Benzow KA, Bird TD, Day JW, Moseley ML, Ranum LPW. 1998. Rapid cloning of expanded trinucleotide repeat sequences from genomic DNA. *Nat Genet* 18:72–75

Kosambi DD. 1944. The estimation of map distances from recombination values. *Ann Eugen* 12:172–175

Kostyu DD, Ober CL, Dawson DV, Ghanayem M, Elias S, Martin AO. 1989. Genetic analysis of HLA in the U.S. Schmiedenleut Hutterites. *Am J Hum Genet* 45:261–269

Kouri RE, Fain PR. 1990. Meiotic mapping panels: An efficient mapping strategy for genetic mapping. *Am J Hum Genet* 47:A186. Abstract

Kruglyak L. 1997. The use of a genetic map of biallelic markers in linkage studies. *Nat Genet* 17:21–24

Kruglyak L, Daly M, Lander ES. 1995. Rapid multipoint linkage analysis of recessive traits in nuclear families, including homozygosity mapping. *Am J Hum Genet* 56:519–527

Kruglyak L, Daly MJ, Reeve-Daly MP, Lander ES. 1996. Parametric and nonparametric linkage analysis: A unified multipoint approach. *Am J Hum Genet* 58:1347–1363

Kruglyak L, Lander ES. 1995. Complete multipoint sib-pair analysis of qualitative and quantitative traits. *Am J Hum Genet* 57:439–454

Kullback S. 1959. *Information Theory and Statistics.* New York: Wiley

Kullback S, Leibler RA. 1951. On information and sufficiency. *Ann Math Statist* 22:79–86

Laan M, Pääbo S. 1997. Demographic history and linkage disequilibrium in human populations. *Nat Genetics* 17:435–438

Lalouel JM. 1977. Linkage mapping from pair-wise recombination data. *Heredity* 38:61–77

———. 1979. GEMINI—A computer program for optimization of general nonlinear functions. University of Utah, Department of Medical Biophysics and Computing. Technical Report No. 14. Salt Lake City, Utah

Lalouel JM, Yee S. 1980. *POINTER: Computer programs for complex segregation analysis of nuclear families with pointers. Popul Genet Lab Tech Rep 3.* Honolulu: University of Hawaii

Lander ES, Botstein D. 1986a. Strategies for studying heterogeneous genetic traits in humans by using a linkage map of restriction fragment length polymorphisms. *Proc Natl Acad Sci USA* 83:7353–7357

———. 1986b. Mapping complex genetic traits in humans: New methods using a complete RFLP linkage map. *Cold Spring Harbor Symp Quant Biol* 51:49–62

———. 1989. Mapping Mendelian factors underlying quantitative traits using RFLP linkage maps. *Genetics* 121:185–199

Lander ES, Green P. 1987. Construction of multilocus genetic maps in humans. *Proc Natl Acad Sci USA* 84:2363–2367

Lander ES, Green P, Abrahamson J, Barlow A, Daly MJ, Lincoln SE, Newburg L. 1987 MAPMAKER: An interactive computer package for constructing primary genetic linkage maps of experimental and natural populations. *Genomics* 1:174–181

Lander E, Kruglyak L. 1995. Genetic dissection of complex traits: Guidelines for interpreting and reporting linkage results. *Nat Genet* 11:241–247

Lang BF, Burger G, O'Kelly CJ, Cedergren R, Golding GB, Lemieux C, Sankoff D, Turmel M, Gray MW. 1997. An ancestral mitochondrial DNA resembling a eubacterial genome in miniature. *Nature* 387:493–497

Lange K. 1997. *Mathematical and Statistical Methods for Genetic Analysis.* Berlin: Springer

Lange K, Boehnke M. 1982. How many polymorphic genes will it take to span the human genome? *Am J Hum Genet* 34:842–845

Lange K, Elston RC. 1975. Extensions to pedigree analysis. I. Likelihood calculations for simple and complex pedigrees. *Hum Hered* 25:95–105

Lange K, Matthysse S. 1989. Simulation of pedigree genotypes by random walks. *Am J Hum Genet* 45:959–970

Lange K, Spence MA, Frank MB. 1976. Application of the lod method to the detection of linkage between a quantitative trait and a qualitative marker: A simulation experiment. *Am J Hum Genet* 28:167–173

Lange K, Weeks DE. 1989. Efficient computation of LOD scores: Genotype elimination, genotype redefinition, and hybrid maximum likelihood algorithms. *Ann Hum Genet* 53:67–83

Lange K, Weeks D, Boehnke M. 1988. Programs for Pedigree Analysis: MENDEL, FISHER, and dGENE. *Genet Epidemiol* 5:471–472

Lathrop GM, Chotai J, Ott J, Lalouel JM. 1987. Tests of gene order from three-locus linkage data. *Ann Hum Genet* 51:235–249

Lathrop GM, Hooper AB, Huntsman JW, Ward RH. 1983. Evaluating pedigree data. I. The estimation of pedigree error in the presence of marker mistyping. *Am J Hum Genet* 35:241–262

Lathrop GM, Lalouel JM, Julier C, Ott J. 1984. Strategies for multilocus linkage analysis in humans. *Proc Natl Acad Sci USA* 81:3443–3446

———. 1985. Multilocus linkage analysis in humans: Detection of linkage and estimation of recombination. *Am J Hum Genet* 37:482–498

Lathrop GM, Lalouel JM, White RL. 1986. Calculation of human linkage maps: Likelihood calculations for multilocus linkage analysis. *Genet Epidemiol* 3:39–52

Lathrop GM, Ott J. 1990. Analysis of complex diseases under oligogenic models and intrafamilial heterogeneity by the LINKAGE programs. *Am J Hum Genet* 47:A188. Abstract

Lawrence S, Giles CL. 1998. Searching the world wide web. *Science* 280:98–100

Lazzeroni LC. 1998. Linkage disequilibrium and gene mapping: An empirical least-squares approach. *Am J Hum Genet* 62:159–170

Lazzeroni LC, Arnheim N, Schmitt K, Lange K. 1994. Multipoint mapping calculations for sperm-typing data. *Am J Hum Genet* 55:431–436

Lazzeroni LC, Lange K. 1998. A conditional inference framework for extending the transmission/disequilibrium test. *Hum Hered* 48:67–81

Leal SM, Ott J. 1990. Expected lod scores in linkage analysis of autosomal recessive traits for affected and unaffected offspring. *Am J Hum Genet* 47:A188. Abstract

———. 1994. A likelihood approach to calculating risk support intervals. *Am J Hum Genet* 54:913–917

———. 1995. Variability of genotype-specific penetrance probabilities in the calculation of risk support intervals. *Genet Epidemiol* 12:859–862

Leal SM, Rabinowitz D, Ott J. 1999. Stratification of families in linkage analysis has its price (in preparation)

Lechler R. 1994. *HLA and Disease.* London: Academic Press

Lehmer DH. 1964. The machine tools of combinatorics. In *Applied Combinatorial Mathematics,* edited by EF Beckenbach. New York: Wiley

Lernmark A, Ott J. 1998. Sometimes it's hot, sometimes it's not. *Nat Genet* 19:213–214

Levy-Lahad E, Bird TD. 1996. Genetic factors in Alzheimer's disease: A review of recent advances. *Ann Neurol* 40:829–840

Lewontin RC. 1964. The interaction of selection and linkage. I. General considerations: Heterotic models. *Genetics* 49:49–67

Li CC, 1987. A genetical model for emergenesis: In memory of Laurence H. Snyder, 1901–86. *Am J Hum Genet* 41:517–523

———. 1988. Pseudo-random mating populations. *Genetics* 119:731–737

Li W. 1997. The complexity of DNA. *Complexity* 3:33–37

Li W, Fann CSJ, Ott J. 1998. Low order trends of female-to-male map distance ratios along human chromosomes. *Hum Hered* 48:266–270

Liberman U, Karlin S. 1984. Theoretical models of genetic map functions. *Theor Popul Biol* 25:331–346

Lin S. 1996. Multipoint linkage analysis via Metropolis jumping kernels. *Biometrics* 52:1417–1427

Lin S, Speed TP. 1996. Incorporating crossover interference into pedigree analysis using the chi^2 model. *Hum Hered* 46:315–322

Lincoln SE, Lander ES. 1992. Systematic detection of errors in genetic linkage data. *Genomics* 14:604–610

Lindenbaum S. 1979. *Kuru Sorcery.* Palo Alto, California: Mayfield

Linder D, Kaiser McCaw B, Hecht F. 1975. Parthenogenetic origin of benign ovarian teratomas. *New Engl J Med* 292:63–66

Louis TA. 1982. Analysis of categorical data: Exact tests and log-linear models. In *Statistics in Medical Research,* edited by V Miké, KE Stanley. New York: Wiley, pp 402–431

Lucek P, Hanke J, Reich J, Solla S, Ott J. 1998. Multi-locus nonparametric linkage analysis of complex trait loci with neural networks. *Hum Hered* 48:275–284

———. 1999. Pattern recognition in multi-locus affected sib pair analysis through neural networks (in preparation)

Lunetta KL, Boehnke M, Lange K, Cox DR. 1996. Selected locus and multiple mapping panel models for radiation hybrid mapping. *Am J Hum Genet* 59:717–725

Lynch M, Walsh B. 1998. *Genetics and Analysis of Quantitative Traits.* Sunderland, Massachusetts: Sinauer Associates

MacLean CJ, Morton NE, Elston RC, Yee S. 1976. Skewness in commingled distribution. *Biometrics* 32:695–699

MacLean CJ, Sham PC, Kendler KS. 1993. Joint linkage of multiple loci for a complex disorder. *Am J Hum Genet* 53:353–366

McClearn GE. 1993. Genetics, systems, and alcohol. *Behav Genet* 23:223–230

McGue M, Gottesman II, Rao DC. 1986. The analysis of schizophrenia family data. *Behav Genet* 16:75–87

McKusick VA. 1990. *Mendelian Inheritance of Man,* 9th edition. Baltimore: Johns Hopkins University Press

McKusick VA, Ruddle FH. 1977. The status of the gene map of the human chromosomes. *Science* 196:390–405

McPeek MS, Speed TP. 1995. Modeling interference in genetic recombination. *Genetics* 139:1031–1044

Mather K. 1936. Types of linkage data and their value. *Ann Eugen* 7:251–264

———. 1938. Crossing-over. *Biol Reviews* (Cambridge Philosophical Society) 13: 252–292

Maynard Smith J. 1989. *Evolutionary Genetics.* Oxford: Oxford University Press

Mein CA, Esposito L, Dunn MG, Johnson GCL, Timms AE, Goy JV, Smith AN, Sebag-Montefiore L, Merriman ME, Wilson AJ, Pritchard LE, Barnett AH, Bain SC, Todd JA. 1998. A search for type 1 diabetes susceptibility genes in families from the United Kingdom. *Nat Genet* 19:297–300

Melki J, Abdelhak S, Sheth P, Bachelot MF, Burlet P, Marcadet A, Aicardi J, Barois A, Carriere JP, Fardeau M, Fontan D, Ponsot G, Billette T, Angelini C, Barbosa C, Ferriere G, Lanzi G, Ottolini A, Babron MC, Cohen D, Hanauer A, Clerget-Darpoux F, Lathrop M, Munnich A, Frézal J. 1990. Gene for chronic proximal spinal muscular atrophies maps to chromosome 5q. *Nature* 344:767–768

Mendel G. 1866. Versuche über Pflanzen-Hybriden. *Verh Naturforsch Ver Brünn* 4:3–47

Mérette C, King M-C, Ott J. 1992. Heterogeneity analysis of breast cancer families by using age at onset as a covariate. *Am J Hum Genet* 50:515–519

Mérette C, Ott J. 1996. Estimating parental relationship in linkage analysis of recessive traits. *Am J Med Genet* 63:386–391

Meyers DA, Conneally PM, Hecht F, Lovrien EW, Magenis E, Merritt AD, Palmer CG, Rivas ML, Wang L. 1975. Linkage group I: Multipoint mapping. *Cytogenet Cell Genet* 14:381–389

Meyers DA, Conneally PM, Lovrien EW, Magenis RE, Merritt AD, Norton JA, Palmer CG, Rivas ML, Wang L, Yu PL. 1976. Linkage group I: The simultaneous estimation of recombination and interference. *Cytogenet Cell Genet* 16:335–339

Miller DA, Miller OJ, Dev VG, Hashmi S, Tantravahi R, Medrano L, Green H. 1974. Human chromosome 19 carries a poliovirus receptor gene. *Cell* 1:167–173

Mitelman F (editor). 1995. *ISCN 1995. An International System for Human Cytogenetic Nomenclature.* Basel: Karger

Mittmann O. 1938. Vererbung durch ein Genpaar und Mitwirkung des Restgenotypes im statistichen Nachweis. *Z Indukt Abst Vererb* 75:191–232

Mohr J. 1954. *A Study of Linkage in Man.* Copenhagen: Munksgaard

———. 1964. Practical possibilities for detection of linkage in man. *Acta Genet Basel* 14:125–132

Moldin SO. 1997a. Detection and replication of linkage to a complex human disease. *Genet Epidemiol* 14:1023–1028

———. 1997b. The maddening hunt for madness genes. *Nat Genet* 17:127–129

Monaco AP, Kunkel LM. 1988. Cloning of the Duchenne/Becker muscular dystrophy locus. In *Advances of Human Genetics Vol 17,* edited by H Harris, K Hirschhorn. New York: Plenum, pp 61–98

Moore JP. 1997. Coreceptors: Implications for HIV pathogenesis and therapy. *Science* 276:51–52

Morgan TH. 1911. Random segregation versus coupling in mendelian inheritance. *Science* 34:384

Morgan TH. 1928. *The Theory of Genes.* New Haven: Yale University Press

Morton NE. 1955. Sequential tests for the detection of linkage. *Am J Hum Genet* 7:277–318

———. 1956. The detection and estimation of linkage between the genes for elliptocytosis and the Rh blood type. *Am J Hum Genet* 8:80–96

———. 1978. Analysis of crossingover in man. *Cytogenet Cell Genet* 22:15–36

———. 1998. Significance levels in complex inheritance. *Am J Hum Genet* 62:690–697

Morton NE, Collins A. 1998. Tests and estimates of allelic association in complex inheritance. *Proc Natl Acad Sci USA* 95:11389–11393

Morton NE, MacLean CJ. 1974. Analysis of family resemblance. 3. Complex segregation of quantitative traits. *Am J Hum Genet* 26:489–503

Motulsky AG, Fraser GR, Felsenstein J. 1971. Public health and long-term genetic implications of intrauterine diagnosis and selective abortion. *Birth Defects* 7(5):22–32

Muller J. 1916. The mechanism of crossing over. *Am Nat* 50:193–207

Murphy EA, Chase GA. 1975. *Principles of Genetic Counseling.* Chicago: Yearbook. (Reprinted 1990 by UMI Out-of-Print Books on Demand.)

Murphy EA, Trojak JL. 1986. The genetics of quantifiable homeostasis: I. The general issues. *Am J Med Genet* 24:159–169

Musarella MA, Weleber RG, Murphey WH, Young RSL, Anson-Cartwright L, Mets M, Kraft SP, Polemeno R, Litt M, Worton RG. 1989. Assignment of the gene for complete X-linked congenital stationary night blindness (CSNB1) to Xp11.3. *Genomics* 5:727–737

Nakamura Y, Leppert M, O'Connell P, Wolff R, Holm T, Culver M, Martin C, Fujimoto E, Hoff M, Kumlin E, White R. 1987. Variable number of tandem repeat (VNTR) markers for human gene mapping. *Science* 235:1616–1622

Nei M, Roychoudhury AK. 1974. Sampling variances of heterozygosity and genetic distance. *Genetics* 76:379–390

Neugebauer M, Baur MP. 1991. A comprehensive pedigree analysis tool: FAP (Family Analysis Package). In *Recent Progress in the Genetic Epidemiology of Cancer,* edited by HT Lynch, P Tautu. Heidelberg: Springer, pp 145–149

Neuman RJ, Rice JP. 1992. Two-locus models of disease. *Genet Epidemiol* 9:347–365

Newman TG, Odell PL. 1971. *The Generation of Random Variates.* New York: Hafner

NIH. 1997. *The Sixth Report of the Joint National Committee on Prevention, Detection, Evaluation, and Treatment of High Blood Pressure (JNC VI).* NIH, National Heart, Lung and Blood Institute. NIH Publication No. 98-4080, November 1997. (Also available from http://www.nhlbi.nih.gov/nhlbi/cardio/hbp/prof/jncintro.htm)

Nijenhuis A, Wilf HS. 1978. *Combinatorial Algorithms for Computers and Calculators.* New York: Academic Press

Nordström S, Thorburn W. 1980. Dominantly inherited macular degeneration (Best's disease) in a homozygous father with 11 children. *Clin Genet* 18:211–216

Nothiger R. 1977. Ernst Hadorn (1902–1976). *Genetics* 86:1–4

O'Brien SJ, Dean M. 1997. In search of AIDS-resistance genes. *Sci Am* 277:44–51

O'Connell JR, Weeks DE. 1995. The VITESSE algorithm for rapid exact multilocus linkage analysis via genotype set-recording and fuzzy inheritance. *Nat Genet* 11:402–408

O'Connell P, Lathrop GM, Law M, Leppert M, Nakamura Y, Hoff M, Kumlin E, Thomas W, Elsner T, Ballard L, Goodman P, Azen E, Sadler JE, Cai GY, Lalouel J-M, White R. 1987. A primary genetic linkage map for human chromosome 12. *Genomics* 1:93–102

Ott J. 1974a. Estimation of the recombination fraction in human pedigrees: Efficient computation of the likelihood for human linkage studies. *Am J Hum Genet* 26:588–597

―――. 1974b. Computer simulation in human linkage analysis. *Am J Hum Genet* 26:64A. Abstract

―――. 1976. A computer program for linkage analysis of general human pedigrees. *Am J Hum Genet* 28:528–529

―――. 1977a. Linkage analysis with misclassification at one locus. *Clin Genet* 12:119–124. Erratum in *Clin Genet* 12:254 (1977)

―――. 1977b. Counting methods (EM algorithm) in human pedigree analysis: Linkage and segregation analysis. *Ann Hum Genet* 40:443–454

―――. 1978a. A simple scheme for the analysis of HLA linkages in pedigrees. *Ann Hum Genet* 42:255–257

―――. 1978b. Some statistical properties of the lod method and the method of scoring known recombination events in linkage analysis. *Cytogenet Cell Genet* 22:702–705

―――. 1979a. Maximum likelihood estimation by counting methods under polygenic and mixed models in human pedigrees. *Am J Hum Genet* 31:161–175

―――. 1979b. Detection of rare major genes in lipid levels. *Hum Genet* 51:79–91

―――. 1979c. Ascertainment in the Seattle lipid studies. In *Genetic Analysis of Common Diseases and Applications to Predictive Factors in Coronary Disease,* edited by CF Sing, M Skolnick. New York: Alan R. Liss, pp 383–388

―――. 1983. Linkage analysis and family classification under heterogeneity. *Ann Hum Genet* 47:311–320

―――. 1986a. Y-linkage and pseudoautosomal linkage. *Am J Hum Genet* 38:891–897

―――. 1986b. The number of families required to detect or exclude linkage heterogeneity. *Am J Hum Genet* 39:159–165

―――. 1986c. Linkage probability and its approximate confidence interval. *Genet Epidemiol Suppl* 1:251–257

―――. 1989a. Statistical properties of the haplotype relative risk. *Genet Epidemiol* 6:127–130

―――. 1989b. Computer-simulation methods in human linkage analysis. *Proc Natl Acad Sci USA* 86:4175–4178

―――. 1990a. Genetic interpretation of disease clustering. In *Convergent Issues in Genetics and Demography,* edited by J Adams, DA Lam, AI Hermalin, PE Smouse. New York: Oxford University Press, pp 245–255

————. 1990b. Invited editorial: Cutting a Gordian knot in the linkage analysis of complex human traits. *Am J Hum Genet* 46:219–221

————. 1991a. Genetic linkage analysis under uncertain disease definition. In *Molecular Genetics and Biology of Alcoholism, Banbury Report 33,* edited by CR Cloninger, H. Begleiter. Cold Spring Harbor, New York: Cold Spring Harbor Laboratory Press

————. 1991b. *Analysis of Human Genetic Linkage,* revised edition. Baltimore: Johns Hopkins University Press

————. 1992. Strategies for characterizing highly polymorphic markers in human gene mapping. *Am J Hum Genet* 51:283–290

————. 1993. Detecting marker inconsistencies in human gene mapping. *Hum Hered* 43:25–30

————. 1994. Choice of genetic models for linkage analysis of psychiatric traits. In *Genetic Approaches to Mental Disorders,* edited by ES Gershon, CR Cloninger. Washington DC: American Psychiatric Press, pp 63–75

————. 1995a. Linkage analysis with biological markers. *Hum Hered* 45:169–174

————. 1995b. How do you compute a lod score? *Nat Genet* 11:354–355

————. 1996. Estimating crossover frequencies and testing for numerical interference with highly polymorphic markers. In *Genetic Mapping and DNA Sequencing, Vol. 81* in ''The IMA Volumes in Mathematics and its Applications,'' edited by T Speed, MS Waterman. New York: Springer, pp 49–63

————. 1997a. Genetic mapping in complex disorders. In *Genetic Mapping of Disease Genes,* edited by I-H Pawlowitzki, JH Edwards, EA Thompson. New York: Academic Press, pp 23–30

————. 1997b. Testing for interference in human genetic maps. *J Mol Med* 75:414–419

Ott J, Bhattacharya S, Chen JD, Denton MJ, Donald J, Dubay C, Farrar GJ, Fishman GA, Frey D, Gal A, Humphries P, Jay B, Jay M, Litt M, Mächler M, Musarella M, Neugebauer M, Nussbaum RL, Terwilliger JD, Weleber RG, Wirth B, Wong F, Worton RG, Wright AF. 1990a. Localizing multiple X chromosome-linked retinitis pigmentosa loci using multilocus homogeneity tests. *Proc Natl Acad Sci USA* 87:701–704

Ott J, Caesar J, Mächler M, Schinzel A, Schmid W. 1990b. Presymptomatic exclusion of myotonic dystrophy in a one-generation pedigree of half-sibs. *Hum Hered* 40:305–307

Ott J, Falk CT. 1982. Epistatic association and linkage analysis in human families. *Hum Genet* 62:296–300

Ott J, Frater-Schröder M. 1981. Absence of linkage between transcobalamin II and ABO. *Hum Genet* 59:164–165

Ott J, Lathrop GM. 1987a. Goodness-of-fit tests for locus order in three-point mapping. *Genet Epidemiol* 45:51–57

————. 1987b. Estimating the position of a locus on a known map of loci. *Cytogenet Cell Genet* 46:674. Abstract

Ott J, Mensink EJBM, Thompson A, Schot JDL, Schuurman RKB. 1986. Heterogeneity in the map distance between X-linked agammaglobulinemia and a map of nine RFLP loci. *Hum Genet* 74:280–283

Ott J, Rabinowitz D. 1997. The effect of marker heterozygosity on the power to detect linkage disequilibrium. *Genetics* 147:927–930

————. 1999. A principal components approach based on heritability for combining phenotype information. *Hum Hered* (in press)

Ott J, Terwilliger JD. 1992. Assessing the evidence for linkage in psychiatric genetics. In *Genetic Research in Psychiatry,* edited by J Mendlewicz, H Hippius. New York: Springer, pp 245–249

Ott J, Terwilliger JD, Lathrop GM. 1998. Testing for interference in incomplete human genetic maps (in preparation)

Ouvrier R. 1996. Correlation between the histopathologic, genotypic, and phenotypic features of hereditary peripheral neuropathies in childhood. *J Child Neurol* 11:133–146

Palmer JD. 1997. The mitochondrion that time forgot. *Nature* 387:454–455

Palotie A, Väisanen P, Ott J, Ryhänen L, Elima K, Vikkula M, Cheah K, Vuorio E, Peltonen L. 1989. Predisposition to familial osteoarthrosis linked to type II collagen gene. *Lancet* i:924–927

Parzen E. 1960. *Modern Probability Theory and Its Applications.* New York: Wiley

Pascoe LL, Morton NE. 1987. The use of map functions in multipoint mapping. *Am J Hum Genet* 40:174–183

Penrose LS. 1935. The detection of autosomal linkage in data which consist of pairs of brothers and sisters of unspecified parentage. *Ann Eugen* 6:133–138

————. 1953. The genetical background of common diseases. *Acta Genet* 4:257–265

Pfanzagl J. 1966. *Allgemeine Methodenlehre der Statistik II. Sammlung Göschen Band 747/747a.* Berlin: Walter de Gruyter

Plášilová M, Feráková E, Kádasi L, Poláková H, Gerinec A. Ott J, Ferák V. 1998. Linkage of autosomal recessive primary congenital glaucoma to the GLC3A locus in Roms (Gypsies) from Slovakia. *Hum Hered* 48:30–33

Plomin R, Owen MJ, McGuffin P. 1994. The genetic basis of complex human behaviors. *Science* 264:1733–1739

Ploughman LM, Boehnke M. 1989. Estimating the power of a proposed linkage study for a complex genetic trait. *Am J Hum Genet* 44:543–551

Prusiner SB. 1997. Prion diseases and the BSE crisis. *Science* 278:245–251

Rabinowitz D. 1997. A transmission disequilibrium test for quantitative trait loci. *Hum Hered* 47:342–350

Rao CR. 1973. *Linear Statistical Inference and Its Application.* New York: Wiley

————. 1989. *Statistics and Truth.* Calcutta: Eka Press

Rao DC, Keats BJB, Lalouel JM, Morton NE, Yee S. 1979. A maximum likelihood map of chromosome 1. *Am J Hum Genet* 31:680–696

Rao DC, Keats BJB, Morton NE, Yee S, Lew R. 1978. Variability of human linkage data. *Am J Hum Genet* 30:516–529

Reeders ST, Breuning MH, Ryynänen MA, Wright AF, Davies KE, King AW, Watson ML, Weatherall DJ. 1987. A study of genetic linkage heterogeneity in adult polycystic kidney disease. *Hum Genet* 76:348–351

Renwick JH. 1969. Progress in mapping human autosomes. *Br Med Bull* 25:65–73

Renwick JH, Bolling DR. 1971. An analysis procedure illustrated on a triple linkage of use for prenatal diagnosis of myotonic dystrophy. *J Med Genet* 8:399–406

Renwick JH, Schulze J. 1961. A computer program for the processing of linkage data from large pedigrees. *Excerpta Medica Int Congr Ser* 32:E145. Abstract

———. 1965. Male and female recombination fraction for the nail-patella: ABO linkage in man. *Ann Hum Genet* 28:379–392

Rice JP, Endicott J, Knesevich MA, Rochberg N. 1987. The estimation of diagnostic sensitivity using stability data: An application to major depressive disorder. *J Psychiatr Res* 21:337–345

Risch N. 1983. A general model for disease-marker association. *Ann Hum Genet* 47:245–252

———. 1988. A new statistical test for linkage heterogeneity. *Am J Hum Genet* 42:353–364

———. 1990a. Linkage strategies for genetically complex traits. I. Multilocus models. *Am J Hum Genet* 46:222–228

———. 1990b. Linkage strategies for genetically complex traits. II. The power of affected relative pairs. *Am J Hum Genet* 46:229–241

Risch N, Claus E. Giuffra L. 1989. Linkage and mode of inheritance in complex traits. In *Multipoint Mapping and Linkage Based upon Affected Pedigree Members: Genetic Analysis Workshop 6.* New York: Liss, pp 183–188

Risch N, Ghosh S, Todd JA. 1993. Statistical evaluation of multiple-locus linkage data in experimental species and its relevance to human studies: Application to nonobese diabetic (NOD) mouse and human insulin-dependent diabetes mellitus (IDDM). *Am J Hum Genet* 53:702–714

Risch N, Giuffra L. 1992. Model misspecification and multipoint linkage analysis. *Hum Hered* 42:77–92

Risch N, Lange K. 1979. An alternative model of recombination and interference. *Ann Hum Genet* 43:61–70

Risch N, Merikangas K. 1996. The future of genetic studies of complex human diseases. *Science* 273:1516–1517

Risch N. Zhang H. 1995. Extreme discordant sib pairs for mapping quantitative trait loci in humans. *Science* 268:1584–1589

Rohde K, Teare MD, Scherneck S, Santibáñez Koref M. 1995. A program using loss-of-constitutional-heterozygosity data to ascertain the location of predisposing genes in cancer families. *Hum Hered* 45:337–345

Romeo G, Devoto M, Costa G, Roncuzzi L, Catizone L, Zuchelli P, Germino G, Keith T, Weatherall DJ, Reeders ST. 1988. A second genetic locus on autosomal dominant polycystic kidney disease. *Lancet* 2:8–11

Root-Bernstein RS, Dillon PF. 1997. Molecular complementarity I: The complementarity theory of the origin and evolution of life. *J Theor Biol* 188:447–479

Rossen RD, Brewer EJ, Sharp RM, Ott J, Templeton JW. 1980. Familial rheumatoid arthritis. Linkage of HLA to disease susceptibility locus in four families where proband presented with juvenile rheumatoid arthritis. *J Clin Invest* 65:629–642

Rotter JI. 1981. The modes of inheritance of insulin-dependent diabetes mellitus. *Am J Hum Genet* 33:835–851

Rotter JI, Landaw EM. 1984. Measuring the genetic contribution of a single locus to a multilocus disease. *Clin Genet* 26:529–542

Rubinstein P, Walker M, Carpenter C, Carrier C, Krassner J, Falk C, Ginsberg F. 1981. Genetics of HLA disease associations. The use of the haplotype relative risk (HRR) and the "haplo-delta" (Dh) estimates in juvenile diabetes from three radical groups. *Hum Immunol* 3:384. Abstract

St George-Hyslop PH, Haines JL, Farrer LA, Polinsky R, Van Broeckhoven C, Goate A, Crapper McLachlan DR, Orr H, Bruni AC, Sorbi S, Rainero I, Foncin J-F, Pollen D, Cantu J-M, Tupler R, Voskresenskaya N, Mayeux R, Growdon J, Fried VA, Myers RH, Nee L, Backhovens H, Martin J-J, Rossor M, Owen MJ, Mullan M, Percy ME, Karlinsky H, Rich S, Heston L, Montesi M, Mortilla M, Nacmias N, Gusella JF, Hardy JA. 1990. Genetic linkage studies suggest that Alzheimer's disease is not a single homogeneous disorder. *Nature* 347:194–197

Sandkuyl LA, Ott J. 1989. Determining informativity of marker typing for genetic counseling in a pedigree. *Hum Genet* 82:159–162

Sasse G, Müller H, Chakraborty R, Ott J. 1994. Estimating the frequency of nonpaternity in Switzerland. *Hum Hered* 44:337–343

Satsangi J, Parkes M, Louis E, Hashimoto L, Kato N, Welsh K, Terwilliger JD, Lathrop GM, Bell JI, Jewell DP. 1996. Two stage genome-wide search in inflammatory bowel disease provides evidence for susceptibility loci on chromosomes 3, 7 and 12. *Nat Genet* 14:199–202

Saunders AM, Strittmatter WJ, Schmechel D, George-Hyslop PH, Pericak-Vance MA, Joo Sh, Rosi BL, Gusella JF, Crapper-MacLachlan DR, Alberts MJ et al. 1993. Association of apolipoprotein E allele epsilon 4 with late-onset familial and sporadic Alzheimer's disease. *Neurology* 43:1467–1472

Sawcer S, Jones HB, Judge D, Visser F, Compston A, Goodfellow PN, Clayton D. 1997. Empirical genomewide significance levels established by whole genome simulations. *Genet Epidemiol* 14:223–229

Schaid DJ, Nick TG. 1990. Sib-pair linkage tests for disease susceptibility loci: Common tests vs. the asymptotically most powerful test. *Genet Epidemiol* 7:359–370

Schildkraut JM, Risch N, Thompson WD. 1989. Evaluating genetic association among ovarian, breast, and endometrial cancer: Evidence for a breast/ovarian cancer relationship. *Am J Hum Genet* 45:521–529

Schork NJ, Boehnke M, Terwilliger JD, Ott J. 1993. Two-trait-locus linkage analysis: A powerful strategy for mapping complex genetic traits. *Am J Hum Genet* 53:1127–1136

Schuler GD. 1997. Sequence mapping by electronic PCR. *Genome Res* 7:541–550

Schuler GD, Boguski MS, Stewart EA, Stein LD, Gyapay G, Rice K, White RE, Rodriguez-Tome P, Aggarwal A, Bajorek E, Bentolila S, Birren BB, Butler A, Castle AB, Chiannilkulchai N, Chu A, Clee C, Cowles S, Day PJ, Dibling T, Drouot N, Dunham I, Duprat S, East C, Hudson TJ et al. 1996. A gene map on the human genome. *Science* 274:540–546

Schwab SG, Albus M, Hallmayer J, Honig S, Borrmann M, Lichtermann D, Ebstein RP, Ackenheil M, Lerer B, Risch N, Maier W, Wildenauer DB. 1995. Evaluation of a susceptibility gene for schizophrenia on chromosome 6p by multipoint affected sib-pair linkage analysis. *Nat Genet* 11:325–327

Seizinger BR, Rouleau GA, Ozelius LJ, Lane AH, Faryniarz AG, Chao MV, Huson S, Korf BR, Parry DM, Pericak-Vance MA, Collins FS, Hobbs WJ, Falcone BG, Iannazzi JA, Roy JC, St George-Hyslop PH, Tanzi RE, Bothwell MA, Upadhyaya M, Harper P, Goldstein AE, Hoover DL, Bader JL, Spence MA, Mulvihill JJ, Aylsworth AS, Vance JM, Rossenwasser GOD, Gaskell PC, Roses AD, Martuza RL, Breakefield XO, Gusella JF. 1987. Genetic linkage of von Recklinghausen neurofibromatosis to the nerve growth factor receptor gene. *Cell* 49:589–594

Shannon CE, Weaver W. 1949. *The Mathematical Theory of Communication.* Urbana: University of Illinois Press

Sherman SL, Jacobs PA, Morton NE, Froster-Iskenius U, Howard-Peebles PN, Nielsen KB, Partington MW, Sutherland GR, Turner G, Watson M. 1985. Further segregation analysis of the fragile X syndrome with special reference to transmitting males. *Hum Genet* 69:289–299

Sherrington R, Brynjolfsson J, Petursson H, Potter M, Dudleston K, Barraclough B, Wasmuth J, Dobbs M, Gurling H. 1988. Localization of a susceptibility locus for schizophrenia on chromosome 5. *Nature* 336:164–167

Shields DC, Collins A, Buetow KH, Morton NE. 1991. Error filtration, interference, and the human linkage map. *Proc Natl Acad Sci USA* 88:6501–6505

Siddique T, McKinney R, Hung W-Y, Bartlett RJ, Burns G, Mohandas TK, Ropers H-H, Wilfert C, Roses AD. 1988. The poliovirus sensitivity (PVS) gene is on chromosome 19q12 → q13.2. *Genomics* 3:156–160

Simonic I, Gericke GS. 1996. The enigma of common fragile sites. *Hum Genet* 97:524–531

Simonic I, Gericke GS, Ott J, Weber JL. 1998. Identification of genetic markers associated with Gilles de la Tourette Syndrome in an Afrikaner population. *Am J Hum Genet* 63:839–846

Sing CF, Haviland MB, Reilly SL. 1996. Genetic architecture of common multifactorial diseases. *Ciba Found Symp* 197:211–229

Sing CF, Rothman ED. 1975. A consideration of the chi-square test of Hardy–Weinberg equilibrium in a non-multinomial situation. *Ann Hum Genet* 39:141–145

Slatkin M, Excoffier L. 1996. Testing for linkage disequilibrium in genotype data using the Expectation–Maximization algorithm. *Heredity* 76:377–383

Slatkin M, Rannala B. 1997. Estimating the age of alleles by use of intraallelic variability. *Am J Hum Genet* 60:447–458

Smith CAB. 1953. The detection of linkage in human genetics. *J Roy Statist Soc* 15B:153–184

———. 1957. Counting methods in genetical statistics. *Ann Hum Genet* 21:254–276

———. 1959. Some comments on the statistical methods used in linkage investigations. *Am J Hum Genet* 11:289–304

———. 1961. Homogeneity test for linkage data. *Proc Sec Int Congr Hum Genet* 1:212–213

———. 1963. Testing for heterogeneity of recombination fraction values in human genetics. *Am Hum Genet* 27:175–182

———. 1975. A non-parametric test for linkage with a quantitative character. *Ann Hum Genet* 38:451–460

———. 1989. Some simple methods for linkage analysis. *Ann Hum Genet* 53:277–283

Smith RJH, Holcomb JD, Daiger SP, Caskey CT, Pelias MZ, Alford BR, Fontenot DD, Hejtmancik JF. 1989. Exclusion of Usher syndrome gene of much of chromosome 4. *Cytogenet Cell Genet* 50:102–106

Snedecor GW, Cochran WG. 1967. *Statistical Methods.* Ames, Iowa: Iowa State University Press

Sneel RG, Lazarou LP, Youngman S, Quarrell OWJ, Wasmuth JJ, Shaw DJ, Harper PS. 1989. Linkage disequilibrium in Huntington's disease: An improved localization for the gene. *J Med Genet* 26:673–675

Sobel E, Lange K, 1996. Descent graphs in pedigree analysis: Applications to haplotyping, location scores, and marker-sharing statistics. *Am J Hum Genet* 58:1323–1337

Southern EM. 1975. Detection of specific sequences among DNA fragments separted by gel electrophoresis. *J Mol Biol* 98:503–517

Spence MA, Bishop DT, Boehnke M, Elston RC, Falk C, Hodge SE, Ott J, Rice J, Merikangas K, Kupfer D. 1993. Methodological issues in linkage analyses for psychiatric disorders: Secular trends, assortative mating, bilineal pedigrees. Report of the MacArthur Foundation Network I Task Force on Methodological Issues. *Hum Hered* 43:166–172

Speed TP, McPeek MS, Evans SN. 1992. Robustness of the no-interference model for ordering. *Proc Natl Acad Sci USA* 89:3103–3106

Spielman RS, Ewens WJ. 1996. The TDT and other family-based tests for linkage disequilibrium and association. *Am J Hum Genet* 59:983–989

———. 1998. A sibship test for linkage in the presence of association: The sib transmission/disequilibrium test. *Am J Hum Genet* 62:450–458

Spielman RS, McGinnis RE, Ewens WJ. 1993. Transmission test for linkage disequilibrium: The insulin gene region and insulin-dependent diabetes mellitus (IDDM). *Am J Hum Genet* 52:506–516

Spotila LD, Caminis J, Devoto M, Shimoya K, Sereda L. Ott J, Whyte MP, Tenenhouse A, Prockop DJ. 1996. Osteopenia in 37 members of seven families: Analysis based on a model of dominant inheritance. *Mol Med* 2:313–324

Stern C. 1973. *Principles of Human Genetics.* San Francisco: Freeman

Stewart I. 1996. *From Here to Infinity. A Guide to Today's Mathematics.* Oxford: Oxford University Press

Stewart J. 1992. Genetics and biology: A comment on the significance of the Elson–Stewart algorithm. *Hum Hered* 42:9–15

Stockert E, Boyse EA, Sato H, Itakura K. 1976. Heredity of the G_{IX} thymocyte antigen associated with murine leukemia virus: Segregation data simulating genetic linkage. *Proc Natl Acad Sci USA* 73:2077–2081

Strachan T, Abithol M, Davidson D, Beckmann JS. 1997. A new dimension for the human genome project: Towards comprehensive expression maps. *Nat Genet* 16:126–132

Strachan T, Read AP. 1996. *Human Molecular Genetics.* New York: Wiley-Liss

Strickberger MW. 1985. *Genetics,* third edition. New York: MacMillan

Stringham HM, Boehnke M. 1996. Identifying marker typing incompatibilities in linkage analysis. *Am J Hum Genet* 59:946–950

Sturt E. 1976. A mapping function for human chromosomes. *Ann Hum Genet* 40:147–163

Sturtevant AH. 1913. The linear arrangement of six sex-linked factors in *Drosophila,* as shown by their mode of association. *J Exp Zool* 14:43–59

Suarez BK. 1978. The affected sib pair IBD distribution for HLA-linked disease susceptibility genes. *Tissue Antigens* 12:87–93

Suarez BK, Hampe CL, Van Eerdewegh P. 1994. Problems of replicating linkage claims in psychiatry. In *Genetic Approaches to Mental Disorders,* edited by ES Gershon, CR Cloninger. Washington, DC, American Psychiatric Press, pp 23–46

Suarez BK, Van Eerdewegh P. 1984. A comparison of three affected-sib-pair scoring methods to detect HLA-linked disease susceptibility genes. *Am J Med Genet* 18:135–146

Sullivan LS, Daiger SP. 1996. Inherited retinal degeneration: Exceptional genetic and clinical heterogeneity. *Mol Med Today* 2:380–386

Sykes B, Ogilvie D, Wordsworth P, Wallis G, Mathew C, Beighton P, Nicholls A, Pope FM, Thompson E, Tsipouras P, Schwartz R, Jensson O, Arnason A, Børresen A-L, Heiberg A, Frey D, Steinmann B. 1990. Consistent linkage of dominantly inherited osteogenesis imperfecta to the type I collagen loci: COL1A1 and COL1A2. *Am J Hum Genet* 46:293–307

Tanzi RE, Watkins PC, Stewart GD, Wexler NS, Gusella JF, Haines JL. 1992. A genetic linkage map of human chromosome 21: Analysis of recombination as a function of sex and age. *Am H Hum Genet* 50:551–558

Tennyson CN, Klamut HJ, Worton RG. 1995. The human dystrophin gene requires 16 hours to be transcribed and is cotranscriptionally spliced. *Nat Genet* 9:184–190

Terwilliger JD, Ding Y, Ott J. 1992. On the relative importance of marker heterozygosity and intermarker distance in gene mapping. *Genomics* 13:951–956

Terwilliger JD, Ott J. 1992a. A multi-sample bootstrap approach to the estimation of maximized-over-models lod score distributions. *Cytogenet Cell Genet* 59:142–144

———. 1992b. A haplotype-based 'haplotype relative risk' approach to detecting allelic associations. *Hum Hered* 42:337–346

———. 1994. *Handbook of Human Genetic Linkage*. Baltimore: Johns Hopkins University Press

Terwilliger JD, Shannon WD, Lathrop GM, Nolan JP, Goldin LR, Chase GA, Weeks DE. 1997. True and false positive peaks in genomewide scans: Applications of length-biased sampling to linkage mapping. *Am J Hum Genet* 61:430–438

Terwilliger JD, Speer M, Ott J. 1993. Chromosome-based method of rapid computer simulation in human genetic linkage analysis. *Genet Epidemiol* 10:217–224

Terwilliger JD, Weeks DE, Ott J. 1990. Laboratory errors in the reading of marker alleles cause massive reductions in lod score and lead to gross overestimates of the recombination fraction. *Am J Hum Genet* 47:A201. Abstract

Terwilliger JD, Zöllner S, Pääbo S. 1998. Mapping genes through the use of linkage disequilibrium generated by genetic drift: 'Drift mapping' in small populations with no demographic expansion. *Hum Hered* 48:138–154

Thode HC, Finch SJ, Mendell NR. 1988. Simulated percentage points for the null distribution of the likelihood ratio test for a mixture of two normals. *Biometrics* 44:1195–1201

Thompson EA. 1984. Information gain in joint linkage analysis. *IMA J Math Appl Med & Biol* 1:31–49

———. 1986. *Pedigree Analysis in Human Genetics*. Baltimore: Johns Hopkins University Press

———. 1996. Likelihood and linkage: From Fisher to the future. *Ann Statistics* 24:449–465

Thompson EA, Deeb S, Walker D, Motulsky AG. 1988. The detection of linkage disequilibrium between closely linked markers: RFLPs at the AI-CIII apolipoprotein genes. *Am J Hum Genet* 42:113–124

Thompson EA, Neel JV. 1997. Allelic disequilibrium and allele frequency distribution as a function of social and demographic history. *Am J Hum Genet* 60:197–204

Thomson G. 1983. Investigation of the mode of inheritance of the HLA associated diseases by the method of antigen genotype frequencies among diseased individuals. *Tissue Antigens* 21:81–104

Thomson G, Robinson WP, Kuhner MK, Joe S, Klitz W. 1989. HLA, insulin gene, and Gm associations with IDDM. *Genet Epidemiol* 6:155–160

Tiwari HK, Elston RC. 1997. Linkage of multilocus components of variance to polymorphic markers. *Ann Hum Genet* 61:263–261

Trembath RC, Clough RL, Rosbotham JL, Jones AB, Camp RDR, Frodsham A, Browne J, Barber R, Terwilliger J, Lathrop GM, Barker JNWN. 1997. Identification of a major susceptibility locus on chromosome 6p and evidence for further disease loci revealed by a two stage genome-wide search in psoriasis. *Hum Molec Genet* 6:813–820

Trevor-Roper PD. 1952. Marriage of two complete albinos with normally pigmented offspring. *Br J Ophthalmol* 36:107–110

Väisänen P, Elima K, Palotie A, Peltonen L, Vuorio E. 1988. Polymorphic restriction sites of type II collagen gene: Their location and frequencies in the Finnish population. *Hum Hered* 38:65–71

Vogel F, Motulsky AG. 1986. *Human Genetics.* New York: Springer

Wald A. 1947. *Sequential Analysis.* New York: Wiley

Wallace DC. 1989. Report of the committee on human mitochondrial DNA. *Cytogenet Cell Genet* 51:612–621

Wallace DC, Singh G, Lott MT, Hodge JA, Schurr TG, Lezza AMS, Elsas II LJ, Nikoskelainen EK. 1988. Mitcochondrial DNA mutation associated with Leber's hereditary optic neuropathy. *Science* 242:1427–1430

Wang DG, Fan JB, Siao CJ, Berno A, Young P, Sapolsky R, Ghandour G, Perkins N, Winchester E, Spencer J, Kruglyak L, Stein L, Hsie L, Topaloglou T, Hubbell E, Robinson E, Mittmann M, Morris MS, Shen N, Kilburn D, Rioux J, Nusbaum C, Rozen S, Hudson TJ, Lipshutz R, Chee M, Lander ES. 1998. Large-scale identification, mapping, and genotyping of single-nucleotide polymorphisms in the human genome. *Science* 280:1077–1082

Wang L, Paradee W, Mullins C, Shridhar R, Rosati R, Wilke CM, Glover TW, Smith DI. 1997. Aphidicolin-induced FRA3B breakpoints cluster in two distinct regions. *Genomics* 41:485–488

Ward R, Stringer C. 1997. A molecular handle on the Neanderthals. *Nature* 388:225–226

Warren AC, Slaugenhaupt SA, Lewis JG, Chakravaarti A, Antonorakis AE. 1989. A genetic linkage map of 17 markers on human chromosome 21. *Genomics* 4:579–591

Watson JD, Hopkins NH, Roberts JW, Argetsinger Steitz J, Weiner AM. 198a. *Molecular Biology of the Gene, Vol 1: General Principles,* 4th edition. Menlo Park California: Benjamin Cummings Publishing Company, Inc

———. 1987b. *Molecular Biology of the Gene, Vol II: Specialized Aspects,* 4th edition. Menlo Park California: Benjamin Cummings Publishing Company, Inc

Weber JL, May PE. 1989. Abundant class of human DNA polymorphisms which can be typed using the polymerase chain reaction. *Am J Hum Genet* 44:388–396

Weber JL, Stephenson M. 1993. Modeling human meiosis. *Am J Hum Genet* 53(suppl):216. Abstract

———. 1994. Patch mapping. In *Abstracts of the 1994 Meeting on Genome Mapping and Sequencing.* Cold Spring Harbor, New York: Cold Spring Harbor Laboratory

Weber JL, Wang Z, Hansen K, Stephenson M, Kappel C, Salzman S, Wilkie PJ, Keats B, Dracopoli NC, Brandriff BF, Olsen AS. 1993. Evidence for human meiotic recombination interference obtained through construction of a short tandem repeat-polymorphism linkage map of chromosome 19. *Am J Hum Genet* 53:1079–1095

Weeks DE. 1991. Human linkage analysis: Strategies for locus ordering. In *Advanced Techniques in Chromosomes Research,* edited by KW Adolph. New York: Marcel Dekker, pp 297–330

Weeks DE, Lange K. 1988. The affected-pedigree-member method of linkage analysis. *Am J Hum Genet* 42:315–326

———. 1990. Linkage methods for identifying genetic risk factors. In *Genetic Variation and Nutrition,* edited by AP Simopoulos, B. Childs. Basel: Karger, pp 35–48

Weeks DE, Lathrop GM. 1995. Polygenic disease: Methods for mapping complex disease traits. *Trends Genet* 11:513–519

Weeks DE, Lathrop GM, Ott J. 1993. Multipoint mapping under genetic interference. *Hum Hered* 43:86–97

Weeks DE, Lehner T, Squires-Wheeler E, Kaufmann C, Ott J. 1990. Measuring the inflation of the lod score due to its maximization over model parameter values in human linkage analysis. *Genet Epidemiol* 7:237–243

Weeks DE, Ott, J. 1989. Risk calculations under heterogeneity. *Am J Hum Genet* 45:819–821

Weeks DE, Ott J, Lathrop GM. 1990. SLINK: A general simulation program for linkage analysis. *Am J Hum Genet* 47:A204. Abstract

Weeks DE, Ott J, Lathrop GM. 1994. Detection of genetic interference: Simulation studies and mouse data. *Genetics* 136:1217–1226

Weinberg W. 1927. Mathematische Gundlagen der Probandenmethode. *Z Indukt Abstamm u Vererb Lehre* 48:179–228

Weir BS. 1989. Locating the cystic fibrosis gene on the basis of linkage disequilibrium with markers? In *Multipoint Mapping and Linkage Based on Affected Pedigree Members: Genetic Analysis Workshop 6,* edited by RC Elston, MA Spence, SE Hodge, JW MacCluer. New York: Liss, pp 81–86

———. 1996. *Genetic Data Analysis II.* Sunderland, Massachusetts: Sinauer Associates

Weissenbach J, Bentolila S. 1996. Integrating maps requires integrated data. *Nat Biotechnology* 14:678

Werner P, Raducha MG, Prociuk U, Henthorn PS, Patterson DF. 1997. Physical and linkage mapping of human chromosome 17 loci to dog chromosomes 9 and 5. *Genomics* 42:74–82

White JA, McAlpine PJ, Antonarakis S, Cann H, Eppig JT, Frazer K, Frézal J, Lancet D, Nahmias J, Pearson P, Peters J, Scott A, Scott H, Spurr N, Talbot Jr C, Povey S. 1997. Guidelines for human gene nomenclature (1997). *Genomics* 45:468–471

White JK, Auerbach W, Duyao MP, Vonsattel JP, Gusella JF, Joyner AL, MacDonald ME. 1997. Huntingtin is required for neurogenesis and is not impaired by the Huntington's disease CAG expansion. *Nat Genet* 17:404–410

White RL, Lalouel J-M, Nakamura Y, Donis-Keller H, Green P, Bowden DW, Mathew CGP, Easton DF, Robson EB, Morton NE, Gusella JF, Haines JL, Retief AE,

Kidd KK, Murray JC, Lathrop Gm, Cann HM. 1990. The CEPH consortium primary linkage map of human chromosome 10. *Genomics* 6:393–412

White R, Leppert M, Bishop DT, Barker D, Berkowitz J, Brown C, Callahan P, Holm T, Jerominski L. 1985. Construction of linkage maps with DNA markers for human chromosomes. *Nature* 313:101–105

Whittemore AS, Halpern J. 1994. A class of tests for linkage using affected pedigree members. *Biometrics* 50:118–127

Whittemore AS, Tu I-P. 1998. Simple, robust linkage tests for affected sibs. *Am J Hum Genet* 62:1228–1242

Williamson JA, Amos CI. 1990. On the asymptotic behavior of the estimate of the recombination fraction under the null hypothesis of no linkage when the model is misspecified. *Genet Epidemiol* 7:309–318

Wichman BA, Hill ID. 1982. Algorithm 183: An efficient and portable pseudo-random number generator. *Applied Statistics* 31:188–190

Wingo PA, Ory H, Layde PM, Lee NC, Cancer and Steroid Hormone Group. 1988. The evaluation of the data collection process for a multicenter, population-based, case-control design. *Am J Epidemiol* 128:206–217

Winkler C, Modi W, Smith MW, Nelson GW, Wu X, Carrington M, Dean M, Honjo T, Tashiro K, Yabe D, Buchbinder S, Vittinghoff E, Goedert JJ, O'Brien TR, Jacobson LP, Detels R, Donfield S, Willoughby A, Gomperts E, Vlahov D, Phair J, O'Brien SJ. 1998. Genetic restriction of AIDS pathogenesis by an SDF-1 chemokine gene variant. *Science* 279:389–393

Woolf B. 1955. On estimating the relation between blood and disease. *Ann Hum Genet* 19:251–253

Wright Jr JE, Johnson K, Hollister A, May B. 1983. Meiotic models to explain classical linkage, pseudolinkage, and chromosome pairing in tetrapoid derivative salmonid genomes. In *Isozymes Current Topics in Biological and Medical Research Vol 10: Genetics and Evolution,* edited by MC Rattazzi, JG Scandalios, GS Whitt. New York: Alan R. Liss, pp 239–260

Wright AF, Teague PW, Bruford E, Carothers A. 1997. Problems in dealing with linkage heterogeneity in autosomal recessive forms of retinitis pigmentosa. In *Genetic Mapping of Disease Genes,* edited by I-H Pawlowitzki, JH Edwards, EA Thompson. New York: Academic Press, pp 255–272

Xie X, Ott J. 1990. Determining the effect of a change in affection status on the lod score. *Am J Hum Genet* 47:A205. Abstract

———. 1993. Testing linkage disequilibrium between a disease gene and marker loci. *Am J Hum Genet* 53:1107. Abstract

Yamamoto F, Clausen H, White T, Marken J, Hakomori S. 1990. Molecular genetic basis of the histo-blood group ABO system. *Nature* 345:229–233

Ying K-L, Ives EJ. 1968. Asymmetry of chromosome number 1 pair in three generations of a phenotypically normal family. *Can J Genet Cytol* 10:575–589

Zapata C, Alvarez G, Carollo C. 1997. Approximate variance of the standardized measure of gametic disequilibrium D'. *Am J Hum Genet* 61:771–774

Zeng ZB, Houle D, Cockerham CC. 1990. How informative is Wright's estimator of the number of genes affecting a quantitative character? *Genetics* 126:235–247

Zhao H, Speed TP, McPeek SM. 1995. Statistical analysis of crossover interference using the chi-square model. *Genetics* 139:1045–1056

Zhao LP, Thompson E, Prentice R. 1990. Joint estimation of recombination fractions and interference coefficients in multilocus linkage analysis. *Am J Hum Genet* 47:255–265

Zigas V. 1990. *Laughing Death. The Untold Story of Kuru.* Clifton, New Jersey: Humana Press

Zlotogora J. 1998. Germ line mosaicism. *Hum Genet* 102:381–386

Index

ABO blood group, 3, 4, 22, 25, 28, 29, 181, 285
Adenomatous polyposis, 61, 71
Affected sib-pair analysis, 273; two-locus, 304
Affinity, 16
Age-of-onset curve, 164
AGFAP method, 272
AIDS-resistance genes, 257, 308
Albinism, 216
Algorithm: Elston-Stewart, 58, 80, 182, 187; Lander-Green, 58, 81; recursive, 185; EM, 189; peeling, 184; quasi-Newton, 190
Allele, 27; definition of, 3; frequency, misspecified, 250
Allelic association, 283
Allozygous, 4
Alzheimer disease, 234, 253
Analysis: affected sib pair, 273; affected-only, 152; basic linkage, 53; exclusion, 279; indirect, 55; neural network, 325; of single sperm cells, 82; of variance, 310; principal components, 318; segregation, 320; survival, 166
Antigen, 25
Ascertainment: bias, 156, 236; correction, 156, 237, 241; deliberately biased, 240
Association, 281; allelic, 8, 265, 283; HLA and disease, 27
Assortative mating, 237
A-test, 223
Autosome, 8
Autozygous, 4

Backcross, 13, 93; phase-known double, 100; phase-unknown double, 104; phase-unknown triple, 122; triple, 119
Bailey's rule, 44
Bayes theorem, 50, 106
Bayesian inference, 37
Bias, 42, 231, 250; ascertainment, 156, 236; asymptotic, 236, 239, 244; in risk, 241; possible in TDT, 241
Bilineal pedigree, 230
Bipolar disease, 299
Blood pressure, 319
Bone mineral density, 175
Bootstrap, 210
BRCA1, 162
Breast cancer, 162, 170, 234, 253, 278, 307, 323
B-test, 220

CAG repeats, 257
Candidate loci, 260
Case-control studies, 291
CASH study, 162
Centromere index, 22
CEPH families, 34, 98, 144, 187, 238, 250
Charcot-Marie-Tooth disease, 54, 164, 216, 265
Chebyshev, 46
Chiasma, 9, 14, 150
Chloroplast, 9
Chromatid, 9
Chromosomal theory, 3
Chromosome: inversion, 10; morphology, 33; nomenclature, 22; strand, 9; strand, homologous, 14
Classification rule, 224

Clock, evolutionary, 9
Codominant, 5
Coefficient of coincidence, 121, 136, 142; marginal, 128
Coefficient of variation, 147
Collagen, 31, 167, 260
Color blindness, 8, 56
Complex system, 306
Complex trait, 2, 306; contribution by single locus to, 316
Computer programs: 2BY2, 197; ANALYZE, 277; ARLEQUIN, 287; ASPEX, 190, 278, 323; ASSOCIATE, 196, 286; BINOM, 49, 74, 113, 196, 326; CHIPROB, 77, 197, 213; CONTING, 293; CRI-MAP, 146, 189, 249; CROSSOVR, 133; EH, 286; EQUIV, 71, 113, 197, 224; FAP, 188; FastSLINK, 205; GENEHUNTER, 58, 81, 190, 278, 323; HAPLO, 287; HET, 197; HOMOG, 146, 221, 233, 266; HOMOG1a, 232; HOMOG2, 226; HOMOG3R, 227, 302; HOMOGM, 227, 229; HOMOZ, 190, 257; IBD, 301; ILINK, 65, 106, 147, 157, 158, 175; LINKAGE, 58, 80, 106, 163, 187; Linkage Utility, 196; LINKMAP, 145; LIPED, 58, 163, 168, 185, 186, 188, 212, 266; LOKI, 191, 323; MAP+, 190; MAPFUN, 21, 126, 137, 197; MAPMAKER, 145, 188; MAPMAKER/SIBS, 278; MENDEL, 168, 185, 189, 302; MFLINK, 158, 323; MLINK, 108, 266; MOSM, 186; MTEST, 217; NOCOM, 174, 198; NORINV, 66, 198, 311; NORPROB, 198; PAP, 81, 187; PC-LIPED, 166; PEDIG, 186; PERMUTE, 115, 209; POINTER, 162; PVALUES, 197; RELATIVE, 250; Renwick's, 186; S.A.G.E., 276; SEXDIF, 188, 214; SIBPAIR, 277; SimIBD, 278; SIMLINK, 205, 326; SIMULATE, 79, 202; SLINK, 205, 326; SOLAR, 178, 323; TLINKAGE, 302, 304; VARCO, 198, 223; VARCO6, 159; VaryPhen, 199; VITESSE, 58, 190
Computer programming, 37

Computer simulation, 35, 110, 147, 201, 257, 302, 323, 324; of normal variables, 208
Concordance rate, 308, 315
Conditional search, 304
Confidence coefficient, 49
Confidence interval, 48, 49, 148, 204; asymptotic, 69; binomial, 50
Consistency, 43, 236
Correlation coefficient, intraclass, 310; for truncated observations, 312
Coupling, 7
Covariate, 173, 233
Creatine kinase, 264
Creutzfeld-Jacob syndrome, 308
Crossover, 9, 12, 13, 139; frequency, 211; frequency, chi-square model, 131
Cystic fibrosis, 253, 287, 296

D numbers, 32
Databases, 1; genetic, 25; of genetic maps, 23
Decision rule, 45
Density, 165
Diabetes, 276, 314, 316
Discordant, sib pairs, 278
Disequilibrium, linkage. *See* Linkage disequilibrium
Disequilibrium mapping, 284, 289, 321, 324
Distance, genetic, 22
Distribution: age-of-onset, 166; binomial, 130; chiasma, 131; chi-square, 174; crossover, 128, 131; invalid crossover, 132; logistic, 164, 207; mixed, 172; mixture of, 198; mixture of two normal, 178; multivariate, 318; negative binomial, 261; overlapping, 175; Poisson, 131; posterior, 59; prior, 37, 59; risk, 242, 267; shifted Poisson, 133; skewed, 174
Distribution function, 165
DNA: chip, 31; fingerprinting, 200; polymorphism, 27; variants, 25
Dominant, 4
Drift, genetic, 6
Drosophila, 3, 129, 131, 141, 211
Duchenne Muscular Dystrophy, 2, 22, 253, 264, 271
Duffy blood group, 33, 265
Dyslexia, 319

ELOD, 88, 97, 99, 111, 155, 203, 205;
    conditional, 106
EM algorithm, 142, 189
Emergent properties, 306
EMLOD, 90, 110, 205
Entropy, 88
Epigenetic inheritance, 9
Epistasis, 9, 285, 298
Epistatic interaction, 317
Equilibrium: Hardy-Weinberg, 6, 84, 285;
    linkage, 8, 122; mutation and drift,
    32; mutation-selection, 267
Error: genome-wide type I, 76; genotyping,
    247; incorporated in analysis, 249;
    mean square, 43; pedigree, 141; rate,
    247; type I, 44, 46, 75; type II, 44;
    typing, 241; undetected, 248
Escherichia coli, 291
Estimate, 40; biased, 124, 159; consistent,
    43; fully efficient, 56; maximum
    likelihood, 38, 40; maximum
    likelihood, biased, 42; maximum
    likelihood, inconsistent, 236;
    maximum likelihood, of a function,
    41; unbiased, 42, 85; iterative
    maximum likelihood, 142
Exclusion: analysis, 279; mapping, 70, 262;
    of theta values, 69
Expectation, 42

Factor-union system, 25
False-positive, 153; results, in TDT, 294
Founder, 15
Fragile site, 33
Fragile X syndrome, 33, 161, 318

Gamete, 5, 9
Gametic drive, 270
Gene: AIDS-resistance, 257; conversion, 16;
    counting, 144; definition, 3; diversity,
    28; frequency, 4; mapping, 13;
    mapping workshops, 25; symbols, 24
Genes: number of, 3; number of disease,
    313; proportion polymorphic, 24
Genetic basis, 320
Genetic epidemiology, 164
Genetic marker, 34
Genocopy, 161
Genomic imprinting, 270
Genomic mismatch scanning, 291
Genotype, 26, 38, 94, 152; definition of, 4;
    inconsistent, 6; multilocus, 115

Gerstmann-Sträussler syndrome, 260, 308
Glaucoma, 12

Hadorn, xx
Haploinsufficiency, 257
Haplotype, 7, 8, 12, 13, 16, 27, 55, 62, 94,
    115, 299; parental origin, 96; relative
    risk method, 292
Haseman-Elston method, 276
Hemophilia, 8, 56
Heritability, 309, 310, 318
Heterogeneity, 146, 212, 215; misspecified,
    245; mixture of families, 220; models
    of, 231; test for, 220
Heterozygosity, 28, 84, 197; biased estimate
    of, 30; loss of, 319
Heterozygotes, selective advantage, 253
Heterozygous, 4
HHRR approach, 293, 327
Hirschsprung disease, 307
Histocompatibility, 27
HLA locus, 27
Hlod, 225, 302
Holliday structure, 14
Homozygosity mapping, 255, 259
Homozygous, 4
Huntington disease, 253
Hutterites, 28
Hypercholesterolemia, 172, 186
Hypertension, 319
Hypothesis, 38; composite 45, 47; simple, 45

IBD, 250, 255, 273, 315; sharing, 324
IBS, 277
Importance sampling, 209
Imprinting, 9, 270
Inbreeding, 28
Infantile neuronal ceroid lipofuscinosis, 195
Information: expected, 84, 91; Kullback-
    Leibler, 88; linkage, 54; matrix, 93;
    statistical, 85; for linkage, 15, 27, 64
Informativeness, 84, 85; expected, 86
Intercross, 93, 98
Interference, 18, 125, 126, 127, 139;
    chromatid, 14; complete, 23, 139,
    142; limiting marginal, 130;
    numerical, 128; positional, 128, 133
Internet, xx, 1
Interval, confidence (*See* Confidence
    interval); support (*See* Support
    interval)

Jackknife, 210

Karyotype, 22
Kugelberg-Welander disease, 232
Kuru, 307

Length-biased sampling, 147
Liability, 309; class, 160
Likelihood, 38, 39; and probability, 39;
    calculated recursively, 80;
    conditional, 64; ratio, 39, 41, 46
Linkage: centromeric, 82; genetic, 15; group,
    16; parameter, 102
Linkage disequilibrium, 8, 280; causes of,
    285; measures of, 288; testing for,
    286
Location score, 117
Locus, 3; ordering, 140; ordering, power for,
    139; orders, 115; orders,
    discrimination between; 138;
    modifier, 300; nomenclature of, 24;
    pseudoautosomal, 191; quantitative
    trait, 171
Lod score, 38, 39, 57; calculated analytically,
    179; correlation at two loci, 303;
    critical, 67, 78, 213; expectation of
    the maximum, 90; expected, 84, 87,
    88, 96; generalized, 117, 121; map-
    specific multipoint, 117; maximum,
    109; maximum of the expected, 89;
    maximum or average, 206; maximum
    possible, 107; observed, 96
Longevity, 309
Loop, 183, 260; consanguinity, 183;
    marriage, 183
Loss of heterozygosity, 319
Lutheran blood group, 26, 273
Lyon hypertensive rat, 319

Map distance, 10; female-to-male ratio of,
    188, 214; sex-specific, 147
Map expansion, 125
Map function: binomial, 20; Carter-Falconer,
    18; Felsenstein's, 19; graph of, 20;
    Haldane, 18; Kosambi, 18, 126, 138,
    150; Morgan's, 17; multilocus-
    feasible, 129; Rao's, 19; Sturt, 19;
    integration, 148; length, 22, 35;
    framework, 116; genetic, 33; radiation
    hybrid, 148
Mapping, homozygosity, 255
Marker, 3; genetic, 24

Markov chain, Monte Carlo, 191
Martin-Bell syndrome, 33
MASC method, 272
Mather, 14
Mating type, 93
MCMC methods, 191
Meiosis, 9
MELOD, 89
Mendel, 2; laws, 38
Method: affected sib-pair, 272; AGFAP, 272;
    APM, 277; direct, 53; disequilibrium
    mapping, 289; Edwards', of
    equivalent numbers, 70; genomic
    mismatch scanning, 291; haplotype
    relative risk, 292; Haseman-Elston,
    276; lod score, 61; MASC, 272;
    maximum likelihood, 56, 62; MCMC,
    191; Monte Carlo, 201;
    nonparametric, 272; peeling, 58;
    possible triangle, 274; proband, 156;
    shared segment mapping, 290;
    SimIBD, 278; two-point, for
    equivalent numbers, 71
MIM, 24
Minisatellite, 31
Misclassification, 27, 176, 242; disregarded
    in analysis, 243, 251
Mitochondria, 8, 9, 25
Mixture of distributions, 173
MNS blood group, 285
Mod score, 323
Mode of inheritance, Mendelian, 254
Model 38; hidden Markov, 81; inheritance,
    321; multiplicative, 317; polygenic
    threshold, 310; realistic, 322;
    regressive, 81, 177; threshold, 299;
    two-locus, 298; wrong analysis, 322
Mohr, 34
Mosaicism, 56, 270
M-test, 217, 220
Multidimensional scaling, 278
Multiple comparisons, 75
Mutation, 5, 16, 32; rate, 266
Myopia, 308

Nail-patella syndrome, 211
NCBI, 2, 24
Neanderthal, 9
Neural networks, 325
Neurofibromatosis, 260

Nomenclature: of DNA polymorphisms, 32; of loci, 24
Nonobese diabetic mouse, 314
Nonpaternity, 247; rate, 201
Nuisance parameter, 158, 225

OMIM, 24
Osteoarthrosis, 167, 260
Osteogenesis imperfecta, 228
Osteoporosis, 172
Ovarian teratomas, 82

p value, 44, 47, 49; approximate, 49; confidence interval for, 204
Papua New Guinea, 307
Parameter, 40, 93; linkage, 102; nuisance, 41, 158, 225
Parkinson disease, 234
Paternity, 200; index, 200
Peak, true, 147
Pedigree 15; bilineal, 230; complex, 184; error, 247; likelihood, 183; simple, 184
Peeling, 58, 184
Penetrance 4, 151; age-dependent, 161, 164; estimation of, 156; factors, 299; incomplete, 153; misspecified, 244; for monozygotic twins, 168; ratio, 153; wide sense and narrow sense, 151
Phase, 7, 8, 16, 101, 180
Phenocopy, 153, 169, 273; genetic, 161; rate, 153
Phenotype, 25, 26, 32, 38, 89, 94, 152, 317; definition of, 4; multivariate, 171; probability, 95; quantitative, 171; unknown, 152
PIC value, 29, 197
Poliovirus, sensitivity, 308
Polycystic kidney disease, 218, 222
Polymorphism, 27; DNA, 30; incomplete marker, 133; information content (PIC), 29; restriction fragment length, 31; single nucleotide, 31
Population, isolated, 5, 28, 321
Positional cloning, 253
Power, 45, 90, 325; of linkage test, 90; transformation, 174, 199
Prion, 308
Probability: generating function, 130; inverse conditional, 51; posterior for linkage, 60, 68; prior, 51

Proband, 264; method, 156
Pseudoautosomal regions, 16, 22, 191
Pseudorandom number, 202

QTL, 171
Quasilinkage, 16

Radiation hybrid mapping, 33, 35
Random numbers, 201
Recessive, 4; trait, parents related, 255
Recombination, 17, 139; definition of, 13
Recombination fraction, 14, 16; and age, 214; direct estimation of, 103; formal parameter, 88; male–female, 15; *n*-fold, 118; sex difference of, 66, 211; unbiased estimate of, 237; probability, 117; somatic, 17; value, 129
Reference families. *See* CEPH families
Regressive model. *See* Model, regressive
Relative risk, 281
Renwick, xx, 11
Repeat, 2; CA, 31; CAG, 257; expansions, 257; trinucleotide, 2, 257
Replicate, 202
Replication study, 321
Repulsion, 7
Resampling, 209
Restriction, secondary, 33
Result, false-negative, 44; false-positive, 44
Retinitis pigmentosa, 5, 216, 227
RFLPs, 31
Risk, 195, 263; distribution, 267; distribution, skewed, 269; ratio, 153; ratio, calculated numerically, 317; ratio, drop-off rate, 315; recurrence, 264, 315; relative, 281; support interval for, 265; under heterogeneity, 266

Sampling: acceptance, 46; length-biased, 147
Santavuori disease, 195
Schizophrenia, 299, 305, 307, 312, 315, 317
Scrapie, 307
Screening of newborns, 269
Segregation: analysis, 161, 162, 320; distortion, 270; irregular, 270
Semirandom, 10
Sensitivity, 45
Severity of disease, 319
Sex-limited, 8
Sex-linked, 8
Shared-segment method, 290

Sib-pair method, 56, 273; equivalence with
    lod score analysis, 279
Significance level, 46, 73, 204; Bonferroni,
    79; empirical, 47, 203
Simpson's paradox, 286
Simultaneous search, 146, 304
SNP, 31
Southern blot, 27
Specificity, 45
Spinal muscular atrophy, 232
Standard error, 92
Statistic, 40
Stratification, 324
Support, 39, 47; global, 116
Support interval, 50, 68, 158; for risks, 265
Survival analysis, 166
Susceptible, 165
Synteny, 16

TDT. *See* Test, TDT
Telomere, 211
Test: *A,* 223; *B,* 220; conservative, 46; exact,
    in simple families, 72; *F,* 47; for
    linkage, 65; for linkage with 1 df
    under sex difference, 67; HHRR, 293;
    likelihood ratio, 47; *M,* 217, 220;
    McNemar, 294; mean, 275; minmax,
    275; multiple marker, 77; one-sided,
    47; power of, 45; proportion, 276; S-
    TDT, 295; sequential, 46, 56;

significance, 44, 48; statistical, 45; *t,*
    47; TDT, 294, 328
Testcross, 93
Tetranucleotide, 32
Tourette syndrome, 291
Trait: oligogenic threshold, 321; X-linked,
    257
Transformation, probability integral, 207
Transmission disequilibrium test. *See* Test,
    TDT
Transposon, 3
Trinucleotide, 32; repeat. *See* Repeat,
    trinucleotide
Twin: dizygotic, 308; monozygotic, 168, 308
Two-stage search, 327

U scores, 56
Uniparental disomy, 270
Usher's syndrome, 220, 238

Variance, asymptotic, 92; components, 177,
    311
VNTR, 31

Wald, 46
Werdnig-Hoffman disease, 232
World-wide web, xx, 1

X-linked: inheritance, 264; lethal trait, 266;
    traits, 257

Y statistic, 55, 57

About the Author

Jurg Ott received a Ph.D. degree in zoology from the University of Zurich in 1967 and an M.S. degree in biomathematics from the University of Washington in 1972. He is a professor at the Rockefeller University, New York, and head of its Laboratory of Statistical Genetics. He serves on various editorial boards, is editor-in-chief of *Human Heredity,* and is a member of HUGO.

In the past twenty-five years, Jurg Ott has developed many new methods in human statistical genetics and implemented them in computer programs. For example, he wrote the first generally available computer program on human linkage analysis (LIPED), introduced the concept of an expected lod score that is now in general use, and developed methods of computer simulation for human families.